Neurocytopathology

Neurocytopathology

JOHN M. ANDREWS, M.D.
Associate Professor of Pathology
Consultant in Neuropathology
Department of Pathology
St. Mark's Hospital and University of Utah School of Medicine
Salt Lake City, Utah

G. BERRY SCHUMANN, M.D.
Professor of Pathology
Director, Cytopathology and Cytotechnology
University of Alberta
Edmonton, Alberta, Canada

SANS TACHE
WILLIAMS & WILKINS
BALTIMORE • HONG KONG • LONDON • MUNICH
PHILADELPHIA • SYDNEY • TOKYO

Editor: Charles W. Mitchell
Managing Editor: Victoria M. Vaughn
Copy Editor: Thomas Lehr
Designer: Norman W. Och
Illustration Planner: Ray Lowman
Production Coordinator: Raymond E. Reter

Printed in the United States of America

Library of Congress Cataloging-in-Publication Data

Andrews, John M. (John Morton), 1936–
Neurocytopathology / John M. Andrews and G. Berry Schumann.
p. cm.
Includes bibliographical references and index.
ISBN 0-683-00227-9
1. Nervous system—Cytopathology. I. Schumann, G. Berry (Gilbert Berry), 1946– . II. Title.
[DNLM: 1. Cytological Techniques. 2. Nervous System—pathology. 3. Nervous System Diseases—pathology. WL 101 A567n]
RC347.A53 1992
616.8′047—dc20
DNLM/DLC
for Library of Congress 91–30226
CIP

92 93 94 95 96
1 2 3 4 5 6 7 8 9 10

To those whose efforts
have provided the knowledge
upon which
this text is based.

Preface

The application of cytologic techniques to the study of nervous system diseases continues to gain popularity. This textbook, entitled *Neurocytopathology*, was created after both authors recognized a need for information that bridged the fields of neuropathology and cytopathology. The authors' backgrounds combine experience gained in clinical medicine, laboratory research, surgical pathology, and cytopathology. Their goal has been to provide a source of information that would accelerate communication between physicians and the medical laboratory regarding cytologic methods used, or being considered, for studying disorders of the nervous system. The theme throughout has been to emphasize key points and potential diagnostic problems, rather than reiterate information that is already well described in many other sources but that may be less relevant to the immediate needs of the cytotechnologist, cytopathologist, and general surgical pathologist.

Chapter 1 outlines the purposes of the book and briefly summarizes further sources of information on neurocytopathology. A list of representative neuropathology, cytopathology, and general references to further assist the reader is included at the end of Chapter 1, and relevant continuing medical education courses are also listed. Chapter 2 provides the reader with cytohistologic correlations of normal neural elements, as a foundation for assessing alterations associated with disease.

Chapter 3 outlines the multiparameter approach to cerebrospinal fluid (CSF) analysis and the type of information obtainable from body fluid, microbiology, and cytology laboratories. Tables provide examples of clinical conditions associated with abnormalities of specific CSF cytologic elements. Chapter 4 describes qualitative CSF methods and their clinical utility. The steps in performing a CSF cytologic examination are reviewed, and color illustrations highlight important morphologic criteria used in identifying normal and abnormal cells. Chapter 5 describes a quantitative CSF approach and discusses the value of this less frequently applied technique in monitoring, for example, neoplastic conditions.

Chapter 6 discusses general aspects of cytologic methods applied to neural tissue biopsies and aspirates. Methods for preparing brain smears are described. Chapter 7 discusses neoplasia and related disorders, and tables relevant to frequently asked questions are provided for quick reference by the reader.

Chapter 8 discusses examples of non-neoplastic neurological disorders that may be encountered by the general surgical pathologist and the cytopathologist. Chapter 9 reviews pitfalls in diagnosis and is a reminder of the limitations of present cytologic methods. Chapter 10 presents a brief discussion of future trends in the field of neurocytopathology. The Appendix provides step-by-step instructions for selected laboratory procedures and stains.

Although not intended as a comprehensive atlas of neurocytopathology, selected color figures are included in the back of the book and are cited in the appropriate chapters. Standardized magnifications have been used, where applicable, to allow the reader quick comparison of important features relating to the size of certain cell types (e.g., normal lymphocytes versus blasts or tumor cells). Magnifications listed in the figure legends refer to the magnifications in the original 35-mm color transparencies produced by the photomicroscope, and are not the precise magnifications of the figures as printed. Separate lists of tables and illustrations are included to facilitate rapid access to the required information.

It has become apparent to us during the course of this project that time and printed space would limit a truly comprehensive presentation of this topic, and we have attempted to emphasize features that would make this a useful resource in the day-to-day challenges in diagnosing nervous system disease in specimens of limited quantity. It is hoped that our clinical colleagues will find it a useful guide in determining when and how to request these procedures, and that they may obtain a greater appreciation for the very real problems pathologists—when restricted by circumstances to morphologic methods alone—may encounter in attempting to provide a rapid answer to the clinical question posed. As diagnostic cytopathology is increasingly accepted as a practical tool, and with health care providers currently searching for reasonable and cost-effective ways to deliver health care, it is our ultimate hope that this book will be seen as a contribution that will further these worthy goals and place the current status of these techniques in proper perspective.

Acknowledgments

The authors wish to thank many who assisted us in this publication. Carol Hamby, Lynda Harrison, Irene Olson, Corrine Reddoor, and Carole Stutz provided secretarial assistance and word processing expertise; Matt Riding and Denise Hardy assisted with the preparation of the appendix; Jane Errion provided assistance and advice concerning library research and retrieval of publications; histotechnological assistance was provided by Pam Ramachandran, Callie Birch, and Amanda Forester. Special thanks also go to illustrator Dick Golda, photographer Tom W. Turner, and others in the Department of Pathology at the University of Alberta.

Several colleagues and friends have shared their case material with us over the years, some of which was subsequently utilized for illustrations included in this publication. We especially thank Uwamie Tomiyasu, M.D. (Figures 7.3**C**, **D**, and **F**; 7.15**A**; and 8.1**A**, **C**, **D**, and **E**), Thomas Abbott, M.D. (Figures 7.6**A** and **B**, 8.1**B**, and 8.2**E**), Jeannette Townsend, M.D. (Figure 8.2**F**), K. Nguyen, M.D. (Figures 7.1**B** and 7.4**B**), Cheryl Harris, M.D. (Figure 7.15**F**, **G**, and **H**), Stacey Garry, M.D. (Figure 7.7**B**), Reuben Doggett, M.D. (Figure 7.3**A** and **B**), and James Murphey, M.D. Lynn Gaufin, M.D., provided us with insights concerning the perspective of the neurosurgeon in the diagnosis and management of many of the entities discussed in this text.

Dr. Jeannette Townsend has provided continued support and advice, and we have been grateful for her extensive experience and expertise in surgical neuropathology on many occasions. Dr. Carl Kjeldsberg's expertise in hematopathology and cerebrospinal fluid analysis has also been most helpful to us. Tim Satterfield, Vicki Vaughn, Raymond Reter, and their colleagues at Williams & Wilkins have guided us through the publication process with patience and professionalism.

Finally, we thank our families for their understanding during this time-consuming task, and we hope to justify their trust that the result would be worthwhile to our colleagues and patients.

Contents

List of Tables

List of Color Plates

Abbreviations

AIDS	acquired immune deficiency syndrome
ALL	acute lymphocytic leukemia
AML	acute myelogenous leukemia
CALLA	common acute lymphocytic leukemia antigen
CMV	cytomegalovirus
CNS	central nervous system
CSF	cerebrospinal fluid
CT	computed tomography
DNA	deoxyribonucleic acid
Glioblastoma	glioblastoma multiforme
ETOH	ethyl alcohol
FNA	fine-needle aspiration
GFAP	glial fibrillary acidic protein
GI	gastrointestinal
GMS	Gomori's methenamine silver
HD	Hodgkin's disease
H&E	hematoxylin and eosin
HSV	herpes simplex virus
LP	lumbar puncture (spinal tap)
MEN	multiple endocrine neoplasia
MPNST	malignant peripheral nerve sheath tumor
MRI	magnetic resonance imaging
MS	multiple sclerosis
N/C	nuclear/cytoplasmic (ratio)
Pap	Papanicolaou
PAS	periodic acid-Schiff
PCR	polymerase chain reaction
PML	progressive multifocal leuko-encephalopathy
PNET	primitive neuroectodermal tumor
PNS	peripheral nervous system
RBC	red blood cell (erythrocyte)
TdT	terminal deoxynucleotidyl transferase
WBC	white blood cell (leukocyte)

1 / Introduction

Initial application of cytologic techniques to the study of diseases of the nervous system (i.e., neurocytopathology) were largely confined to cerebrospinal fluid (CSF), and this remains an area of considerable importance (see Chapters 3, 4, and 5). More recently, cytologic techniques as applied to neural tissue biopsy specimens have become increasingly emphasized. We can appreciate the reluctance expressed by some of our surgical pathology colleagues to embrace the use of smear-imprint techniques in the context of intraoperative consultations. The morphologic diversity of normal neural tissue and the heterogeneity of many neuropathologic entities, both neoplastic and non-neoplastic, can conspire to make the occasional neurosurgical specimen in a general community hospital setting a diagnostic challenge even with a generous tissue sample. Further, just as proficiency in advanced cardiac resuscitation techniques may deteriorate with time, diagnostic skills in neuropathology acquired during one's training years might be expected to decrease without regular practice (5). To complicate an already difficult problem would be nonsensical if no advantage in comparison to traditional frozen section methods accrued. We believe, however, that the available data now supports the view that cytologic methods do have a specific and important role to play in this context, when properly applied.

This trend in the use of cytologic techniques in intraoperative consultations has evolved, and continues to gain momentum, for several reasons. There has been remarkable success in the use of the cervicovaginal (Pap) smears in early diagnosis of female genital tract cancer, and this has prompted efforts to apply such cytologic methods to other organ systems. There is a desire by all health care professionals to explore techniques that are perceived as having the potential to reduce the cost of, and thus improve access to, the best possible health care of our patients.

Ongoing efforts to devise techniques that combine precision in diagnosis with the least possible patient morbidity and mortality have led to dramatic progress in neuroimaging techniques and new neurosurgical stereotactic techniques that allow retrieval of very small fragments of tissue from small or deep-seated central nervous system (CNS) sites with a high degree of accuracy and minimal disturbance of intervening normal tissue (i.e., decrease in operative risk) (2). The poor regenerative capacity of CNS tissues also provides strong motivation to establish a diagnosis and institute treatment as soon as possible, in order to preserve maximum function.

Sufficient data exists, we believe, to warrant an attempt at providing an overview and assessment of the current status of this field. Several of the most comprehensive monographs on CSF cytology (see General Reference list) are no longer in print, and much of the recent literature regarding the use of cytology techniques in cerebrospinal fluid and in intraoperative consultations is found in relatively brief reviews in widely diverse sources.

Our major goals, therefore, include the following. First, to present in brief and accessible format, items from the neuropathologic and cytopathologic literature we consider of most immediate practical importance to surgical pathologists, cytologists, and clinicians who are expanding (or planning to expand) the cytologic techniques they apply in their routine practice. Second, to provide technical data sufficient to permit implementation of the more important techniques in an existing surgical/cytopathology laboratory setting, as may be deemed appropriate by the responsible staff members. Third, to provide a representative list of both published material and continuing medical education sources on these topics. This last goal reflects our recognition that our own choice of balance between brevity and detail on any given topic will not necessarily be appropriate to all readers, and we have attempted to minimize this deficiency by providing appropriate references. It also reflects our appreciation of the dynamic character of this field and the relatively brief half-life of any effort to capture its current state. We hope this will also encourage and facilitate active participation in this discipline by those who share our view that the role of cytopathology in this and many other subspecialties within the broader field of pathology is yet to be fully realized, and will be a fascinating and productive career opportunity for both clinical and basic science investigators for the foreseeable future.

We have found the information sources listed at the end of this chapter to be useful, and they are representative of the types of library materials we would recommend to any laboratory involved in neurocytopathology. Authors of several of these publications are also currently active as lecturers in the continuing medical education courses listed.

As a final introductory comment, the need for good communication between the various members of the diagnostic and therapeutic team has been frequently emphasized by authors on these topics, and we believe it should continue to be emphasized until it is universally applied. We place the primary responsibility for demonstrating the importance of this type of communication on the pathologist, who is in the best position to inform other members of the team concerning issues critical to arriving at a proper tissue diagnosis. The importance to the pathologist of relevant data from the clinical history and examination, imaging techniques, other laboratory studies, etc., can only be appreciated by other team members if they are made fully aware of, for example, the frequency and scope of "look-alikes" in pathology.

The format of the tumor atlas of differential diagnosis by Toker (6) provides one of many potential means by which the pathologist may graphically demonstrate that there are, for example, more than 30 tumors in which the dominant cell type is oncocytic in appearance, more than 50 tumors (including many neural tumors) composed of small round cells, etc. It follows that the spectrum of differential diagnostic possibilities can be immediately reduced by the type of clinical information noted above. In addition, the marked morphologic heterogeneity of certain neural tumors, compounded by varying degrees of reactivity of the surrounding brain tissue, can be demonstrated by making available to coworkers the illustrations mapping cytologic variation within a given glial tumor, such as those described in several recent publications (1, 3, 4). Consultation among team members prior to obtaining a CSF or tissue specimen will also tend to ensure that test priorities, particularly in small specimens, are consistent with clinical priorities and are handled in a manner that minimizes technical artifacts.

References to Chapter 1

1. Burger, P.C., Scheithauer, B.W., and Vogel, F.S. Surgical Pathology of the Nervous System and its Coverings. Churchill Livingstone, New York, 1991, pp. 216–230.
2. Kelly, P.J. Tumor Stereotaxis. W.B. Saunders Co., Philadelphia, 1991.
3. Okazaki, H., and Scheithauer, B.W. Slide Atlas of Neuropathology. Gower Medical Publishing, New York, 1988.
4. Paulus, W., and Pfeiffer, J. Intratumoral histologic heterogeneity of gliomas. A quantitative study. Cancer 64:442–447, 1989.

5. Stross, J.K. Maintaining competency in advanced cardiac life support skills. JAMA 249:3339–3341, 1983.
6. Toker, C. Tumors. An Atlas of Differential Diagnosis. University Park Press, Baltimore, 1983.

General References

General Neuropathology—Neoplastic and/or Non-neoplastic Disorders

1. Adams, J.H., Corsellis, J.A.N., and Duchen, L.W. (Eds.): Greenfield's Neuropathology, Ed. 4. John Wiley and Sons, New York, 1984.
2. Burger, P.C., Scheithauer. B.W., and Vogel, F.S. Surgical Pathology of the Nervous System and its Coverings. Ed. 3. Churchill Livingstone, New York, 1991.
3. Davis, R.L., and Robertson, D.M. (Eds.): Textbook of Neuropathology, Ed. 2. Williams & Wilkins, Baltimore, 1991.
4. Esiri, M.M., and Oppenheimer, D.R. Diagnostic Neuropathology: A Practical Manual. Year Book Medical Publishers, Chicago, 1989.
5. Friede, R.L. Developmental Neuropathology. Ed. 2. Springer-Verlag, New York, 1989.
6. Glenner, G.G., and Grimley, P.M. Tumors of the Extra-Adrenal Paraganglion System (Including Chemoreceptors). Second Series, Fascicle 9. Atlas of Tumor Pathology. Armed Forces Institute of Pathology, Washington, D.C., 1974.
7. Harkin, J.C., and Reed, R.J. Tumors of the Peripheral Nervous System. Second Series, Fascicle 3. Atlas of Tumor Pathology. Armed Forces Institute of Pathology, Washington, D.C., 1969.
8. Kepes, J.J. Meningiomas. Biology, Pathology and Differential Diagnosis. Masson Publishing USA, Inc., New York, 1982.
9. Kovacs, K., and Horvath, E. Tumors of the Pituitary Gland. Second Series, Fascicle 21. Atlas of Tumor Pathology. Armed Forces Institute of Pathology, Washington, D.C., 1986.
10. Reed, R.J., and Harkin, J.C. Tumors of the Peripheral Nervous System. Supplement. Second Series, Fascicle 3. Atlas of Tumor Pathology. Armed Forces Institute of Pathology, Washington, D.C., 1983.
11. Rubinstein, L.J. Tumors of the Central Nervous System. Second Series, Fascicle 6. Atlas of Tumor Pathology. Armed Forces Institute of Pathology, Washington, D.C., 1972.
12. Rubinstein, L.J. Tumors of the Central Nervous System. Supplement. Second Series, Fascicle 6. Atlas of Tumor Pathology. Armed Forces Institute of Pathology, Washington, D.C., 1982.
13. Russell, D.S., and Rubinstein, L.J. Pathology of Tumours of the Nervous System. Ed. 5. Williams & Wilkins, Baltimore, 1989.
14. Weller, R.O. (Ed.): Nervous System, Muscle and Eyes. Ed. 3, Vol. 4 of: W. St. C. Symmers (General Editor): Systemic Pathology. Churchill Livingstone, New York, 1990.

General Neuropathology: Atlases

1. Hirano, A. (Ed.): Color Atlas of Pathology of the Nervous System. Ed. 2. Igaku-Shoin Medical Publishers, Inc., New York, 1988.
2. Kepes, J.J. Pathology of Brain Tumors. Ed. 2. Part I: Astrocytomas and Oligodendrogliomas; Part II: Other Neuroectodermal and Germinal Cell Tumors; Part III: Nonglial Neoplasms of the Central Nervous System and its Coverings; Part IV: Neurolemmomas, Neurofibromas, Epithelial Tumors, Metastases and Dysgenetic Syndromes (255 35-mm slides plus audiocassettes). Available through: Medcom/Trainex, P.O. Box 3225, Garden Grove, CA 92642, U.S.A. Phone (800) 877-1443; FAX (714) 898-4852.
3. Okazaki, H., and Scheithauer, B.W. Slide Atlas of Neuropathology (997 35-mm slides with 285 text pages), 1988. Available through: Gower Medical Publishing, 101 Fifth Avenue, New York, NY 10003, U.S.A. Phone (212) 929-6290.
4. Weller, R.O. Colour Atlas of Neuropathology. Miller and Oxford University Press, Oxford, 1984.

General References with Emphasis on Neuropathology Frozen Sections, Smears, Imprints, and/or Cerebrospinal Fluid Cytology

1. Adams, J.H., Graham, D.I., and Doyle, D. Brain Biopsy, the Smear Technique for Neurosurgical Biopsies. J.B. Lippincott Co., Philadelphia, 1981.
2. Bigner, S.H. Central Nervous System. Chapter 18 in: Bibbo, M. (Ed.): Comprehensive Cytopathology. W.B. Saunders Co., Philadelphia, 1991, pp. 468–483.
3. Bigner, S.H., and Johnston, W.W. Cytopathology of the Central Nervous System. In: Johnston, W.W. (Ed.): Masson Monographs in Diagnostic Cytopathology, Vol. 3. Masson Publishing USA, Inc., New York, 1983.
4. Chandrasoma, P.T., and Apuzzo, M.L.J. Stereotactic Brain Biopsy. Igaku-Shoin, New York, 1989.

5. den Hartog Jager, W.A. Color Atlas of C.S.F. Cytopathology. J.B. Lippincott Co., Philadelphia, 1980.
6. Fishman, R.A. Cerebrospinal Fluid in Diseases of the Nervous System. W.B. Saunders Co., Philadelphia, 1980.
7. Franks, A.J. Diagnostic Manual of Tumors of the Central Nervous System, Churchill Livingstone, New York, 1988.
8. Garcia, J.H. Brain Biopsy. Chapter 6 in: Garcia, J.H., Escalona-Zapata, J., Sandbank, U., and Cervós-Navarro, J. (Eds.): Diagnostic Neuropathology. Vol. II. Field and Wood Medical Publishers, Inc., W.W. Norton and Company, Inc., Scranton, PA, 1990.
9. Herndon, R.M., and Brumback, R.A. (Eds.): The Cerebrospinal Fluid. Kluwer Academic Publishers, Boston, 1989.
10. Jane, J.A., and Yashon, D. Cytology of Tumors Affecting the Nervous System. Charles C. Thomas, Publishers, Springfield, IL, 1969.
11. Kjeldsberg, C.R., and Knight, J.A. Body Fluids. Laboratory Examination of Amniotic, Cerebrospinal, Seminal, Serous and Synovial Fluids: A Textbook Atlas. American Society of Clinical Pathologists Press. Ed. 2. Chicago, 1986.
12. Koss, L.G. Cerebrospinal Fluid, Miscellaneous Fluids, the Eye, and the Skin. Chapter 27 in: Diagnostic Cytology and Its Histopathologic Bases. Ed. 3, J.B. Lippincott Co., Philadelphia, 1979, pp. 971–988.
13. Kölmel, H.W. Atlas of Cerebrospinal Fluid Cells. Ed. 2. Springer-Verlag, New York, 1977.
14. Liwnicz, B.B., and Rodriguez, C.A. The Central Nervous System. Chapter 16 in: Koss, L.G., Woyke, S., and Olszewski, W. (Eds.): Aspiration Biopsy. Cytologic Interpretation and Histologic Bases. Igaku-Shoin, New York, 1985.
15. Nochomovitz, L., Sidawy, M., Silverberg, S.I., Jannotta, F., and Schwartz, A. Intraoperative Consultation. A Guide to Smears, Imprints and Frozen Sections. American Society of Clinical Pathologists Press, Chicago, 1989.
16. Oehmichen, M. Cerebrospinal Fluid Cytology. An Introduction and Atlas. W.B. Saunders Co., Philadelphia, 1976.
17. Rosenthal, D.L. Cytology of the Central Nervous System. In: Wied, G.L. (Ed.): Monographs in Clinical Cytology, Vol. 8. S. Karger, New York, 1984.
18. Scheithauer, B.W. Central Nervous System and Pituitary. Chapter 8 in: Silva, E.G., and Kraemer, B.B. (Eds.): Intraoperative Pathologic Diagnosis. Frozen Section and Other Techniques: Williams & Wilkins, Baltimore, 1987.
19. Schultenover, S.J. Cerebrospinal Fluid and Central Nervous System. Chapter 14 in: Ramzy, I. Clinical Cytopathology and Aspiration Biopsy. Fundamental Principles and Practice. Appleton and Lange, Norwalk, CT, 1990.
20. Takahashi, M. Color Atlas of Cancer Cytology, Ed. 2. Igaku-Shoin, New York, 1981.
21. Wied, G.L., Keebler, C.M., Koss, L.G., and Reagan, J.W. Compendium on Diagnostic Cytology. Ed. 6. (Second Printing). Tutorials in Cytology, Chicago, IL, 1990.

Appendix

Selected Examples of Continuing Medical Education Sources in General Cytopathology and Neurocytopathology

1. **Tutorials on Clinical Cytology**
   Contact: The University of Chicago
   Continuing Education in Cytology
   Tutorials of Cytology
   5941 Maryland Ave. H.M. #449
   Chicago, Il 60637, USA
   Telephone (312) 702-6569
   Fax Phone (312) 955-8873
2. **Annual Postgraduate Institute for Pathologists in Clinical Cytopathology**
   Contact: Yener S. Erozan, M.D., Director,
   or Betty Ann Pemley, M.S., Administrator
   111 Pathology Bldg.
   600 N. Wolfe Street
   Baltimore, MD 21205, USA
   Telephone (301) 955-8594
3. **Advances in Cytology**
   Contact: Harvard Medical School
   Department of Continuing Education
   P.O. Box 825
   Boston, MA 02117, USA
   Telephone (617) 432-1525
4. **Cytology Review Course**
   Contact: Joseph H. Selliken, Jr., M.D.
   The Osler Institute
   1094 Dawn Lane
   P.O. Box 2218
   Terre Haute, IN 47802, USA
   Telephone (800) 356-7537 or (812) 299-5658

5. **American Society of Clinical Pathologists**
P.O. Box 12075
Chicago, IL 60612, USA
Telephone (800) 621-4142
In Illinois call: (312) 738-4890
6. **American Association of Neuropathologists, Inc.**
Office of the Secretary-Treasurer
Department of Pathology
State University of New York at Buffalo
School of Medicine and Biomedical Sciences
204 Farber Hall
Buffalo, NY 14214, USA
Telephone (716) 898-3114
7. **American Registry of Pathology Armed Forces Institute of Pathology**
Education Division (EDE)
Washington, DC 20306-6000, USA
Telephone: Commercial (301) 427-5231
Autovon 291-5208
8. **American Society of Cytology**
Contact: Office of the Secretary-Treasurer
American Society of Cytology
1015 Chestnut Street, Suite 1518
Philadelphia, PA, USA
Telephone (215) 922-3880
9. **United States and Canadian Academy of Pathology**
Contact: The United States-Canadian Division
International Academy of Pathology
3643 Walton Way Extension
Augusta, GA 30909, USA
Telephone (404) 733-7550
10. **International Academy of Cytology**
Contact: Office of the Membership Committee
William W. Johnston, M.D., F.I.A.C., Chairman
Division of Cytopathology
Box 3712, Duke University Medical Center
Durham, NC 27710, USA
Telephone (919) 684-2486
Fax phone (919) 684-6306
OR
Contact: Manuel Hilgarth, M.D., F.I.A.C., Secretary
Professor of Obstetrics and Gynecology
University of Freiburg
Hugstetterstrasse 55
D-7800 Freiburg, Germany
Telephone (49) (761) 270-3076
Telefax (49) (761) 270-3122
Telex 4972334 ACTACYT
11. **Courses on Fine Needle Aspiration Cytology**
Contact: Heinz K. Grohs, M.D.
International Institute for Applied Cyto Sciences
P.O. Box 377
Manchester, MA 01944, USA
Telephone (508) 741-1215, Ext. 4101

2 / Cytohistologic Correlations

The curricula of medical students, cytotechnology students, and pathology residents are not, in our experience, characterized by an overexposure to histology of the nervous system. Further, teaching sets of glass slides in most cytology laboratories understandably emphasize the samples most commonly encountered (e.g., gynecologic, respiratory tract, pleural and peritoneal fluids), and artifacts imposed on specimens by the techniques employed may vary from tissue to tissue.

For these reasons, and others which are also self-evident, we recommend that each laboratory develop not only a reference library reflecting each of the major subjects pertinent to this topic (see General References in Chapter 1), but also a basic glass slide reference set in which various nervous system structures obtained as rapidly as possible postmortem are exposed to techniques identical to those utilized in the study of pathologic material. A suggested list of structures to be examined is provided in Table 2.1, and can be modified to best reflect the spectrum of neurological specimens seen in each laboratory.

We have found it helpful to subject such tissues to imprints (touch preparations) and smear techniques (for comparison with intraoperative biopsy specimens) as well as cytocentrifuge and membrane filter methods (for comparison with CSF cytology material), and then correlate such findings with routinely processed paraffin sections obtained from the fresh brain slice facing the zone sampled for cytologic study. To this is added, for the pathology portion of the teaching set, neuropathological biopsy specimens and CSF cytologies, as opportunity allows.

Interlaboratory exchange of extra teaching slides may be a mutually advantageous means to acquire examples of the more commonly encountered entities. By such means, a useful and readily accessible teaching set can be provided for all personnel involved in the screening and final reporting of such specimens.

Before approaching the cytology of various neural structures, a few comments on staining methods are in order. We do not minimize the value of various special stains in the examination of neural tissues, much of our current understanding of its structure and function being a result of such methods. Our emphasis in this volume, however, is on current applications of cytology to nervous system disorders, in which the major areas of practical application in clinical medicine focus on CSF cytology and intraoperative consultation of wet tissue specimens. Characteristics of both of these applications include cost-effective procedures and, particularly for the latter, a maximum turn-around time of a few minutes from acquisition of the specimen to telephone report. This precludes, in most settings, routine use of other than the Papanicolaou (Pap) and Wright's (Diff-Quik) stains for CSF cytology and hematoxylin and eosin (H&E) staining for tissue biopsy materials. The former are already standardized in most surgical and cytopathology laboratories, and the latter has the advantage of wide familiarity among pathologists in the context of frozen and paraffin sections stained with similar dyes. H&E staining also demonstrates most cytoplasmic and neuropil structures in greater detail than either the Pap or Diff-Quik methods. Although rapid methods for several other stains have been developed (e.g., reticulin stain), they have relatively limited application, and difficulties encountered in the continuous maintenance of fresh solutions for the occasional neural tissue specimen tends to discourage their use. Use of all appropriate special stains and markers, however, is encouraged in the portion of the specimen that is subsequently processed for routine and/or special study.

Points we have found useful for facilitating the study of such material follow. It is generally appreciated that cell sizes may vary with the fixation method employed as well as with various cell preparation methods. A useful means of estimating the size of any particular structure is by extrapolation from the nearly ubiquitous normal peripheral blood elements, which have a fairly uniform size, in the same preparation. The approximate cell (not nuclear) diameters of the most commonly encountered elements are as follows: erythrocytes, 7 μm; neutrophils, 10 to 12 μm; eosinophils, 13 μm; monocytes, 14 to 20 μm; small lymphocytes, 6 to 10 μm, and large lymphocytes, 10 to 15 μm. The nucleus of the small lymphocyte averages 5 μm in diameter.

Table 2.1.
Suggested Sites for Normal Neurocytology Teaching Sets

Cerebral cortex	Brain stem
Frontal	Substantia nigra
Lateral temporal	Inferior olive
Uncus (Ammon's horn)	Basis pontis
Parietal	
Occipital	Spinal cord
	Anterior horn
Deep nuclei	Clarke's column
Caudate	Posterior horn
Putamen	
Globus pallidus	Ependyma
Thalamus	
Amygdala	Choroid plexus
White matter	Pia-arachnoid
Centrum semiovale	
Spinal cord	Pineal body
Cerebellum	Pituitary
Cortex	Anterior
Dentate nucleus	Posterior
	Infundibulum

Neurons

Normal neurons vary in maximum size from 4 to 5 μm to approximately 100 μm, depending on the area of nervous system sampled. Considerable variation is present even within a small zone of neocortex, for example, with the largest neurons being concentrated in layers 3 (layer of pyramidal cells) and 5 (ganglionic layer). Most neurons in surgical biopsy specimens will not exceed 60 to 70 μm in diameter, since areas containing the largest neurons (e.g., motor cortex, anterior horn of spinal cord) are less likely to be purposely sampled, to minimize postoperative motor deficits. Small neurons with inconspicuous nucleoli may not be readily distinguished from astrocytes by light microscopy unless special staining techniques are employed. Larger neurons typically contain a centrally placed nucleus with a single prominent nucleolus (red with Pap stain, blue with H&E), finely distributed chromatin, and a round to angular soma with finely granular cytoplasm (lightly eosinophilic background containing Nissl substance with H&E; pale green with Pap stains) (Fig. 2.1).

There is often a conspicuous extension of soma as an apical dendritic root that merges with the surrounding neuropil in larger neurons, whereas axons exiting from such neurons are devoid of Nissl substance at their origin (i.e., axon hillock). Exceptions to these general characteristics include the more dense chromatin of cerebellar granular layer neurons and certain situations in which cytoplasmic pigments are more conspicuous (both discussed below). In addition, the neurons of Clarke's column in the spinal gray matter may normally contain more eccentrically placed nuclei as well as central cytoplasmic clearing, the latter resembling "chromatolysis."

Astrocytes

Nuclei of protoplasmic (predominant in gray matter) and fibrous (predominant in white matter) astrocytes are indistinguishable by light microscopy using H&E, Pap, or Diff-Quik stains. Their single (rarely paired) nucleus is approximately 7 to 10 μm in diameter, round to ovoid, and contains rather fine, homogeneously distributed chromatin (18). In normal neural tissue they appear as isolated nuclei without a well-defined cell soma distinguishable from the surrounding neuropil (Fig. 2.2**A**). In certain areas where astrocytes normally accumulate more fibrillar material with aging (e.g., subpial, subependymal, perivascular, inferior olivary nuclei), a more distinct separation of the cytoplasm and proximal processes associated with a given astrocyte nucleus can be appreciated against the neuropil background. Generally, however, conspicuous astrocyte perikarya and processes are more frequently encountered in reactive (and sometimes neoplastic) astrocyte populations.

Although the electrical impulse-conducting properties of neurons are well known, efforts to define astrocyte functions have yielded a rather complex array of possibilities. Functions attributed to astrocytes include structural support, insulation, metabolic functions including fluid and electrolyte balance, interactions with endothelial cells related to blood-brain barrier functions, limited phagocytic capability, and a role as a key component in the reaction of the nervous system to a variety of types of injury. Of these, only the reactive changes are of major importance morphologically, and will be dealt with in subsequent chapters.

Oligodendrocytes

As with astrocytes, normal oligodendrocytes appear as apparently "bare" nuclei on a background of neuropil, without its cytoplasm being clearly distinguishable from the latter with commonly utilized stains and preparation methods. The "fried egg" appearance caused by a clear zone completely surrounding the nucleus, as typically seen in autopsy-derived tissues or other circumstances in which fixation is delayed and/or otherwise inadequate, is not seen in rapidly frozen and/or fixed tissue, normal or neoplastic. The oligodendrocyte nucleus is very similar to that of a lymphocyte nucleus, both in size (about 5 to 7 μm) and chromatin content and distribution (Fig. 2.2**A** and **B**). Those that occur in gray matter (e.g., cerebral cortex, deep nuclei) may be seen as perineuronal satellite oligodendrocytes, one or a few such cells closely applied to, or even indenting, the soma of larger neurons. This normal appearance, seen in both sections and smears, is not to be confused with Scherer's secondary structures. The latter are seen in certain central nervous system (CNS) neoplasms and are discussed further in Chapters 7 and 8. Oligodendrocytes are also present in random distribution in the gray matter neuropil, presumably in relation to myelin internodes of nearby axons. In white matter, oligodendrocytes are seen in apparently random distribution and also in "indian-file" array between adjacent axons. The latter are referred to as interfascicular oligodendrocytes. Large oligodendrocyte nuclei cannot be reliably distinguished from small astrocyte nuclei in normal tissue without special stains or ultrastructural study.

The major function ascribed to oligodendroglia cells is genesis and maintenance of the myelin sheath of CNS axons. Its role as a perineuronal satellite cell is less clear. It tends to succumb readily to a wide variety of pathologic insults and plays little role in reactive phenomena in most disease processes, in contrast to the astrocyte.

Microglia

Traditionally, this term has been applied to a putative third glial element, originally separated from astrocytes and oligodendrocytes by means of metallic impregnation techniques. Microglia have been regarded as resting macrophages that give rise to a substantial population of rod-shaped and/or plump phagocytic cells (or lipid macrophages), as well as some multinucleated reactive cells, seen in a variety of neuropathologic processes. The origin of such cells has, in recent years, been variously ascribed to neuroectodermal sources, pericytes, migratory blood-derived elements of the monocyte-macrophage system, or some combination of these. A thoughtful and thorough review of this complex subject has recently been published by Dolman (4), who suggests that (*a*) there is presently no persuasive evidence to support the notion that there exists a resident cell population within the CNS related to the mononuclear phagocytic system; (*b*) reactive cells participating in the "glial nodules" or "stars" (more recently referred to as glial-mesodermal nodules, or monocyte nodules) and forming the lipid phagocytes in CNS tissues are derived primarily, if not exclusively, from monocytes of bone marrow origin; and (*c*) the term microglia, which implies a single distinct cell system, is misleading and no longer applicable.

Lipofuscin

Lipofuscin is a yellow to yellow-brown cytoplasmic pigment derived from lysosomes and is more conspicuous in neurons than in other neural constituents. In the normal nervous system it increases with age, and is more prominent within certain populations (e.g., dentate nucleus, inferior olivary nucleus, dorsal root ganglia, and anterior horn cells) (Fig. 2.1**B**).

Corpora Amylacea

These round bodies generally stain gray to pale blue to purple with H&E stains, and varying shades of violet with the Pap stain (Fig. 2.3**A** to **C**). Their outer border typically has a soft or fluffy appearance. The central portion of the corpora amylacea is not refractile by usual bright field microscopy, nor does it appear as a maltese cross with polarization; both of these features distinguish corpora amylacea from contaminating talc crystals (Fig. 2.3**D**). They are composed of a glycogen-like carbohydrate with a protein component and are morphologically identical with polyglucosan bodies of axons and Lafora bodies in neurons. They are situated within astrocyte processes, usually do not exceed 15 to 30 μm in diameter, and vary in number in different brains but become increasingly prominent with age. In normal brains they demonstrate preferential accumulation in certain sites, including subpial and subependymal areas, Ammon's horn, globus pallidus, perivascular zones, and spinal cord posterior columns.

Neuropil

This term refers to the rather amorphous, by light microscopy, feltwork composed of processes of neurons, astrocytes, and oligodendrocytes, within which the more obvious nuclei (and, in the case of the larger neurons, parakarya) reside. It is eosinophilic in H&E stains and pale blue-green with the Pap stain. Clear vacuoles resulting from alcohol extraction of CNS lipids are common in neuropil smears. With the exception of astrocyte processes in certain areas (see above), light microscopically resolved fibers in this zone in normal brains are generally neuronal, and not glial, in origin.

Vasculature

Blood vessels encountered in brain tissue smears initially give the impression of hypervascularity, in comparison to one's preconceived notions derived from routine paraffin sections. Adjustment to the more accurate reflection of their true prominence in normal CNS gray matter is quickly acquired, however. Vascular size in parenchymal brain biopsy material seldom exceeds that of small muscular arteries and arterioles. The latter are generally in the 20 to 100 μm diameter range and are readily identified by their bidirectional nuclear orientation (longitudinally disposed endothelial nuclei and circumferentially oriented smooth muscle nuclei (Fig. 2.4**A**). Venules, 20 μm and greater in diameter, demonstrate a more haphazard orientation of nuclei than arterioles of similar size. The nuclei are derived from endothelial cells, fibroblasts, and (at 45 μm diameter and larger) smooth muscle elements (Fig. 2.4**B**). Capillaries average 8 to 10 μm in diameter. They (as well as the immediate postcapillary venules) are composed of only two cellular elements, endothelial cells and pericytes (Fig. 2.4**C**). The latter reside in a more peripheral location compared to the endothelial cell, within a split in the basement membrane upon which the endothelium rests. Pericytes tend to have a more ovoid shape (Fig. 2.4**D**). The functions of the endothelial cell are legion and beyond the scope of this review, but their role in the blood-brain barrier is of particular importance in this context. The role of the pericyte is less clear, with functions as varied as regulation of microvascular growth (2) and migration into neural tissue as an activated phagocyte in certain disease processes (see microglia, above) being among those suggested. Familiarity with the normal appearance of CNS vessels in smear preparations is especially useful as an aid to determining, for example, the presence or absence of endothelial proliferation, which may be present in certain primary and secondary CNS neoplasms (see Chapter 7).

White Matter

Aside from the relative hypocellularity, prominence of large axons (tinted red with both H&E and Pap stains), and absence of neurons, the description of cellular constituents above also applies to this brain component (Fig. 2.2**A**). The nuclei of oligodendrocytes, whose cell processes are connected to multiple myelin internodes by tenuous processes easily disrupted by smear techniques, exhibit no consistent or intimate relationship to the myelin sheaths of the axons, in contrast to the close relationship of Schwann cell nuclei to a single myelin internode in peripheral nerve smears. The white matter of spinal cord will be similar in smears, reliably distinguished from large cerebral white matter bundles only if the numbers of Clarke's column or anterior horn neurons, with the nuclear and cytoplasmic peculiarities of the former and/or the large size of the latter, are sufficient to provide a clue.

Deep Cerebral Nuclei

Brain tissue smears from these zones exhibit numerous similarities with those of cerebral cortex, including the spectrum of neurons, astrocytes, oligodendrocytes, and vascular structures described above. Also similar is the shaggy or mossy appearance of neuron cell surfaces in smears (Fig. 2.1**A**), due to the adherent remnants of synaptic knobs and probably astrocyte processes (the latter more likely a significant contributor to this appearance in smeared Purkinje cells from cerebellar cortex).

Prominent axons are more visible in smears of deep nuclei such as thalamus than in most of the cerebral cortex (with the exception of the visual cortex, with its large-axon population from the visual radiations found in layer 4 as the outer stripe or line of Baillarger, also termed the line of Gennari). We have also encountered binucleate neurons more commonly in deep nuclei (e.g., thalamus) than in cortex of normal brains. Thus, the occasional binucleate neuron in an otherwise normal smear should not tempt one to diagnose a gangliocytoma or ganglioglioma, for example. The degree of cohesion between neurons and neuropil also varies in smears from different locations, with relatively intact neurons smearing in thin layers more readily from, for example, the amygdala than from cortex or from some other deep nuclei.

Finally, there are neurons in certain locations that contain neuromelanin (brown with H&E stain, olive green with Pap stain). A few neuromelanin-containing neurons, with their large size and conspicuous nucleolus, might easily bring to mind a malignant melanoma, emphasizing the constant need for application of all cytologic criteria for malignancy (Fig. 2.5). Table 2.2 summarizes the locations in normal neural tissue in which melanin-containing cells have been described. Parenthetically, even in the context of prominent melanin-containing cells within a cerebral mass lesion, caution is appropriate before a diagnosis of metastatic melanoma is made. There are a number of primary central and peripheral nervous system neoplasms in which melanin pigment may infrequently occur (see Table 7.11). In the substantia nigra, microscopic pigment within neurons appears at about 2 to 5 years of age but is not grossly apparent until the mid-teens. Melanin accumulation ("true" melanin derived from melanophores, unlike neuromelanin) has also been described in the normal leptomeninges, especially in the vicinity of the ventral medulla and rostral cervical areas; it is more commonly seen in dark-skinned races. It may also be accentuated in pregnancy, and can be found in normal choroid plexus (21).

Table 2.2.
Normal Sites of Melanin-containing Cells in the Nervous System

Zona compacta of the substantia nigra
Locus ceruleus
Dorsal motor nucleus of the vagus
Neurons of the red nucleus capsule
Tegmentum of brainstem
Fourth ventricle roof neurons
Dorsal root ganglia
Sympathetic ganglia
Leptomeninges

Cerebellar Cortex

The discrepancy between the true complexity of cellular arborization and interconnections, and the apparent simplicity of structure as seen by routine H&E and Pap stained neural tissue is striking throughout the nervous system, and no less so in cerebellar cortex (Fig. 2.6**A** to **C**). Even when this complex structure is architecturally disordered by smear preparations or other cytologic techniques, however, certain major cell lines can be readily distinguished (Fig. 2.6**D** to **F**). We cannot appreciate differences between nuclei of stellate or basket cells from astrocytes (unless the former contain a more prominent nucleolus than would be typical of an astrocyte). The more widely distributed astrocyte and oligodendrocyte nuclei are essentially identical to those described above. The Bergmann astrocytes, within the Purkinje cell layer, also give the appearance of bare nuclei against the neuropil unless stimulated to undergo reactive change in various pathologic processes. Their proliferation and elaboration of fibrous processes is, however, a very useful indicator that sparseness of Purkinje cells in a given area is the result of a pathologic process and not simply an artifact of the plane of section. In the latter instance, of course, the Bergmann glia are not unusually prominent. Similarly, earlier comments on vasculature are equally applicable here.

Two neural populations are very conspicuous in cerebellar cortex. Purkinje cells are obvious due to both their substantial size and their flask-shaped perikaryon. Granule cells from the deeper granular layer of the cortex are among the smallest of neurons, with a diameter of only 5 to 6 μm, nearly all of which is nucleus. While similar in size to the lymphocyte, and having rather dense chromatin, the majority are readily distinguishable from lymphocytes by a characteristic, central aggregation of chromatin and a relative aggregation of chromatin near the inside of the nuclear envelope, separated by a zone with more sparse chromatin. This gives the granule cell nucleus a "targetoid" profile, which remains in cells subjected to smear, cytocentrifuge, or filter techniques (Fig. 2.6**C** to **F**). An intermediate sized, clearly neuronal-type cell is infrequently seen in smears of cerebellar cortex, and its presence requires some search even in paraffin sections, but corresponds to the Golgi type II neuron population (Fig. 2.6**C**).

Review of Figure 2.6**A** to **F** reveals that the cerebellar cortex is the most cellular zone of normal brain tissue on smears, due to the dense granule cell population, and thus is the normal area that would most readily lend itself to misinterpretation as a small-cell neoplasm or chronic inflammatory infiltrate. This is particularly true in infants, in which a subpial layer of small, primitive-appearing cells is normally present at birth (the fetal or external granular layer of Obersteiner). This external granular layer gradually disappears over the first 6 to 12 months of age as its cells migrate through the molecular and Purkinje cell layers to their permanent location in the granular cell layer, maturing en route into granule cells. Cerebellar cortex cellular distribution essentially reaches the adult appearance by 18 months of age (15).

Ependyma

Ependymal cells surface the ventricular system, cerebral aqueduct, and central canal of the spinal cord. They are cuboidal to columnar, approximately 10 μm in cell diameter, and form a single layer of cells with the exception of a few areas that may demonstrate stratification (e.g., where ventricular surfaces form sharp angulations, etc.). They are occasionally encountered in the immediate subependymal neural parenchyma as single cells, small groups, or even rosettes. They are directly applied to the underlying neural tissue without interposition of a basement membrane (Fig. 2.7**A** and **B**). Their free surface is ciliated, the prominence of cilia by light microscopy demonstrating regional variation and a general decrease with age. Smear techniques support the conclusion that cell-to-cell junctions between ependymal cells are more resistant to mechanical forces than those between choroid plexus epithelial cells, a point that is helpful in distinguishing these two cell populations in smear preparations and other types of cytopreparations (Fig. 2.7**C** and **D**). (Also see choroid plexus discussion below.)

Smears of ependymal surfaces reveal sheets or small groups of cells one layer thick, or bare nuclei of ependymal cells, but very infrequent profiles of individual ependymal cells with what appears to be a relatively intact perinuclear cytoplasm and cell membrane. As bare nuclei, they resemble those of astrocytes more than other neural components. Nucleoli, as a rule, are not conspicuous. We have noted that occasional normal ependymal cell fragments may tend to condense, in cytocentrifuge and membrane filter preparations, with resultant mildly increased chromatin density and/or nuclear molding (Fig. 2.7**E** and **F**). This appearance is a potential pitfall for misinterpretation as a medulloblastoma, small-cell undifferentiated metastatic carcinoma, or other morphologically similar neoplasm (see Fig. 7.7).

A second ependymal cell type, the tanycyte, is a bipolar, elongate cell more readily recognized in comparative neuroanatomical and mammalian neuroembryonic studies than in adult human brains (5). Its primary significance from the standpoint of the surgical pathologist is as a proposed cell of origin for ependymomas that have a prominent fibrillary architecture resembling astrocytomas, since this potential diagnostic error (more likely to occur in spinal than in cranial sites) could theoretically affect therapeutic decisions adversely (6).

With aging, ependymal cytoplasmic arc- or ring-shaped structures may appear, enhanced with silver impregnation methods, periodic acid-Schiff (PAS) and Congo red stains, and are termed "silver rings of Biondi" (16).

Choroid Plexus

The choroid plexus consists of four aggregates of complex vascular fronds protruding into the ventricular system (right and left lateral ventricles and third and fourth ventricles, respectively) and is functionally the source for the majority of the cerebrospinal fluid. The surface epithelium is cuboidal to low columnar, averages 15 μm in cell diameter, and is dispersed as a single layer with infrequent exceptions (Fig. 2.8). The nuclei are centrally to basally situated, more round than ovoid, and contain more dense and coarse chromatin distribution than the ependymal cells, with which they are in continuity. The transition zone between the ependyma and choroid plexus epithelium is along grossly discernible lines called taenia (e.g., taenia choroidea of the fourth ventricle, taenia thalami of the third ventricle, etc.). This transition zone is rather abrupt, being only a few cell diameters in width (Fig. 2.9**A**), and the distinction between the two types of epithelium is typically readily apparent in normal brains on paraffin sections and in both H&E and Pap stained smears and cytocentrifuge and membrane filter preparations (Fig. 2.9**B**). Focal ependymal differentiation may occasionally be seen within the choroid plexus proper (11). Binucleate cells are rare in choroid plexus epithelium, as are cilia, but microvilli are common. The epithelium rests on a basement membrane (in contrast to ependyma) beneath which are blood vessels, connective tissue elements (including pia-arachnoid, fibroblasts, and collagen), lymphocytes, bone marrow-derived elements of the monocyte-macrophage system, and nerve fibers. With aging, commonly encountered additional structures in choroid plexus papillary fronds include epithelial cytoplasmic silver rings of Biondi, stromal fibrous tissue proliferations (Fig. 2.9**C** and **D**), hyalin plaques, mulberry bodies (aggregates of hyalinized endothelial cells), xanthogranulomas, and psammoma bodies. The latter appear to arise from mineralization of the stromal fibrillar aggregates (Fig. 2.9**C** and **D**) and contain calcium salts and cholesterol. The choroid plexus epithelial cytoplasm is eosinophilic with H&E, and green to purple with the Pap stain. It appears granular in well-fixed preparations but may also demonstrate vacuolization (Fig. 2.8**D**). Choroid plexus epithelium resembles ductal epithelium in other tissues (e.g., breast), presenting a pavement or mosaic-like appearance en face due to the polyhedral outlines of the fairly distinct cell membranes.

This epithelium is more discohesive than ependyma in smears, and characteristically smears as small groups and individual cells with intact-appearing cell membranes and cytoplasm and a central dense nucleus (Fig. 2.8**B**). In smears, cytocentrifuges, and membrane filter preparations from fresh brain coronal slices, they become deposited on surfaces by the knife as each section is made and tend to be nearly ubiquitous in smears prepared from a variety of sites unless care is taken to remove the intended sample from just beneath the exposed surface.

Meninges

The meninges include dura mater (pachymeninges), arachnoid mater, and pia mater (the last two collectively termed pia-arachnoid or leptomeninges). The dura mater is composed of dense fibrous connective tissue (fibroblasts associated with collagen and some elastic fibers) with associated blood supply. The outer layer of the dura merges with the periosteum of the inner table of the skull, and the inner layer abuts the arachnoid mater. The interconnecting space between the arachnoid mater and pia mater (the latter being the more condensed portion of cells and connective tissue directly applied to the astrocyte processes surfacing the neural parenchyma) is traversed by delicate trabeculae and comprises the subarachnoid space, occupied by cerebrospinal fluid. Architectural characteristics of the connections between the dura and arachnoid are less resistant to mechanical stresses than the connections within each respective layer, making this zone a potential space within which blood, pus, or other fluids may dissect as a result of various disease processes. Extensions of pia mater accompany penetrating leptomeningeal vessels for some distance into the neural parenchyma. Recent data suggest that the space so created (Virchow-Robin space) may be in continuity with the subpial space rather than the subarachnoid space as has been traditionally taught (20), but wc maintain the traditional viewpoint at the time of this writing.

The pia-arachnoid consists of delicate collagen fibers, a few elastic fibers, and flattened cells with round to ovoid to elliptical nuclei, reminiscent of mesothelial cells. A few fibroblasts and macrophages, as well as the leptomeningeal vasculature, are present. The nuclei of meningothelial (pia-arachnoid) cells have a rather distinct nuclear membrane, fine chromatin, and a small, inconspicuous nucleolus (Fig. 2.10). Nuclear pseudoinclusions (cytoplasmic spurs) and nuclear clefts or folds are variably prominent. The external layer of arachnoid cells (most closely applied to dura, and thus termed arachnoidal cap cells) is intimately associated with the formation of arachnoid villi (through which cerebrospinal fluid reaches the intravascular compartment of the dural sinuses), and these cells have a pronounced tendency to form aggregates and whorls. These latter structures may hyalinize and become mineralized, forming laminated, ovoid basophilic structures (psammoma bodies) rich in calcium apatite crystals with iron, and with concentrically arranged collagen fibers (Fig. 2.10**A**; also see Fig. 7.9**A** and **B**) (21). Not to be confused are pseudopsammoma bodies, which are hyalinized, eosinophilic intracellular bodies seen in secretory meningiomas (12). The arachnoidal cap cell is considered the cell of origin of meningiomas. Its cytoplasm is lightly eosinophilic with H&E and pale green with the Pap stain (Fig. 2.10).

Pineal Body (Epiphysis)

Pinealocytes, comprising an estimated 90 to 95% of the cell population of the pineal body, are neurosecretory cells arranged in cords and nests surrounded by capillaries (Fig. 2.11). Processes extending from the pinealocyte soma have knob- or club-shaped terminal expansions, which end in intimate relationship to the surrounding capillaries but may also terminate in the connective tissue septae (extensions of the pia mater surfacing the pineal body) separating nests and cords of pinealocytes. The cellular elements of the pineal also includes sparse fibrous astrocytes, unmyelinated sympathetic nerve twigs, and larger myelinated aberrant habenular and posterior commissure nerve fibers. Very rarely, a more typical ganglion cell is found in otherwise normal pineal bodies. Functions attributed to the pineal body include secretion of melatonin by pinealocytes, the effects of which include suppression of gonadotrophin secretion. It may thus prevent the development of precocious puberty. Some support for this theory is provided by observations that the onset of normal puberty is accompanied by involution of the pineal body and that precocious puberty may occur in the presence of mass lesions encroaching on the pineal body and presumably reducing its normal functional capacity.

The nuclei of pinealocytes average approximately 10 to 12 μm in diameter, have a stippled "salt and pepper" chromatin distribution, and display a tendency to form nuclear clefts and folds, which may result in a rather striking convoluted appearance to the nucleus that is reminiscent of certain neoplastic cells (Figs. 2.11 and 2.12). These nuclear characteristics, together with the club-shaped terminal expansions of their cytoplasmic processes, make the pinealocyte unique among the normal neuronal elements we have examined with cytopreparatory techniques. Although they are visible with routine as well as metallic impregnation techniques (3), one more readily appreciates these features in cytopreparatory techniques. As pointed out by Russell and Rubinstein (21, p. 381), the terminal expansions on pinealocyte cell processes are very scant before 8 years of age. Inclusion of this structure in study sets has the additional benefit of refamiliarizing one with the normal anatomy of this infrequently sampled structure, and avoiding the pitfall of its confusion with a neoplasm. Laminated or amorphous calcifications (psammoma bodies, brain sand, acervulus, calcospherites) in the pineal body parenchyma and immediately adjacent tissue (pineal pial capsule, habenular commissure, and habenular trigone) are a regular accompaniment of aging, usually present by the late teens and increasing in numbers thereafter (Fig. 2.12D). Other accompaniments of aging include the development of pineal body cysts and astroglial Rosenthal fibers and plaque-like aggregates (gliosis).

In this brief review of pineal body cytologic features, the discrepancy between the cell lines listed and the most common primary tumor of the pineal body, the germinoma, warrants comment. This point is dealt with in most texts by statements indicating that germ cells (the presumptive source of germinomas) originate in the yolk sac endoderm and migrate to the region of the future gonadal ridge, where subsequent development leads to the formation of the mature gonads. In addition, germ cells are also described as migrating or disseminating widely throughout many tissues and organs in the early embryonic stages, including the hindgut, neural crest derivatives such as peripheral ganglia and adrenal, spleen, liver, brain, optic cup, notochord, heart, and thymus. Although the initial migration (i.e., from yolk sac to gonadal ridge) is said by some authors (17) to occur by direct ameboid movement of individual germ cells, Meyer's careful studies in chick embryos describe migration of germ cells via vascular channels to both gonadal and extragonadal sites (including brain), with subsequent penetration of vascular walls and invasion of extravascular embryonic tissues accompanied by development of prominent pseudopodial processes (14). While this provides a more satisfactory explanation for the presence of germ cell tumors in such diverse extragonadal sites as pineal body, suprasellar area, mediastinum, retroperitoneum, spinal cord, sacrococcygeum, nasopharynx, and orbit, we are not aware of reports unequivocally demonstrating such "resting" germ cell elements in, for example, normal human pineal body or diencephalic tissue. Nor are we aware of a convincing explanation for the favored sites, midline preponderance, or occasional simultaneous multifocal occurrence of germ cell tumors in brain, mediastinum, and testis (2, 7-9, 13). Should such resting germ cell elements exist in normal tissues, it would seem theoretically possible that some of the more sophisticated, recently developed cell marker techniques might be utilized to reveal their presence.

Pituitary Gland

Anatomic regions of the pituitary gland include the anterior pituitary (pars anterior, pars distalis), the pars intermedia, and the posterior pituitary (neurohypophysis, pars nervosa). Traditionally, the median eminence (at the rostral end of the pituitary stalk) is included as a region of the neurohypophysis, and the pars anterior, tuberalis, and intermedia are collectively referred to as the adenohypophysis. The slender pituitary stalk, composed in part by a rostral extension continuous with both the anterior (pars tuberalis) and posterior (infundibular stem) pituitary, connects the intrasellar portion of the pituitary gland with the hypothalamus.

Anterior Pituitary (Pars Anterior, Pars Distalis)

Studies in recent years have greatly expanded the precision with which anterior pituitary neoplasms and their functional products can be elucidated. With the time and stain selection restraints imposed by intraoperative consultation requirements, however, reliance on more crude distinctions between the presence or absence of a heterogeneous versus homogeneous cell population in a pituitary mass will most often be adequate to allow appropriate decisions concerning both surgical procedures and proper tissue utilization for diagnostic purposes (also see section on pituitary neoplasms, Chapter 7).

The normal anterior pituitary is composed of a rich network of capillaries and sinusoids with the usual accompanying connective tissue components. The latter are in continuity with a dense collagenous capsule surrounding the gland. This capsule is separated from the dural surface of the sella by a less dense layer of connective tissue containing numerous veins, and by variable amounts of pia-arachnoid, which typically passes through the diaphragma sellae with the pituitary stalk. The subarachnoid space, in contrast, indents the roof of the sella only slightly below the level of the diaphragma sellae in most individuals. The endocrine cells of the anterior pituitary are arranged as irregular cords, masses, and acini. They are, with either H&E or Pap stains, roughly separable into three groups based on tinctorial qualities: acidophiles (eosinophilic with H&E, green with Pap), basophiles (a vague blue tint on H&E, tan to brown with Pap) and chromophobes (that population not clearly separable into either eosinophilic or basophilic categories due to poor affinity for stains) (Fig. 2.13**A** and **B**). The relative overall percentages of these three populations are 40% acidophiles, 10% basophiles, and 50% chromophobes. However, in a given small sample such a cell spectrum is unlikely due to a somewhat uneven distribution of cell types in the normal gland. Acidophiles are preferentially situated laterally (i.e., acidophilic wings) and basophiles medially (including the pars tuberalis) as well as anteriorly (i.e., mucoid wedge). The mucoid wedge terminology derives from the PAS positivity of the glycoprotein-rich secretory product of basophiles (thyrotrophin, lactogenic hormone, and follicle-stimulating hormone). Basophiles may also produce adrenocorticotrophic hormone and melanocyte-stimulating hormone. The functional products of acidophiles are growth hormone and prolactin. Chromophobes are the remaining cells in which less prominent stored hormone granules, and resultant lack of distinguishing tinctorial (or even ultrastructural) features are present, and thus can represent quiescent, degranulated, or otherwise hormone-poor cells or more than one type. The focal preponderance of a given cell type in normal glands may mimic an adenoma in very small biopsy specimens, especially in frozen tissue, and cautious interpretation is appropriate in such circumstances. Squamous metaplasia of adenohypophyseal cells may be prominent in some normal glands, particularly in the pars tuberalis. This may raise the question of other squamous cell-containing lesions in the vicinity of the sella (e.g., craniopharyngioma, epidermoid cyst, dermoid cyst) particularly in sparse smear preparations. Smear preparations of normal anterior pituitary demonstrate a greater degree of cell pleomorphism with or without chromatin coarseness, and also multinucleation, than is readily appreciated in normal paraffin sections, and does not in itself warrant a diagnosis of neoplasia (a principle well recognized in endocrine organs in general by the surgical pathologist) (Fig. 2.13). The appearance of acidophiles, basophiles, chromophobes, and a large population of predominantly bare nuclei on a rather "dirty" granular background in smear preparations of the anterior pituitary reflects the fragility of these cells when subjected to cytopreparatory techniques and should not be confused with "tumor diathesis."

Pars Intermedia

The pars intermedia, which is rudimentary in humans, is composed of cysts of variable size containing a colloid-like substance and occasional cellular debris and is lined by simple cuboidal epithelium that includes some ciliated cells. Small groups of clear cells that may surround a lumen and resemble salivary gland tissue may occur in this zone, as may a few cells with an oncocytic appearance and cells resembling one or another anterior pituitary glandular cell population, particularly basophiles.

Posterior Pituitary

The spectrum of structures in this portion of the pituitary are relatively few. Blood vessels are common, with their accompanying mesodermal derivatives (e.g., collagen, reticulin, fibroblasts). Predominantly unmyelinated axons of the hypothalamohypophyseal tract (primarily derived from the periventricular and supraoptic nuclei of the hypothalamus) are conspicuous. Their contained neurosecretory granules (composed of oxytocin, and antidiuretic hormone or vasopressin) occasionally form basophilic (with H&E), globular aggregates termed Herring bodies. The predominant cell population is the pituicyte, regarded as a modified astrocyte, which may accumulate a lipofuscin-like pigment with age and may also demonstrate some phagocytic properties, but whose main role is assumed to be structural support (Fig. 2.13**E** and **F**). The degree of nuclear pleomorphism and very fibrillar background of the normal posterior pituitary could, on routine stains and without knowledge of the exact source of the tissue, raise the question of gliosis or even a low-grade astrocytoma in a small tissue fragment (Figs. 2.13**E** and **F**). Its fibrillar content also results in generally poor smear preparations and a low yield of cells with other cytopreparatory techniques. Anterior pituitary-type basophiles are also found in the posterior pituitary zone in many normal glands.

Peripheral Nerves, Dorsal Spinal Root and Autonomic Ganglia, and the Extra-Adrenal Paraganglion System

This group of normal structures is not conducive to smear preparations or other commonly utilized cytopreparatory techniques, their respective cell populations being encased in a rather fibrous, rubbery tissue background. Frozen sections remain the standard approach to most such specimens requiring intraoperative verification (e.g., confirmation of neural rather than vascular fibrous-appearing tissue in a presumed vagotomy specimen). Since the inclusion of such structures may unavoidably occur in specimens such as mass lesions submitted from a variety of sites, however, a few comments concerning their cytologic features follows.

Dorsal root ganglia of spinal nerves contain a wide spectrum of neuronal sizes, ranging from approximately 15 to 120 μm, with larger neurons predominating. Individual ganglion cells are surrounded by a layer of flattened satellite or capsule cells, the latter somewhat analogous to CNS astrocytes. The ganglion cell processes, both proximal and distal, have an axonal appearance due to investment in a myelin sheath formed by the Schwann cell. Although the Schwann cell is the peripheral nervous system counterpart of the oligodendrocyte, among the more important structural differences between these two (in myelinated as opposed to unmyelinated nerves) is the association of each Schwann cell with a single myelin internode, the Schwann cell nucleus being included in the outermost layer of a given internode wrapping. The oligodendrocyte, in contrast, sends delicate processes that terminally expand to form as many as 30 to 50 internodes of myelin on multiple axons coursing through the neuropil in the vicinity of its soma.

A peripheral ganglion is invested by a dense connective tissue capsule, portions of which accompany the penetrating vessels. This connective tissue capsule is in continuity with (from without inward) the epineurium, (fibrovascular sheath around the peripheral nerve trunk as a whole), perineurium (the sheath of similar tissue surrounding individual nerve fascicles—bundles of axons—within the nerve trunk), and endoneurium (delicate loose fibrovascular connective tissue surrounding individual axons within a fascicle) of the peripheral nerve. For a more complete discussion of central versus peripheral myelin sheaths and general nerve structure, see reviews by Johnson (10) and Raine (19).

Autonomic ganglia, while structurally similar in many respects to spinal nerve ganglia, do demonstrate features which may allow light microscopic differentiation from the latter. In comparison to spinal ganglia, autonomic ganglion cells are multipolar (rather than pseudounipolar), tend to be smaller in size, contain an eccentric rather than centrally situated nucleus and tend to have a less uniform, more discontinuous layer of flattened satellite cells surrounding each ganglion cell.

Structures known as paraganglia are generally regarded as arising from the neural crest, migrating to their eventual location in widely disseminated sites where they form a system of cellular aggregates linked to one another—and to the adrenal medulla—by certain structural and functional characteristics. Structurally, in addition to the expected connective tissue and vascular elements, there are two major cellular components. The first are chief cells (type I cells, epithelioid or glomus cells), typically arranged in discrete nests (Zellballen) with finely granular (pink with H&E) cytoplasm, and round to ovoid nuclei with fine chromatin, a small nucleolus, and a distinct nuclear membrane. The cytoplasm may vary in staining density among the chief cells in different paraganglia and within the same cell aggregate, depending in part on their content of neurosecretory granules.

The second major cell component consists of sustentacular (type II) cells, oval or lenticular in shape and with a generally more dense nuclear chromatin. Sustentacular cells surround the nests of chief cells, reminiscent of the satellite cells of autonomic ganglia, and do not contain neurosecretory products. Due to their wide distribution, paraganglia may unexpectedly appear in, for example, radical neck dissection specimens for neoplastic disease. In this setting, close attention to the architecture, biphasic cell population, and nuclear characteristics will usually resolve any suspicion that they represent infiltrating carcinoma cells without the need for histochemical markers (e.g., chromogranin).

Occasionally, aggregates of epithelioid cells bearing some resemblance to paraganglia, in that they consist of nests of cells associated with prominent vasculature, are of yet another source. Glomus bodies, a specialized arteriovenous anastomosis more familiar to pathologists in a distal extremity location, may cause confusion with neoplasms when found in unfamiliar sites. Albrecht and Zbieranowski (1) have recently reviewed this potential diagnostic pitfall relative to the glomus coccygeum, normally found in front of, or immediately below, the tip of the coccyx and measuring up to 2.5 mm in diameter. It is generally oval in shape, and smaller nodules may be found near the main mass. Coccygectomy specimens removed for coccydynia have, in our hands, been one source of readily accessible teaching material for the demonstration of such normal structures.

References

1. Albrecht, S., and Zbieranowski, I. Incidental glomus coccygeum. When a normal structure looks like a tumor. Am. J. Surg. Pathol. 14:922–924, 1990.
2. Antonelli-Orlidge, A., Smith, S.R., and D'Amore, P.A. Influence of pericytes on capillary endothelial cell growth. Am. Rev. Respir. Dis. 140:1129–1131, 1989.
3. del Rio-Hortega, P. Pineal gland. Section XIV in: Penfield, W. (Ed.): Cytology and Cellular Pathology of the Nervous System. Hafner Publishing Co., New York, 1965, 2:637–703.
4. Dolman, C.L. Microglia. Chapter 4 in: Davis, R.L., and Robertson, D.M. (Eds.): Textbook of Neuropathology. Ed. 2. Williams & Wilkins, Baltimore, 1991, pp. 141–163.
5. Flament-Durand, J., and Brion, J.P. Tanycytes: Morphology and functions: A Review. Int. Rev. Cytol. 96:121–155, 1985.
6. Friede, R.L., and Pollak, A. The cytogenetic basis for classifying ependymomas. J. Neuropathol. Exp. Neurol. 37:103–118, 1978.
7. Friedman, N.B., and Van de Velde, R.L. Germ cell tumors in man, pleiotropic mice, and continuity of germplasm and somatoplasm. Hum. Pathol. 12:772–776, 1981.
8. Hisa, S., Morinaga, S., Kobayashi, Y., Ojrina, M., Chikoaka, H., and Sasano, N. Intramedullary spinal cord germinoma producing HCG and precocious puberty in a boy. Cancer 55:2845–2849, 1985.
9. Jennings, M.T., Gelman, R., and Hochberg, F. Intracranial germ-cell tumors: natural history and pathogenesis. J. Neurosurg. 63:155–167, 1985.
10. Johnson, P.C. Peripheral nerve. Chapter 18 in: Davis, R.L., and Robertson, D.M. (Eds.): Textbook of Neuropathology. Ed. 2. Williams & Wilkins, Baltimore, 1991, pp. 1004–1087.
11. Kasper M., and Karsten, U. Focal ependymal differentiation in the choroid plexus of human newborn brain confirmed by immunohistochemistry with monoclonal antibodies. Acta Neuropathol. 73:409–410, 1987.
12. Kepes, J.J. Meningiomas. Biology, Pathology and Differential Diagnosis. Masson Publishing USA, Inc., New York, 1982.
13. Lewis, P.D. Pineal gland. Chapter 17 in: Weller, R.O. (Ed.): Nervous System, Muscle and Eyes. Vol. 4 in: Symmers, W. St. C. (Ed.): Systemic Pathology. Churchill Livingstone, New York, 1990, p. 508.
14. Meyer, D.B. The migration of primordial germ cells in the chick embryo. Dev. Biol., 10:154–190, 1964.
15. Minkowski, A., Larroche, J.C.L., Vignaud, J., Dreyfus-Brisac, C., and Dargassies, S.S.A. Development of the nervous system in early life. Chapter 11 in: Falkner, F. (Ed.): Human Development. W.B. Saunders Co., Philadelphia, 1966, pp. 254–285.

16. Nag, S. The ependymoma and choroid plexus. Chapter 2 in: Davis, R.L., and Robertson, D.M. (Eds): Textbook of Neuropathology. Ed. 2. Williams & Wilkins, Baltimore, 1991, pp. 95–114.
17. Pansky, B. Review of Medical Embryology. Macmillan Publishing Co., Inc., New York, 1982, p. 256.
18. Pittella, J.E.H., and Brasileiro-Filho, G. The significance of paired astrocyte nuclei in normal human nervous tissue. J. Anat. 151:101–105, 1987.
19. Raine, C.S. Oligodendrocytes and central nervous system myelin. Chapter 3 in: Davis, R.L., and Robertson, D.M. (Eds.): Textbook of Neuropathology. Ed. 2. Williams & Wilkins, Baltimore, 1991, pp. 115–140.
20. Ramsay, D.A., and Robertson, D.M. Meninges and their reaction to injury. Chapter 5 in: Davis, R.L., and Robertson, D.M. (Eds.): Textbook of Neuropathology. Ed. 2. Williams & Wilkins, Baltimore, 1991, pp. 164–174.
21. Russell, D.S., and Rubinstein, L.J. Pathology of Tumours of the Nervous System. Ed. 5. Williams & Wilkins, Baltimore, 1989, p. 403.

Additional General References

22. Burger, P.C., Scheithauer, B.W., and Vogel, F.S. Surgical Pathology of the Nervous System and its Coverings. Ed. 3. Churchill Livingstone, New York, 1991, pp. 503–546.
23. Cormack, D.H. Ham's Histology. Ed. 9, J.B. Lippincott Co., Philadelphia, 1987.
24. Crosby, E.C., Humphrey, T., and Lauer, E.W. Correlative Anatomy of the Nervous System. The Macmillan Co., New York, 1962.
25. Duchen, L.W. General pathology of neurons and neuroglia. Chapter 1 in: Adams, J.H., Corsellis, J.A.N., and Duchen, L.W. (Eds.): Greenfield's Neuropathology. Ed. 4. John Wiley & Sons, New York, 1984, pp. 1–52.
26. Glenner, G.G., and Grimley, P.M. Tumors of the Extra-adrenal Paraganglion System (Including Chemoreceptors). Fascicle 9 in: Atlas of Tumor Pathology, Second Series. Armed Forces Institute of Pathology, Washington, D.C., 1974.
27. Hirano, A. Neurons and Astrocytes. Chapter 1 in: Davis, R.L., and Robertson, D.M. (Eds.): Textbook of Neuropathology. Ed. 2. Williams & Wilkins, Baltimore, 1991, pp. 1–94.
28. Kovacs, K., and Horvath, E. Tumors of the Pituitary Gland. Fascicle 21 in: Atlas of Tumor Pathology, Second Series, Armed Forces Institute of Pathology, Washington, D.C., 1986.
29. Peters, A., Palay, S.L., and de F. Webster, H. The Fine Structure of the Nervous System. Neurons and their Supporting Cells. Ed. 3. Oxford University Press, New York, 1991.
30. Sternberg, S.S. (Ed.): Histology for Pathologists. Raven Press, New York, 1992.

3 / CSF Cytopathology—General Aspects

Examination of cells from the cerebrospinal fluid (CSF) plays an important role in clinical medicine (4, 9, 19, 25, 46, 48, 58). Data obtained by such laboratory analysis is integrated with the rest of the clinical picture (9), which includes a careful history and physical examination and radiographic and laboratory studies.

Indications

As with other medical tests, information provided by CSF cytological analysis may be of value for the following reasons: (*a*) to confirm a clinical impression or establish a diagnosis; (*b*) to rule out a diagnosis; (*c*) to monitor therapy; (*d*) to establish prognosis; and (*e*) to screen for or detect occult disease (58, 61). Coordination between clinical and laboratory personnel is mandatory. Clinicians should provide a specimen of adequate volume that has been collected and stored properly and that is accompanied by the appropriate clinical information. The laboratory should report results promptly, with direct communication to the responsible physician when particularly aberrant results are obtained (9). The laboratory should also provide information on normal findings and values, reliability (accuracy) of the interpretation and results, and confounders that could potentially interfere with the cytologic evaluation (e.g., chemotherapeutic effects) (9, 20, 58). Clinician and laboratory personnel interaction is also needed to determine if additional samples might be helpful in the case of ambiguous results.

When properly performed, neurocytopathologic examination can assist the clinician in formulating and prioritizing a list of clinical differential diagnoses and, in certain conditions, assist the clinician in following the results of therapy. One example of the latter situation in modern practice is that of a patient with leptomeningeal leukemia for whom the frequency of therapy will be altered by the results of serial CSF determinations (see Chapters 4 and 5).

Repeated laboratory assessment of fluid may also be indicated by an unexplained poor response to therapy and may identify secondary complications such as opportunistic infection or development of a new neoplastic cell line, which must then be treated (30). Indications for spinal fluid examination are legion and are undergoing change as other diagnostic methods (e.g., imaging techniques) are being improved. Some of the general categories of indications are summarized in Table 3.1. The relative usefulness of the CSF examination in various disorders has also recently been summarized (see Table 3.2) (4, 23).

Comparison with Other Body Fluids

Several features distinguish the clinical evaluation of the CSF from pleural, pericardial, or ascitic fluid (1, 5, 9). First, symptoms suggestive of CNS disease are relatively nonspecific (Table 3.3). Second, CSF is a normal body cavity constituent rather than a transudate or exudate, and the clinician usually cannot determine if there is a qualitative abnormality of the CSF until a specimen has been obtained (9). Third, the removal of pleural or ascitic fluid will often relieve symptoms for a time. In contrast, removal of CSF is much more likely to be performed for diagnostic rather than for therapeu-

Table 3.1.
Selected Examples of Indications for Lumbar Puncture[a]

Suspected conditions
Infections—(meningitis, encephalitis, syphilis)
Subarachnoid hemorrhage
Multiple sclerosis; Guillain-Barré syndrome
Neoplasms with suspected CSF involvement
Therapy/diagnosis
Chemotherapy for leukemia, lymphoma, and fungal infections
Introduction of anesthetics
Introduction of radiographic contrast media

[a] Modified from Kjeldsberg, C.R., and Knight, J.A. Body Fluids. Laboratory Examination of Amniotic, Cerebrospinal, Seminal, Serous, and Synovial Fluids: A Textbook Atlas. Ed. 2. American Society of Clinical Pathologists Press, Chicago, 1986.

Table 3.2.
Disease detected by the spinal tap[a,b]

High sensitivity, high specificity
Bacterial, tuberculous, and fungal meningitis
High sensitivity, moderate specificity
Viral meningitis
Subarachnoid hemorrhage
Multiple sclerosis
Central nervous system syphilis
Infectious polyneuritis
Paraspinal abscess
Moderate sensitivity, high specificity
Meningeal malignancy
Moderate sensitivity, moderate specificity
Intracranial hemorrhage
Viral encephalitis
Subdural hematoma

[a] From Health and Public Policy Committee, American College of Physicians: Position paper: The diagnostic spinal tap. Ann. Intern. Med. 104:880–885, 1986.
[b] Sensitivity is the ability of a test to detect disease when it is present; specificity is the ability of a test to exclude disease when it is not present.

tic reasons, and has a greater potential for risk (e.g., patients with incipient herniation syndromes, local infections in the needle path, presence of a complete spinal block, patients receiving anticoagulant therapy, etc.) (39).

Appearance

Normal CSF is clear and colorless. Turbid CSF may indicate a high protein concentration, increased numbers of erythrocytes or leukocytes, or the presence of numerous microorganisms. Table 3.4 lists the appearances of CSF, causes, and potential clinical implications.

A pink-tinged or frankly bloody sample may result from a traumatic procedure or from pre-existing blood in the CSF. To differentiate these two possibilities, it is customary to count the number of erythrocytes in the first and subsequent tubes, with a substantial decrement suggesting a traumatic tap (see also Chapter 4). In addition, blood introduced by the procedure may clot, whereas blood pre-existing in CSF usually does not. Finally, when a sample of CSF from a traumatic tap is centrifuged immediately after obtaining the sample, the fluid becomes clear and colorless. With pre-existing blood in the CSF, the fluid retains an orange to pink color (xanthochromia) postcentrifugation due to lysis of erythrocytes (Table 3.4). Xanthochromia may be subtle, but can usually be detected at the bedside by comparing CSF with water against a white background. Despite these various strategies traumatic lumbar puncture can be a confounding factor, and methods of calculating the influence of blood on CSF cell counts using peripheral blood samples, assessment of other (non-cytologic) CSF parameters, and the clinical picture must all be carefully assessed to reduce the

Table 3.3.
Symptoms Leading to Cerebrospinal Fluid Evaluation[a]

Headache	Mental nerve paresthesias
Dizziness	Fever of unexplained origin
Altered mentation	Change in affect or memory
Visual disturbances	Seizures
Difficulty with coordination or motor function	Trouble with speech
Unexplained nausea or vomiting	Bladder dysfunction

[a] From Cheson, B.D. Clinical utility of body fluid analyses. Symposium on Body Fluid Analysis. Clin. Lab. Med. 5:155–208, 1985; with permission.

Table 3.4.
Clinical Significance of CSF Appearance

Appearance	Cause	Major Significance
Crystal clear		Normal
Hazy, turbid, cloudy, smoky, milky	WBCs	Meningitis
	RBCs	Hemorrhage (RBC lysis generally begins within 4 hours) Traumatic tap
	Microorganisms	Meningitis
	Protein	Disorders that affect blood-brain barrier Production of IgG within CNS
Oily	X-ray contrast material	Previous radiographic diagnostic procedure
Bloody	RBCs	Hemorrhage
Xanthochromic	Hemoglobin	Old hemorrhage Lysed cells from traumatic tap
	Bilirubin	RBC breakdown Elevated serum bilirubin
	Merthiolate	Contamination
	Carotene	Increased serum levels
	Protein	(SEE ABOVE)
	Melanin	Melanin-containing tumors, melanosis cerebri
Clotted	Protein	(SEE ABOVE)
	Clotting factors	Introduced by traumatic tap
Pellicle formation	Protein Clotting factors	Tubercular meningitis
Green	Myeloperoxidase	Purulent fluid; theoretically, CNS chloroma
Viscous	Capsular polysaccharide	Cryptococcosis
	Mucus	Metastatic mucin-producing carcinomas

potential errors in diagnosis resulting from blood contamination of CSF (40).

There are also some infrequent conditions that may alter the appearance of CSF (e.g., oil from myelogram contrast material, fat droplets from a fat embolism, chylous fluid from accidental sampling of a lymphatic, etc. [see Table 3.4]).

Cytologic Components

Reference values for normal CSF are listed in Table 3.5. Selected CSF cytologic findings are also in the illustrations section of this text. CSF cytologic abnormalities occur in a wide variety of neurological disease categories, neoplastic and non-neoplastic. Although it is dealt with in greater detail in subsequent chapters, the nonspecificity of elevations of one or more cytologic component is briefly summarized in Table 3.6. The recent work of Hayward et al. (22) suggests that most, if not all, neutrophils appearing in the CSF of normal individuals may result from blood contamination, although this is still controversial (50).

The question of whether pia-arachnoid cells (''PAM'' cells) and other CSF components such as astrocytes are present in normal CSF is also controversial, having been reported by some authors (58) but with more recent evidence providing a convincing argument for interpreting such cells as hematogenous elements based on marker studies (see Bigner [4], page 470). When cerebrospinal fluid is obtained by ventricular aspiration (where the needle path traverses CNS tissue en route) or by cisternal puncture (where

Table 3.5.
Reference Values for Normal Cerebrospinal Fluid

Physical Characteristics:		
	Volume:	90–160 ml (adult)
	Color:	Colorless
	Appearance (transparency):	Clear
	Specific Gravity:	1.006–1.008
Routine Chemistry:		
	Conventional Units	*S.I. Units*
Glucose	50–80 mg/dl	2.8–4.4 mmol/liter
Protein	15–45 mg/dl	0.15–0.45 g/liter
Albumin	10–30 mg/dl	100–200 mg/liter
Cell Counts:		
	Chamber Count Method	
Adults	0–5 mononuclear cells/ml: 0–0.005 × 10^9/liter	
Neonates	0–30 mononuclear cells/ml: 0–0.030 × 10^9/liter	
	Membrane Filtration Method	
Adults	0–5000 mononuclear cells/ml	
Cell Differential Count:		
	Adults	*Neonates*
Lymphocytes	60% ± 20%	20% ± 15%
Monocytes	30% ± 15%	70% ± 20%
Neutrophils	2% ± 4%	4% ± 4%
Histiocytes	Rare	5% ± 4%
Eosinophils	Rare	Rare
Ependymal cells	Rare	Rare

the possibility of the needle tip touching adjacent CNS structures is enhanced), or when CNS cyst aspirates are examined, depending on the needle path chosen virtually any normal neural structure may be included in the fluid sample submitted (see Chapter 2). Thus, neurons, glia, ependyma, choroid plexus, or pia-arachnoid-derived cells as well as structures such as corpora amylacea are more frequently reported in samples obtained by such techniques.

A number of reports describing CSF abnormalities exist in the literature that do not readily lend themselves to tabular summary. For example, a lower than normal percentage of T-lymphocytes in the CSF (30% compared to 90%) has been reported in the presence of epilepsia partialis continua (21). Mitotic figures may be present in CSF cells in a wide variety of circumstances (16). Non-neoplastic conditions in which CSF cell mitoses have been described include bacterial and viral meningitis, multiple sclerosis, Guillain-Barré syndrome, subacute sclerosing panencephalitis, ischemic stroke, hypoxic/ischemic encephalopathy due to carbon monoxide intoxication, radionecrosis of the spinal cord, and Alzheimer's disease. In non-neoplastic conditions where the mitotic cell was identifiable, mitotic figures have been described in macrophages, monocytes, and rarely plasma cells (16). With regard to neoplasia involving the CSF, various types of lymphoma, carcinoma and sarcoma have been reported in which tumor cell mitoses were described.

CSF pleocytosis with neutrophils, lymphocytes, erythrocytes, and many bizarre, immature, pleomorphic mononucleated cells containing cytoplasmic vacuoles has been reported following intrathecal diagnostic studies with the radiographic contrast material Metrizamide, which has enjoyed increased use in comparison to oil-based

Table 3.6.
Examples of Disease Associations with Elevated CSF Cell Counts[a]

INCREASED LYMPHOCYTES/MONOCYTES

Infections
- Viral meningoencephalitis (including SSPE) (46a)
- Bacterial (particularly late or partially treated; unusual organisms including *Leptospira, Listeria monocytogenes*; tuberculosis, syphilis, *Borrelia burgdorferi* (44)
- Fungal meningitis
- Parasites (cysticercosis, trichinosis, toxoplasmosis)
- Aseptic meningitis associated with septic foci adjacent to the meninges

Multiple sclerosis
Myasthenia gravis (26)
Guillain-Barré syndrome
Acute disseminated encephalomyelitis
Drug therapy
Sarcoidosis of meninges
Polyneuritis
Vasculitis
Benign migraine-like syndrome in children (47)

INCREASED NEUTROPHILS

Normals (probably due to contamination with blood) (22, 48)
Infections
- Bacterial (including tuberculosis, early and during treatment (53); syphilis; *Leptospira*)
- Fungal (early)
- Viral (early)
- Parasitic (amoebic encephalomyelitis, cysticerosis) (60)
- Meningitis associated with septic foci adjacent to meninges (cerebral abscess; subdural empyema)

Following:
- Seizures (17)
- CNS hemorrhage
- Infarction
- Repeated lumbar puncture
- Injection of foreign materials into subarachnoid space (methotrexate, radiographic contrast media)
- Drug therapy (OKT-3) (18)
- In association with metastatic tumor cells

INCREASED EOSINOPHILS

Infections
- Bacterial (e.g., pneumococcal, tuberculosis, syphilis)
- Viral meningoencephalitis
- Fungal (e.g., coccidioidomycosis)
- Rickettsial (e.g., Rocky Mountain spotted fever) (13)

Parasites
- *Angiostrongylus cantonensis*
- Cysticercosis
- Echinococcosis (hydatid disease)
- *Gnathostoma spinigerum*
- *Schistosoma* species
- *Paragonimus westermani*
- *Fasciola hepatica*
- *Hypoderma bovis* (larval migrans)
- Toxocariasis
- Trichinellosis
- Ascariasis
- Onchocerciasis

Table 3.6—*Continued*

INCREASED EOSINOPHILS (*Cont'd*)

In presence of:
- Intrathecal injections of foreign protein (radioiodinated serum albumin, radiographic contrast media)
- Immunizations (e.g., rabies)
- Intracranial shunts
- Vasculitis
- Hypereosinophilic syndrome (28)
- Acute polyneuritis
- Drug reactions (41)
- Food allergies
- Urticaria
- Bronchial asthma
- Trauma (34)
- Neoplasia[b]
  - CNS chloroma (24)
  - Lymphocytic leukemia with CNS spread
  - ALL conversion to acute eosinophilic leukemia (30)
  - Leptomeningeal carcinomatosis (11)
  - Disseminated glioblastoma (14)
  - Neurosarcoidosis (49)

INCREASED PLASMA CELLS

Infections
- Bacterial (syphilis, tuberculosis; Lyme disease) (44)
- Viral meningoencephalitis
- Parasitic infestations
- Subacute sclerosing panencephalitis (SSPE)

Multiple sclerosis (18-97% of cases) (10)
Gullain-Barré syndrome (early)
Sarcoidosis of CNS
Vasculitis
In presence of:
- CSF hemorrhage
- CSF malignancies

INCREASED BASOPHILS

CNS involvement by chronic granulocytic leukemia

INCREASED MACROPHAGES (±GIANT CELLS)

Infections
- Tuberculous meningitis
- Viral meningoencephalitis
- Fungal meningoencephalitis

CSF blood (macrophages may contain erythrocytes, hemosiderin [dark brown pigment granules], or hematoidin [brownish yellow or red crystals]).
Reaction to foreign materials in CSF (radiographic contrast media, shunts, Ommaya reservoir) (6, 56)
In presence of:
- Tissue necrosis (trauma, infarction, abscess)

INCREÁSED EPENDYMAL AND/OR CHOROID PLEXUS EPITHELIAL CELLS (15, 25)

Presence in normals controversial (see text)
Infections
- Viral (mumps meningoencephalitis; enterovirus meningitis)
- Bacterial (treated tuberculous and chronic pneumococcal meningitis)

Table 3.6—*Continued*

INCREASED EPENDYMAL AND/OR CHOROID PLEXUS EPITHELIAL CELLS (*Cont'd*)

In presence of:
- Ventricular shunts (6)
- Hydrocephalus
- Brain stem infarction
- Cervical spondylotic myelopathy
- Acoustic neurilemmoma
- Transverse myelitis
- Intrathecal administration of chemotherapeutic agents
- Post-pneumoencephalography
- Post-traumatic

CONTAMINANTS IN CSF

Cartilage cells (usually from intervertebral disc) (8)
Bone marrow elements, including osteoblasts (from vertebral body marrow) (12, 27, 32, 37)
Squamous cells (from skin, or as laboratory glass slide contaminant)
Soft tissue elements (in needle track, including adipose tissue, connective tissue, striated muscle, capillaries) (5)
Erythrocytes and leucocytes (traumatic tap)
Talc or starch powder (from rubber gloves)[c] (25)
Radiographic contrast media (e.g., Pantopaque)
Debris (stain artifact, pollen spores, cellulose fibers, bacteria, etc.) (45)
Other (e.g., respiratory epithelium in presence of basilar skull fracture, corpora amylacea) (45)

[a] Modified from Krieg, A.F., and Kjeldsberg, C.R. Cerebrospinal fluid and other body fluids. Chapter 18 in: J.B. Henry (Ed.): Clinical Diagnosis and Management by Laboratory Methods. W.B. Saunders Co., Philadelphia, 1991, pp 445–473.
[b] Cases of CNS chloroma with peripheral blood eosinophilia have also been reported; the presence or absence of CSF eosinophilia not determined (24).
[c] Talc may be phagocytosed by CSF macrophages and be confused with, for example, cryptococci (5).

agents in recent years (3). CSF pleocytosis (up to 12 WBCs per mm^3, not over 2% neutrophils or 190 RBCs per mm^3) has been reported following epileptic seizures (17). Caution should always be exercised in interpreting such findings in cases in which erythrocyte contamination is also present (22). A mixed-cellularity pleocytosis (lymphocytes, monocytes, and granulocytes) has been described in relapsing polychondritis (7); occasional LE cells may be seen in CSF in cases of systemic lupus erythematosus (31); and a mixed-cellularity CSF pleocytosis (predominantly eosinophils, but with elevated lymphocytes, basophils, and numerous siderophages) has also been described following craniocerebral trauma (34).

Mollaret's meningitis is a rare clinical syndrome of recurrent benign meningitis in which a given episode is typically characterized by an early neutrophilic CSF pleocytosis followed by mononuclear inflammatory cells, including macrophages. Although most cases are idiopathic, in some cases the etiology has been identified as viral infections of various types, systemic lupus erythematosus and epidermoid cysts (presumably in the latter, secondary to recurrent leakage of cyst contents with resultant chemical meningitis (35).

Finally, a recent study indicates that CSF pleocytosis is a common postmortem event and is more pronounced in children than in adults, particularly in cases of sudden infant death syndrome (43). This postmortem pleocytosis occurred in the absence of histologic evidence of inflammation in brain sections, and all cases had negative CSF cultures for bacteria. The cause of this finding is unclear at present, but this observation suggests that caution in the interpretation of CSF pleocytosis in postmortem specimens is warranted.

The cell count of normal spinal fluid varies with patient age and with the preparation method employed (see Table 3.5 and Chapters 4 and 5). Neonates should not exceed 30 cells per micrometer (60% neutrophils, 40% mononucleated), and values similar to adults occur by about 1 month of age. Whether a proposed use of reagent strips as a screening test for CSF leucocytosis will supplant routine counting chamber methods remains to be seen (36).

Noncytologic Aspects of CSF

The physiology, clinical chemistry, immunology, application of microbiologic techniques, and use of intrathecal therapeutic agents, while outside the scope of our emphasis in this review, are briefly referred to in subsequent chapters and are important topics that must be assimilated in order to have a comprehensive perspective of the role of CSF analysis in clinical medicine. Several excellent reviews are available (19, 25, 29, 31, 38, 42). Textbooks generally indicate that normal adults have a CSF volume of 90 to 150 ml and that the entire volume is renewed four to five times daily (1).

Specimen Handling Protocol

Several suggested protocols and/or flow charts for laboratory processing of CSF specimens are available in the literature (2, 5, 33, 46) and can facilitate the planning of specimen handling (57).

Most physicians have been instructed to collect three 1- to 3-ml CSF specimens in separate sterile tubes. The three samples or aliquots are submitted to the laboratory labeled as illustrated in Figure 3.1.

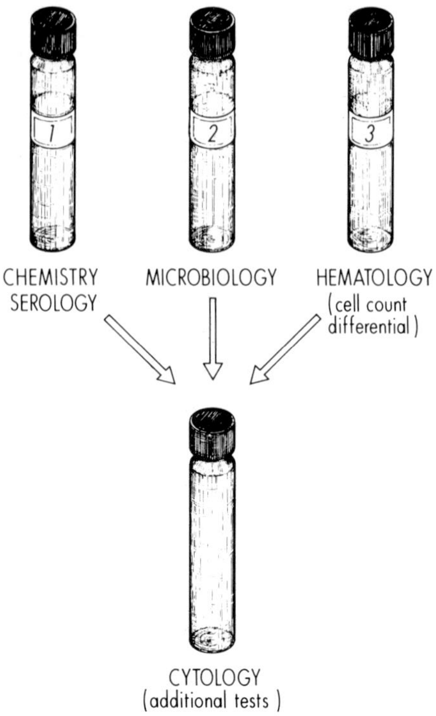

Figure 3.1. Labeling method for processing CSF specimens.

Typically, material submitted for cytologic examination is collected and brought to the laboratory directly. Table 3.7 outlines our recommended procedure for CSF specimen handling.

The need for prioritizing specimen dispersal to various laboratory areas based on the clinical question being asked, the amount of fluid necessary for various studies, and time-sensitive procedures (51, 52) are among the points typically emphasized in such protocols. Quality assurance guidelines pertinent to anatomic pathology in general, and cytopathology in particular, also apply to this area and provide a helpful means of evaluating the role of these techniques in clinical practice (54, 55, 59).

Table 3.7.
Sample Flow Chart for CSF Specimen Handling[a]

CSF		
Specimen receiving		
Routine screening (all specimens)		
Hematology lab: Cell count and differential (1 ml)		
Chemistry lab: Protein and glucose (1 ml)		
Clinical question template example:		
A.	Infection?	
	Microbiology lab:	2-10 ml, depending on agents suspected and tests requested.
	Cytology lab:	3 ml minimum (tube #2 or #3), confirm positive results as indicated with special stains or markers.
B.	Malignancy?	
	Cytology lab:	3 ml minimum (tube #2 or #3); Papanicolaou and Wright's stains (see text). Presence of "atypical" lymphocytes may require 10 ml of fresh CSF for marker studies, etc.
C.	Vascular disease?	
	Hematology lab:	Cell count in tube #1 and #4 to aid differential diagnosis of traumatic LP versus preexisting subarachnoid hemorrhage.
	Cytology lab:	Routine processing versus lyse RBCs to screen for underlying malignant cells, etc.
D.	Demyelinating disease?	
	Chemistry lab:	3 ml plus serum sample: oligoclonal bands, IgG synthesis rate, IgG/albumin ratio, etc.
E.	Other?	
	Electron microscopy, tissue culture for cytogenetics, etc.	
SAVE ALL CSF NOT USED IN INITIAL REQUIRED TESTS		
Specify storage method, site, duration, etc.		

[a] From Andrews, J.M., and Schumann, G.B. Laboratory processing of cerebrospinal fluid specimens. Diagn. Cytopathol. 6(2):139–143, 1990; with permission.

References

1. Adams, R.D., and Victor, M. Principles of Neurology. Ed. 3. McGraw-Hill Book Co., 1985, pp 461–462.
2. Andrews, J.M., and Schumann, G.B. Laboratory processing of cerebrospinal fluid specimens. Diagn. Cytopathol. 6:139–143, 1990.
3. Barrett, T.L., Downey, E.F. Jr., and Garvin, D.F. A bizarre mononuclear cell response in CSF following myelography. Military Medicine 151: 108–109, 1986.
4. Bigner, S.H. Central Nervous System. Chapter 18 in: Bibbo, M. (Ed.): Comprehensive Cytopathology. W.B. Saunders Co., Philadelphia, 1991, pp 468–483.
5. Bigner, S.H., and Johnston, W.W. Cytopathology of the Central Nervous System. In: Johnston, W.W. (Ed.): Masson Monographs in Diagnostic Cytopathology, Vol. 3. Masson Publishing USA, Inc., New York, 1983.
6. Bigner, S.H., Elmore, P.D., Dee, A.L., and Johnston, W.W. The cytopathology of reactions to ventricular shunts. Acta Cytol. 29:391–396, 1985.
7. Brod, S., and Booss, J. Idiopathic CSF pleocytosis in relapsing polychondritis. Neurology 38:322–323, 1988.
8. Chen, K.T.K., and Moseley, D. Cartilage cells in cerebrospinal fluid. Arch. Pathol. Lab. Med. 114: 212, 1990.
9. Cheson , B.D. Clinical utility of body fluid analysis. Symposium on Body Fluid Analysis. Clin. Lab. Med. 5:195–208, 1985.
10. Confavreux, C., Candie, C., Touraine, F., Ventre, J.J., Aimard, G., and Devic, M. Plasma cells in cerebrospinal fluid and multiple sclerosis: diagnostic yield and clinicobiological correlations. Acta Neurol. Scand. 74:432–438, 1986.
11. Conrad, K.A., Gross, J.L., and Trojanowski, J.Q. Leptomeningeal carcinomatosis presenting as eosinophilic meningitis. Acta Cytol. 30:29–31, 1986.
12. Craver, R.D., and Carson, T.H.: Hematopoietic elements in cerebrospinal fluid in children. Am. J. Clin. Pathol. 95:532–535, 1991.
13. Crennan, J.M., and VanScoy, R.E. Eosinophilic meningitis caused by Rocky Mountain spotted fever. Am. J. Med. 80:288–289, 1986.
14. DeFendini, R., Hunter, S.B., Schlesinger, E.B., Leifer, E., and Roland, L.P. Eosinophilic meningitis in a case of disseminated glioblastoma. Arch. Neurol. 38:52–53, 1981.

15. deReuck, J., and Vanderdonckt, P. Choroid plexus and ependymal cells in CSF cytology. Clin. Neurol. Neurosurg. 88:177–179, 1986.
16. deReuck, J., Vanderdonckt, P., de Bleecker, J., Mareels, H., and Vanderwalle, V. Mitotic activity in cerebrospinal fluid cells. Clin. Neurol. Neurosurg. 90:117–119, 1988.
17. Devinsky, O., Nadi, N.S., Theodore, W.H., and Porter, R.J. Cerebrospinal fluid pleocytosis following simple, complex partial, and generalized tonic-clonic seizures. Ann. Neurol. 23:402–403, 1988.
18. Emmons, C., Smith, J., and Flanigan, M. Cerebrospinal fluid inflammation during OKT 3 therapy. Lancet 2:510–511, 1986.
19. Fishman, R.A. Cerebrospinal Fluid in Diseases of the Nervous System. W.B. Saunders Co., Philadelphia, 1980.
20. Frost, J.K. The Cell in Health and Disease. Karger, New York, 1986.
21. Gaggero, R., Cornaglia Ferraris, P., and DeNegri, M. CSF anomalies in children affected by epilepsia partialis continua (EPC). Neuropediatrics 21:143–145, 1990.
22. Hayward, R.A., and Oye, R.K. Are polymorphonuclear leukocytes an abnormal finding in cerebrospinal fluid? Arch. Intern. Med. 148:1623–1624, 1988.
23. Health and Public Policy Committee, American College of Physicians: Position paper: The diagnostic spinal tap. Ann. Intern. Med. 104:880–885, 1986.
24. Hensen, J.W., and Wiley, R.G. CNS chloromas in patients presenting with eosinophilia. Neurology 39:1386–1388, 1989.
25. Herndon, R.M., and Brumback, R.A. The Cerebrospinal Fluid. Kluwer, Academic Publishers, Boston, 1989.
26. Kam-Hansen, S. Asymptomatic oligoclonal CSF IgG and progressive increase of intrathecal IgG synthesis in a patient with myasthenia gravis treated with thymectomy—a 4-year follow-up. J. Neurol. Sci. 75:285–292, 1986.
27. Kapff, C.J., and Jandl, J.H. Blood. Atlas and Sourcebook of Hematology. Little, Brown and Co., Boston, 1981.
28. Kaplan, P.W., Waterbury, L., Kawas, C., Bolla-Wilson, K., and Aurack, D. Reversible dementia with idiopathic hypereosinophilic syndrome. Neurology 39:1388–1391, 1989.
29. Kjeldsberg, C.R., and Knight, J.A. Body Fluids. Laboratory Examination of Amniotic, Cerebrospinal, Seminal, Serous, and Synovial Fluids: A Textbook Atlas. Ed. 2. American Society of Clinical Pathologists Press, Chicago, 1986.
30. Kollegger, H., Preis, P., Maida, E., Zielinski, C.C., Linkesch, W., Bettelheim, P., and Aiginger, P. CSF cytology of a patient with conversion of an acute lymphatic leukemia to an acute eosinophilic leukemia. Eur. Neurol. 25:320–326, 1986.
31. Krieg, A.F., and Kjeldsberg, C.R. Cerebrospinal fluid and other body fluids. Chapter 18 in: Henry, J.B. (Ed.): Clinical Diagnosis and Management by Laboratory Methods. W.B. Saunders Co., Philadelphia, 1991, pp 445–473.
32. Kruskall, M.S., Carter, S.R., and Ritz, L.P. Contamination of cerebrospinal fluid by vertebral bone marrow cells during lumbar puncture. N. Engl. J. Med. 308:697–700, 1983.
33. Kölmel, H.W. Atlas of Cerebrospinal Fluid Cells. Ed. 2. Springer-Verlag, New York, 1977.
34. Kölmel, H.W., and Skotzek, B. Eosinophilic meningoradiculitis following cranio-cerebral trauma. Infection 16:28, 1988.
35. Leestma, J.E. Viral infections of the nervous system. Chapter 15 in: Davis, R.L., and Robertson, D.M. (Eds.): Textbook of Neuropathology, Ed. 2. Williams & Wilkins, Baltimore, 1991, pp. 804–903.
36. Lopez, A., Valera, C., Ródenas, V., Pedromingo, A., and Martinez-Hernandez, P. Suitability of solid-phase chemistry for quantification of leucocytes in cerebrospinal and peritoneal fluid. Clin. Chem. 33:1475–1476, 1987.
37. Luban, N.L.C., Alessi, R.M., Gold, B.G., and Kapur, S. Cerebral spinal fluid pleocytosis with bone marrow contamination. J. Pediatr. 104:254–256, 1984.
38. Lyons, M.K., and Meyer, F.B. Cerebrospinal fluid physiology and the management of increased intracranial pressure. Mayo Clin. Proc. 65:684–707, 1990.
39. Marton, K.I., and Gean, A.D. The spinal tap: A new look at an old test. Ann. Intern. Med. 104: 840–848, 1986.
40. Mehl, A.L. Interpretation of traumatic lumbar puncture. Predictive value in the presence of meningitis. Clin. Pediatr. 25:575–577, 1986.
41. Mine, S., Sato, A., Yamaura, A., Tamachi, S., Makino, H., and Tomioka, H. Eosinophilia of the cerebrospinal fluid in a case of shunt infection: Case report. Neurosurgery. 19:835–836, 1986.
42. Moriarty, G. Central nervous system. Chapter 39 in: Kaplan, L.A., and Pesce, A.J. (Eds.): Clinical Chemistry. Theory, Analysis, and Correlation. C.V. Mosby Co., St. Louis, 1989, pp 594–606.
43. Platt, M.S., McClure, S., Clarke, R., Spitz, W.U., and Cox, W. Postmortem cerebrospinal fluid pleocytosis. Am. J. Forensic Med. Pathol. 10:209–212, 1989.
44. Pohl, P., Schmutzhard, E., and Stanek, G. Cerebrospinal fluid findings in neurological manifestations of Lyme disease. Zentralbl. Bakteriol. Hyg. A, 263:314–320, 1986.
45. Prussig, S.H., and Buhaug, J. Corpora amylacea in cerebrospinal fluid. A source of possible diagnostic error. Acta Cytol. 22:511–514, 1978.

46. Rosenthal, L.D. Cytology of the Central Nervous System. S. Karger, New York, 1984.
46a. Ross, J.S., Magro, C., Szyfelbein, W., and Sorensen, S. Cerebrospinal fluid pleocytosis in aseptic meningitis. Cytomorphic and immunochemical features. Diagn. Cytopathol. 7:532–535, 1991.
47. Rossi, L.N., Vassella, F., Bajc, O., Tönz, O., Lütschg, J., and Mumenthaler, M. Benign migraine-like syndrome with CSF pleocytosis in children. Dev. Med. Child. Neurol. 77:192–198, 1985.
48. Schumann, G.B., and Crisman, L.G. Cerebrospinal fluid cytopathology. Symposium on body fluid analysis. Clin. Lab. Med. 5:275–302, 1985.
49. Scott, T.F. A new cause of cerebrospinal fluid eosinophilia: neurosarcoidosis. Am. J. Med. 84: 973–974, 1988.
50. Simon, R.P., and Koerper, M.A. PMN's in normal spinal fluid examined by cytocentrifuge technique. Ann. Neurol. 7:380–381, 1980.
51. Stark, E., and Wurster, U. Preparation procedure for cerebrospinal fluid that yields cytologic samples suitable for all types of staining, including immunologic and enzymatic methods. Acta Cytol. 31: 374–376, 1987.
52. Steele, R.W., Marmer, D.J., O'Brien, M.D., Tyson, S.T., and Steele, C.R. Leukocyte survival in cerebrospinal fluid. J. Clin. Microbiol. 23:965–966, 1986.
53. Teoh, R., O'Mahony, G., and Yeung, V.T.F. Polymorphonuclear pleocytosis in the cerebrospinal fluid during chemotherapy for tuberculous meningitis. J. Neurol. 233:237–241, 1986.
54. Travers, H. Quality assurance indicators in anatomic pathology. Arch. Pathol. Lab. Med. 114:1149–1156, 1990.
55. Travers, H., Deppisch, L.M., and Loring, G.J. Surgical Pathology/Cytopathology Quality Assurance Manual. College of American Pathologists. Skokie, Ill., 1988.
56. Traynelis, V.C., Willison, C.D., Follett, K.A., Chambers, J., Schochet, S.S. Jr., and Kaufman, H.H. Millipore analysis of valvular fluid in sterile valve malfunctions. Neurosurgery 28:848–852, 1991.
57. Tutuarima, J.A., Hische, E.A.H., Sylva-Steenland, R.M.R., and van der Helm, H. A cytopreparatory method for cerebrospinal fluid in which the cell yield is high and the fluid is saved for chemical analysis. Acta Cytol. 32:425–427, 1988.
58. Wertlake, P.T., Markovits, B.A., and Stella, R.S. Cytologic evaluation of cerebrospinal fluid with clinical and histologic correlation. Acta Cytol. 16:224–239, 1972.
59. Wied, G.L. Clinical cytology: past, present, and future. Beitr. Onkol. 38:1–58, 1990.
60. Wilber, R.R., King, E.B., and Howes, E.L. Jr. Cerebrospinal fluid cytology in five patients with cerebral cysticercosis. Acta Cytol. 24:421–426, 1980.
61. Woo, J., and Henry, J.B. Clinical pathology/laboratory medicine purposes and practice. Chapter 1 in: Henry, J.B. (Ed.): Clinical Diagnosis and Management by Laboratory Methods. W.B. Saunders Co., Philadelphia, 1991, pp. 1–26.

4 / Qualitative CSF Cytopathology

Over the last 10 years CSF cytopathology has gained increased recognition as a valuable medical laboratory test in patients with non-neoplastic as well as neoplastic CNS conditions (see Chapters 7 and 8). However, in many medical institutions it remains, in our opinion, an underutilized diagnostic method. While there are excellent textbooks (6, 15, 18, 29, 39, 45), atlases (13, 27, 41), and articles (7, 8, 17, 19, 24, 40, 49) on the subject of CNS cytopathology (see Chapter 1), new observations and methods for studying neural disease continue to evolve. This chapter discusses some principles of qualitative CSF cytopathology with the hope that this will encourage continued growth of this important laboratory procedure. The clinical utility and more general aspects of CSF examination are reviewed in Chapter 3.

The information presented here is directed primarily toward the cytopathology laboratory and individuals in clinical pathology/laboratory medicine who may wish a review on the practical value of CSF cytopathology and cytologic methods that may be used in providing a diagnostic service. Table 4.1 provides a general outline of qualitative CSF cytopathology work flow for directors and managers who are responsible for this area of laboratory activity. Before a microscopic interpretation of CSF cytology can be initiated, decisions are necessary regarding the type of specimen, storage, inspection of the specimen, and selection of the appropriate cytopreparatory method. The cytology laboratory manual should accurately describe these protocols to obtain the highest possible diagnostic yield from each procedure.

The principles of CSF exfoliative cytopathology and accuracy of the method are briefly reviewed; this information is included primarily for noncytologists. Chapter 1 provides additional references and continuing education activities for the neophyte. Emphasis in this chapter will be on specimen collection and storage, methods of cytopreparation, routine staining, microscopic interpretation of normal and abnormal CSF cytologic samples and reporting of results. Chapter 5 describes a quantitative approach to CSF cytopathology, which we recommend for consideration by medical institutions involved with monitoring and treatment of CNS malignancies.

Principles of CSF Exfoliative Cytopathology

Exfoliation of malignant cells into the CSF depends on the cohesiveness of the tumor cells and their accessibility to the subarachnoid space (Fig. 4.1) (9, 46). Thus, many intracranial tumors, vascular and degenerative diseases, and infectious/inflammatory conditions of CNS tissues are not detectable by exfoliative CSF cytopathology. Direct radiation, chemotherapy, or surgical manipulation may dislodge epithelial lining cells or tumor cells, thereby temporarily resulting in higher diagnostic yields. Since the number of exfoliated benign or malignant cells shed at any given time may be low, multiple specimens may be needed to establish the true origin of the recovered cells (2, 4, 25).

Accuracy

The general detection rate of CNS neoplasms is extremely variable (20.9 to 83.3%)

Table 4.1.
Outline of Qualitative CSF Cytopathology Work Flow

Test request
Specimen collection
Specimen storage
Gross inspection of specimen
Cytopreparatory methods
Sedimentation chamber
Membrane filtration
Cytocentrifugation
Cell block
Cell culture
Microscopic interpretation
Statement of adequacy
Cytodiagnosis
Recommendations
Adjunctive studies
Special stains
Immunocytochemical markers
Electron microscopy

(8, 45). The significance of a positive CSF cytologic finding was studied by Glass et al. (16), who correlated the presence of malignant cells in the CSF with pathologic findings at autopsy. They found that 26% of 117 patients with brain tumors (chiefly secondary, i.e., metastatic) had positive cytologic findings. Their data indicate that positive CSF results are a reliable indication of CNS malignancy, reflecting leptomeningeal or ependymal involvement by tumor. Tumors that directly communicate with the CSF spaces are usually readily diagnosed by CSF cytopathology. Malignant lymphomas and leukemias, because of their tendency for diffuse meningeal involvement, are also readily diagnosed using conventional cytologic methods. Primary CNS tumors such as astrocytomas, ependymomas, and pinealomas are detected with only 30% accuracy because they are parenchymal tumors with limited communication with the CSF (Table 4.2). CSF cytologic studies are more likely to be positive when the neoplastic cells originating in deeper structures invade the subarachnoid space, in the rare cases when the primary site of tumor origin adjoins the CSF spaces, and following surgery. The overall sensitivity of CSF cytopathology can be summarized as follows: 70% for CNS leukemia; 20 to 60% for metastatic meningeal carcinomatosis; and approximately 33% for primary tumors of the CNS (40, 45). Table 4.2 lists the prevalence of positive CSF findings in common CNS tumors. Additional statistical studies are needed to determine the "true" accuracy of CSF cytopathology. In the past, major conclusions of cytologic studies were based on the correlation of cytopathologic results with confirmatory histopathologic material (6, 18, 29, 37, 39, 45). With improved radioimaging techniques and close clinical follow-up after therapy, this traditional cytohistologic correlation may not always be achievable or practical. However, when possible, we believe cytopathology laboratories should make tissue correlation studies a routine part of their quality assurance program.

Currently, there is a dearth in the literature regarding false-positive and false-negative results of CSF cytopathology. Bigner and Johnston (5, 9) reported 5/255 false-positive cases and described the following conditions that may mimic neoplasia:

1. Specimen contamination
2. Herpes interpreted as adenocarcinoma
3. Foreign-body reaction
4. Infectious meningitis
5. Reactive lymphocytes
6. Misinterpretation of ependymal-choroid cells

They suggested that immunologic marker studies may reduce the aforementioned diagnostic pitfalls (see Chapter 10). However, at present, experienced cytologists find reliable morphologic criteria are the most helpful diagnostic assets in improving the accuracy of CSF cytopathology results. Identification of tumor cells can be greatly enhanced when large volumes of CSF are available for analysis. In addition, several lumbar punctures (sometimes as many as

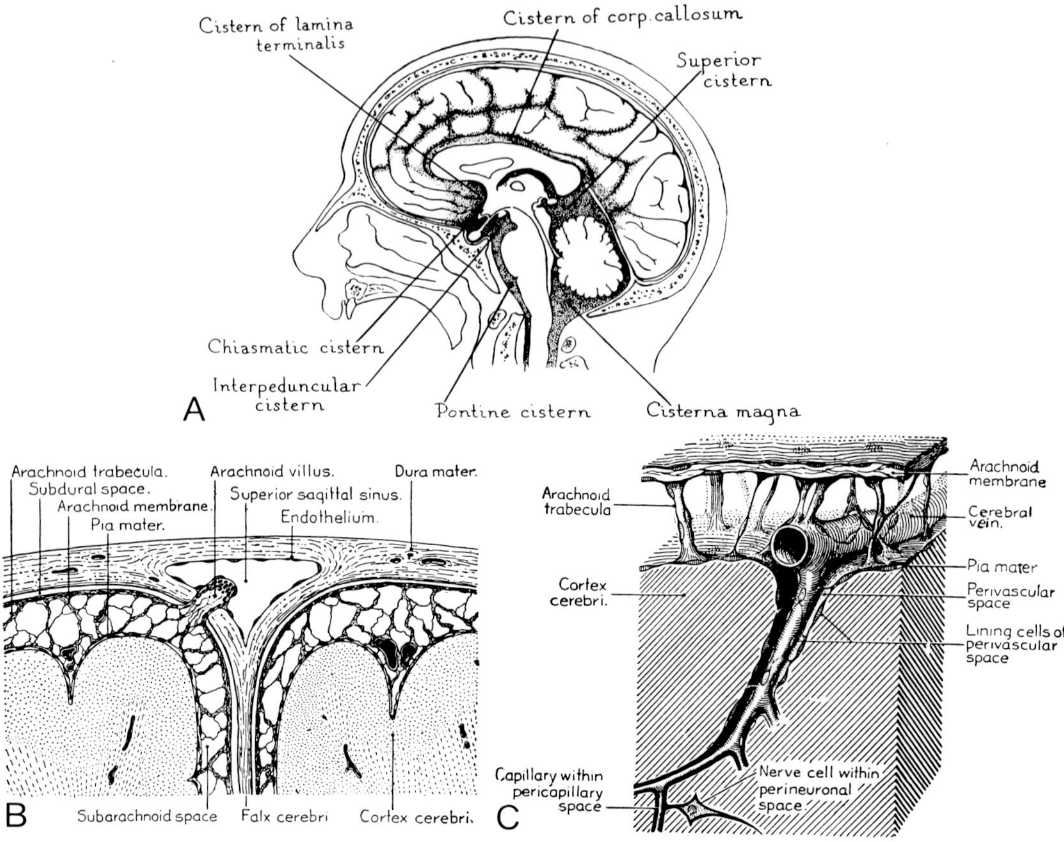

Figure 4.1. **A,** Diagrammatic view of the main subarachnoid cisterns. **B,** Diagram of meninges surrounding cerebral cortex, showing relation of arachnoid villus to dural venous sinus. **C,** Diagram of cerebral pia-arachnoid, showing relations of subarachnoid space, perivascular channels, and nerve cells. (**A** modified from Bailey P. Intracranial tumors. 2nd ed. Springfield, IL: Charles C. Thomas, 1948: 212. **B, C** from Weed L.H. The cerebrospinal fluid. Physiol Rev 1922;2:171–203.)

six or more) may be required before a cytodiagnosis of malignancy can be confirmed in patients with carcinomatous meningitis (15).

Test Request

In CSF cytopathology, as in all diagnostic cytopathology tests, the requesting physician should be aware of the variety of laboratory examinations available. The principal focus of CSF cytopathology laboratories is in the detection of abnormal and malignant cells. Unlike the microbiological or clinical (medical) laboratory examination for infectious conditions (which require rapid determinations, often achieved by automated methods), cytologic examination of CSF represents a time-intensive microscopic assessment of various cellular and morphologic elements by expert observers.

As in virtually all other areas of medicine, good communication between the pathologist, the laboratory, and the clinician will maximize the chance that clinically relevant information will be obtained (1). CSF is most frequently obtained by lumbar puncture (LP). While this minimally invasive procedure is relatively simple, there re-

Table 4.2.
Prevalence of Positive CSF Findings in CNS Tumors[a]

Tumor	%
Primary	
Meningioma	2–5
Astrocytoma, grades I and II	5–25
Astrocytoma, grades III and IV[b]	13–45
Oligodendroglioma	40–55
Medulloblastoma	30–65
Ependymoma	23–50
Pinealoma	37–57
Pituitary adenoma	4
Secondary (with clinical symptoms)	
Leukemia	70–74
Non-Hodgkin's lymphoma	61
Metastatic lung cancer	23–70
Metastatic breast cancer	14
Melanoma	14

[a] From Schumann, G.B., and Colon, F.V. The Clinician's Guide to Diagnostic Cytology. Year Book, Chicago, pp. 236–250, 1982.
[b] Astrocytoma, grades III and IV: glioblastoma multiforme. (See more current astrocytoma classification in Chapter 7.)

mains considerable patient resistance to repeated LPs. Even under ideal circumstances, a suboptimal specimen may be obtained for reasons that are not readily controlled (e.g., severe patient obesity, spinal arthritis, improper positioning, patient motion, and lack of examiner experience). It follows that both patient and physician benefit from proper laboratory strategies in dealing with such specimens. Clinicians are encouraged to contact the laboratory if there are questions regarding CSF cytology before initiating the procedure, or to inform the laboratory concerning suspected diagnostic possibilities that may be under consideration. The latter information may lead to a more rapid diagnosis (i.e., wet mounts for amoebic meningitis, india ink preps for suspected cryptococcus, etc.).

Specimen Collection

Standard sterile techniques for obtaining CSF for cytology are identical to those utilized for any type of CSF study. Because the brain and spinal cord are encased in the skull and vertebrae, respectively, CSF specimens must be obtained by LP or occasionally by suboccipital or other routes. During radiologic and surgical procedures CSF may be obtained directly from the ventricles or from the surrounding subarachnoid space (e.g., cisterns) (Fig. 4.1). Lumbar puncture should be performed only after a thorough clinical evaluation of the patient and serious consideration of the potential value and hazards of this procedure (15). Fishman provides an excellent discussion of the clinical indications and contraindications of LP (15). The specimen is fractionated into separate collection tubes based on the tests specified, with one being designated for cytologic study (see Chapter 3).

We feel that laboratories should provide the clinician with guidelines on the minimal amounts of CSF required in various procedures (1). We recommend that the physician submit at least 3 ml of CSF for routine cytologic studies and an additional 5 to 10 ml if immunologic tumor marker studies are anticipated (see Table 3.7).

Specimen Storage

Cytolysis depends on the temperature at which the CSF is stored. If there is an anticipated delay of several hours, refrigeration is necessary to minimize cellular degeneration. When specimens are left at room temperature there is a significant decrease in cell count. After 24 hours, the cells are no longer vital (that is, they no longer exclude trypan blue) (38). Cell structure can be relatively preserved for 48 hours after LP by storage at 4°C; the addition of fixatives is therefore encouraged only when refrigeration is not available.

Neutrophils and eosinophils are most vulnerable to cytolysis, probably reflecting their high lysosomal enzyme content (38).

Allowing CSF to be held at room temperature for extended periods may decrease the total neutrophilic leukocyte count as much as 50% in the first half hour due to cellular lysis and cell adherence to the tube walls (38). The lymphocyte cell count does not decrease proportionately. This is why we emphasize prompt delivery and processing of the sample as soon as it is obtained.

When one anticipates that sample processing will be delayed and there is no reasonable alternative to keeping the specimen at room temperature, we recommend Saccomanno's fixative for CSF cytologic studies. Laboratory instructions should be provided to ambulatory facilities to add an equal volume of Saccomanno's fixative with CSF and to record the original volume on the specimen tube or requisition slip. Saccomanno's fixative (50% ethanol and 2% Carbowax) is commercially available, and one can contact the cytopathology laboratory for ordering information. Specimens should be gently mixed after adding fixative. Assisting the clinician in obtaining proper specimen-packing materials and courier services will also maximize cooperation in this critical phase of CSF specimen handling. To summarize, available evidence supports the following conclusions:

1. The larger the volume of CSF submitted, the more likely an abnormal CSF will yield a positive microbiological and/or cytological diagnosis
2. The incidence of post-LP headache in patients is not significantly increased by the removal of 20 to 30 ml of CSF (1, 15).
3. Further improvements in the storage and collection of CSF include the following:
   a. Collect the cells in silicon-coated tubes.
   b. Use refrigeration instead of room temperature.
   c. When a delay in transporting the specimen to the laboratory is anticipated, place the CSF directly into a tube and add an equal volume of Saccomanno's fixative. This allows storage for several days. This should be considered for ambulatory facilities where refrigerated storage is not available.

Gross Inspection of Specimen

Fluid inspection is a routine part of the CSF examination procedure. CSF should be immediately spun down, decanted into a separate tube, and compared with a similar tube of water (38). One should look through the tube onto a white background using daylight or artificial lighting. If the CSF is clear one should be able to read fine newspaper print. Slightly cloudy CSF makes the print appear fuzzy and cloudy, and turbid CSF obscures the print (38). Normal CSF is colorless. Yellowish, greenish, and other tints may be caused by a variety of etiologies (see Table 3.4).

Cytopreparation

Selection of cytopreparatory methods for optimal cell recovery and use of techniques that improve morphologic detail are ongoing processes in laboratories interested in maximizing the yield of CSF cytopathology (3, 21, 26). Table 4.3 lists the number of positive CSF cytopathologic findings examined between 1981 and 1986 at the University of Utah. Approximately 12% were positive, 4% suspicious, and 4% atypical or abnormal. The majority of cases were normal or negative (80%). Although it is true that positive CSF yields are not as frequent as in other body cavity fluid studies, cytologic examination may occasionally be the only practical means of establishing the presence

Table 4.3.
Diagnostic Categories for CSF Cytopathologic Results at the University of Utah[a]

Year	Number of CSF Specimens	Unsatisfactory	Negative	Abnormal		
				Atypical[b]	Suspicious[c]	Positive
1981	233	4 (1.7%)	180 (77.2%)	11 (4.7%)	3 (1.3%)	35 (15.1%)
1982	302	0 (0%)	259 (85.8%)	6 (2.0%)	4 (1.3%)	32 (10.6%)
1983	501	17 (3.4%)	408 (81.4%)	18 (3.6%)	11 (2.2%)	47 (9.4%)
1984	441	16 (3.6%)	336 (76.2%)	30 (6.8%)	11 (2.5%)	48 (9.4%)
1985	486	35 (7.2%)	341 (70.1%)	20 (4.1%)	29 (5.9%)	61 (12.5%)
1986	600	39 (6.5%)	406 (67.6%)	20 (3.3%)	37 (6.1%)	98 (16.3%)
Total	2563	111 (4.3%)	1930 (75.3%)	105 (4.1%)	95 (3.7%)	321 (12.5%)

[a] From Schumann, G.B., Crissman, L.G. Diagn. Cytopathol. Vol 2, No 3, September 1986; with permission.
[b] Atypical epithelial or ependymal cells, degenerative changes, and enlarged cells with lobulated nuclei.
[c] Atypical reactive lymphoid cells.

Table 4.4.
Abnormal CSF Interpretations Grouped by Cellularity Observed at the University of Utah

	Atypical	Suspicious	Positive	Total
Normal cellularity <5000 cells/ml or 5 cells/mm^3	33 (13.2%)	13 (5.2%)	106 (42.6%)	152 (61.0%)
Hypercellularity >5000 cells/ml or 5 cells/mm^3	30 (12.0%)	16 (6.4%)	51 (20.5%)	97 (39.0%)
Total	63 (25.3%)	29 (11.6%)	157 (63.1%)	249 (100%)

of infection, neoplasm, or other pathologic process involving the CNS. This is particularly true when definitive clinical or radiographic evidence cannot be obtained. Precise enumeration and identification of mononuclear cells in CSF is important to neurological diagnosis. Frequently, CSF samples with normal cell counts (<5 mononuclear cells per mm^3) contain blastic (i.e., immature hematopoietic) cells or malignant cells (Table 4.4). Because CSF samples are typically smaller in volume than most other body fluid samples, increased care and planning in specimen handling is warranted.

Obviously, improved technological developments are needed to aid cytopathology laboratories in examining this "typically hypocellular specimen" and to reliably diagnose the rare malignant cells. In the mean time a variety of methods have been suggested for CSF cytopreparation and staining (6, 13, 15, 17, 26, 31, 35, 36, 41, 42, 45, 50). Routinely described and debated preparatory techniques in current use are (*a*) sedimentation, (*b*) membrane filtration, and (*c*) cytocentrifugation. Less commonly advocated are methods such as centrifugal bucket cytology, direct smears of a centrifuged specimen, and cell culture. This topic was the subject of an earlier symposium on body fluid analysis (47). The following section briefly describes each of these cytopreparation methods. Readers are encouraged to study the original reference for more technical detail regarding these cell recovery methods.

Cell Recovery Methods

Sedimentation Chamber

The sedimentation chamber is a popular method employed in Europe to cytologically examine the CSF (10, 12, 13, 27, 41). The chamber consists of a plastic cylinder (approximately 14 mm in diameter) that is pressed firmly against a glass slide by a spring, by external weights, or by its own weight. Filter paper is placed around the base of the cylinder to provide suction. CSF (3 to 5 ml) is poured into the cylinder and the cells are spontaneously deposited on the glass slide by gravity. As the liquid portion of the CSF is drawn off onto the paper filter, the cells are thinly spread on the glass slide. The entire process requires 1 to 3 hours, depending on the aliquot size and the consistency of the fluid (41). The slide is then removed, allowed to air dry, and stained with an appropriate stain (e.g., Giemsa). The reported advantage of this method for an air-dried specimen is the optimum cytomorphological result obtained. The disadvantages of the technique include the length of time required for processing, the significant cell loss (30 to 90%) (41), and the fact that the chambers are not commercially available but rather must be constructed by the individual laboratory.

Membrane Filtration

Cerebrospinal fluid can be readily prepared for cytologic study using a membrane filtration method (3, 35, 36, 43, 44), which has the highest rate of cellular recovery (5, 6, 15, 17, 46, 47). Commercially available membrane filters include Millipore and Gelman (cellulose filters), and Nucleopore (a polycarbonate filter).

Preparation of the CSF on a membrane filter begins by labeling the filter with the appropriate laboratory accession number with an indelible electrophoresis pen. The cellulose filters are pre-expanded in 95% ethanol to avoid wrinkling of the filter during specimen preparation. Nucleopore filters are pre-moistened in physiologic saline solution. The frit or grid of the filtration apparatus is moistened using sterile saline, and the pre-expanded, pre-moistened membrane filter is placed on the frit, label side up. The funnel is then placed on the base of the filter apparatus and clamped in place. Two to five ml of sterile saline is added to keep the filter moist while the spinal fluid is poured into the funnel (see Modified Membrane Filtration Technique, below).

Suction is then applied (suction of up to 100 mm Hg has been shown not to cause cellular damage or distortion of the larger cellulose filters). The force of gravity is usually sufficient for the smaller Millipore (25 mm diameter) and Nucleopore filters. Following filtration, the suction is disconnected, leaving a thin covering (approximately 1/8 inch) of fluid over the filter. Care is taken not to let the filter dry out completely. Next, 3 to 5 ml of 95% ethanol is added to the funnel and then drawn through the filter. The clamp and funnel are removed, and the filter is fixed for 15 minutes in a Petri dish containing 95% ethanol. After fixation the filters are stained using a modified Papanicolaou method and are coverslipped. Nucleopore filters are often dissolved with chloroform prior to coverslipping.

In general, filters are more expensive, technically time consuming, and require that individuals be trained in the preparatory techniques. However, results are far superior to those of direct smears, sedimentation techniques, or cytocentrifugation because of the almost complete cell recovery and the excellent cell morphology (6, 15, 47). Equipment is available that allows processing of multiple specimens using a manifold and two to six funnels with filter apparatus attachments. The latter is ideal for high-volume laboratories. The major disadvantages of membrane filters are technical and vary with the type of filter used (31, 47). In addition, Romanowsky-type stains cannot be used because of their affinity for the filter material. A disadvantage of the Gelman and Millipore filters is also the presence of nonspecific background staining. The Nucleopore filter eliminates this problem, but additional technical steps are required (38).

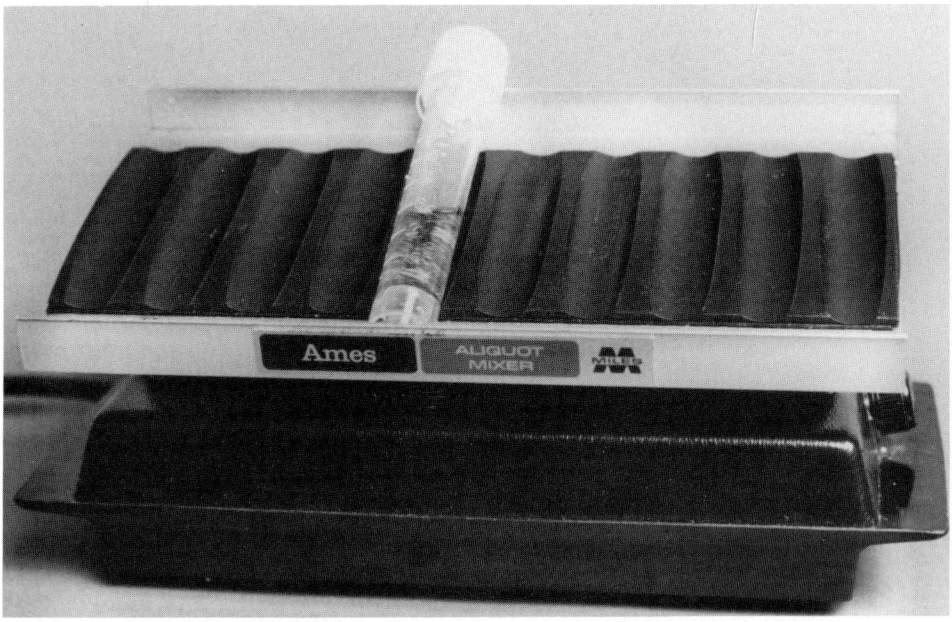

Figure 4.2. Test tube containing 3 ml of CSF on a test tube agitator.

Modified Membrane Filtration Technique

The CSF specimen is mixed for 5 minutes using a test tube agitator (Fig. 4.2). Specimens determined by prior gross inspection to be normal in color and character and that consist of 3 ml or less are placed over a small (25 mm diameter Millipore) membrane filter with a pore size of 5 or less (Figs. 4.3 to 4.5). Any remaining specimen is refrigerated until the final microscopic assessment has been completed (allowing additional preparations to be made in cases suspicious for malignancy).

A 1.0-ml aliquot is used in specimens obtained from patients with previous hypercellular counts (>5000 cells/ml), or in specimens with abnormal color or character (i.e., bloody, milky, xanthochromic, or containing mucoid or other precipitate). These specimens are individually assessed for determination of the aliquot to be examined.

Following preparation, all filters are fixed for 15 minutes in 95% ethyl alcohol, stained with a modified Papanicolaou method (Fig. 4.6), and coverslipped (Fig. 4.7) (also see Fig. 5.1**A**).

Cytocentrifugation

An increasingly popular method for preparing CSF specimens is the cytocentrifugation technique utilizing the Shandon Cytospin (Figs. 4.8 and 4.9) (3, 11, 14, 20, 23, 28, 47, 51, 52). Laboratories using the cytocentrifugation method advocate a wide range of aliquot amounts, centrifugal forces, and spin times (i.e., 0.15 to 1.5 ml, 500 to 1500 rpm, and 4 to 10 minutes). Use of low speed may reduce air drying artifacts.

General steps used in the cytocentrifugation procedure are listed below:

1. Identify each slide by labeling with pencil on the frosted end of the slide (e.g., the laboratory's accession number and/or patient name).
2. Assemble each cytocentrifuge chamber (Fig. 4.9). To accomplish this, place the plastic chamber against the filter paper

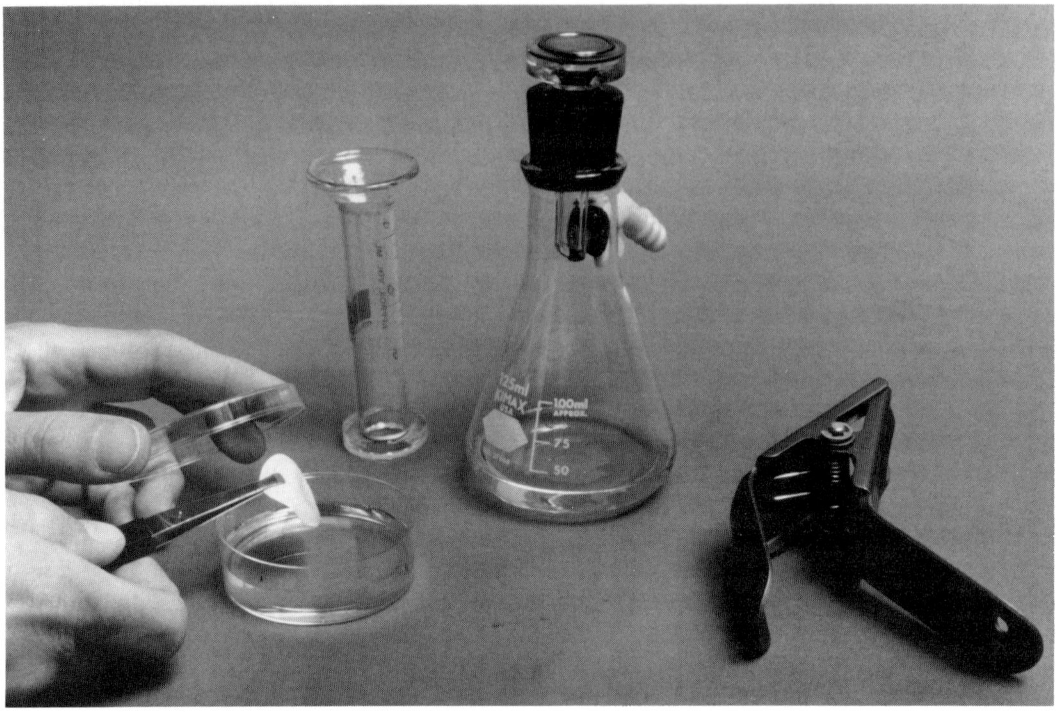

Figure 4.3. Filter apparatus (center) is assembled. Millipore filter (left) is premoistened in 95% ethanol to prevent wrinkling of the filter. (Note: Nucleopore filters are premoistened in physiological saline solution.)

strip or pad (the area around the hole in the filter paper is moistened with 1 to 2 drops of sterile saline) with the textured side against the chamber. A glass slide is held against this unit by means of a spring, and it is then ready to be placed in the cytocentrifuge. Special filter paper strips (brown) are especially recommended for CSF because of their reduced absorption characteristics. One should contact the manufacturer for more information. Disposable chambers are also available for laboratories that prefer this method in handling infectious agents.

3. Insert the assembled unit in the rotor by making sure the chamber, blotter, and slide are pressed to the bottom of the rotor. It should lie flat against the outside wall. The sample chambers must be symmetrically distributed in the machine so that proper balance is achieved during centrifugation (Fig. 4.8).
4. Transfer the aliquot of CSF to the base of the entry port immediately in front of the horizontal chamber. (Bigner recommends placing a drop of sterile saline in the chamber before adding the aliquot of CSF [7]). A drop of bovine albumin may also be used as an aid to cell adherence to the slide.
5. The specimen is then centrifuged at 700 rpm for 5 minutes. Laboratories must ensure that this equipment is periodically calibrated and is part of a routine cleaning and equipment maintenance program.

After centrifugation has been completed, the slides are permitted to air dry or may be alcohol fixed, depending on the desired staining method. If alcohol fixation is chosen, it is important to work quickly in removing and disassembling the chamber assembly so that the specimen is not subjected

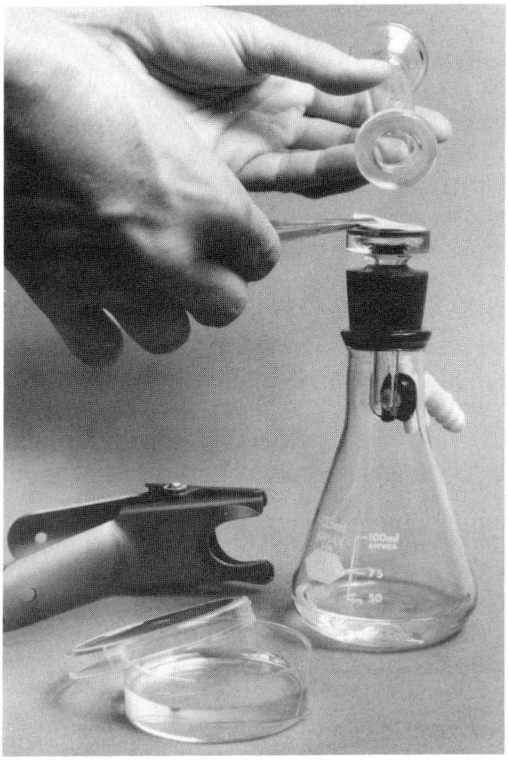

Figure 4.4. Pre-expanded filter placed on frit.

to the detrimental effects of air drying artifacts.

An advantage of cytocentrifugation is not speed, but rather that CSF specimens can be processed by either wet alcohol fixation and Papanicolaou staining or air drying for Wright's staining (38). Additional smears for immunologic marker studies can readily be processed with this technique. A disadvantage of the cytocentrifugation method is the cost of the instrument. Because the instrument is popular for other types of specimens, many laboratories share equipment between cytology and hematology laboratories.

Centrifugal Bucket Cytology

The centrifugal bucket, designed to concentrate cells from dilute body fluids, has been suggested as a means to examine the CSF (32). The apparatus (manufactured by Coulter Electronics, Inc.) is used in conjunction with any laboratory centrifuge with 1⅞-inch rotor spacing. The bucket, when assembled, consists of a carrier that supports a foam pad, a microscopic slide, and a three-dimensional sample block. Each chamber includes a fixative cup with a frit to control the passage of the fixative into the chamber during centrifugation. The specimen is inserted in the sample chamber using a syringe or pipette, the rotors are balanced with saline, and the assembled unit is then centrifuged at 1500 rpm for 10 minutes.

After initial centrifugation, a syringe fitted with a 20-gauge needle is used to remove the supernatant. A fixative is then deposited in the fixative cup and the bucket is centrifuged for 15 minutes at 1200 rpm. The bucket is then disassembled, and the glass slide is ready for staining using a Papanicolaou staining method. Although it is not recommended, non-fixed or air-dried samples may be used. An advantage of this technique is a large cell button or concentrated area of cellular material. A major disadvantage is the high cost and limited availability of the equipment.

Dried Smears

Direct smears are prepared by centrifuging the specimen for 10 minutes at 1500 rpm (490G), decanting the supernatant, and depositing the sediment button on a glass slide (6, 47). The button/sediment can be smeared by using a second slide to disperse the material or by using a metal loop. The prepared smear is then alcohol fixed or air dried, depending on the staining method to be employed. Albuminized slides may enhance cellular recovery, although this is not required routinely. Parlodion is recommended as an excellent cell adhesive (see Appendix). Poly-L-lysine (PLL)-coated slides are another alternative if Parlodion is not available. Krantz (30) reports that immunocytochemistry on PLL-coated slides constitutes

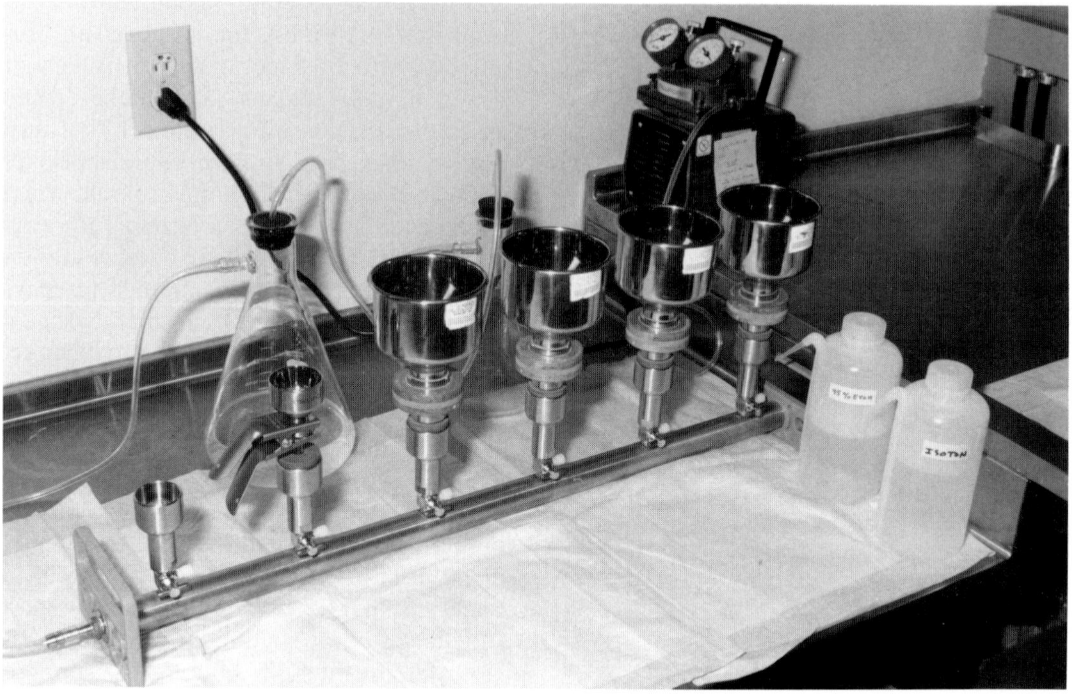

Figure 4.5. Multiple filter apparatus with manifold.

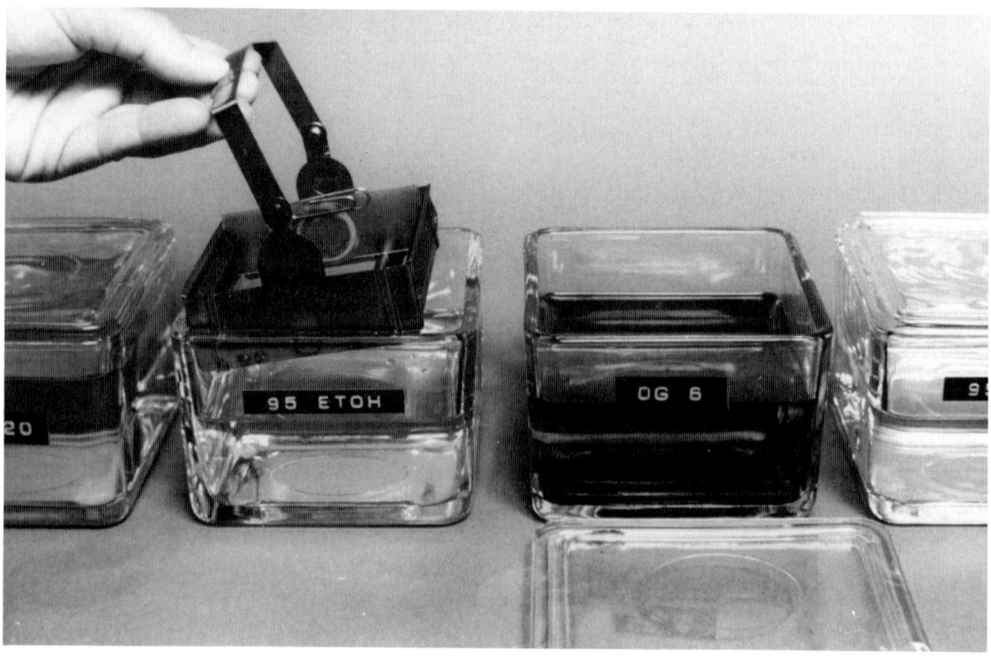

Figure 4.6. Staining the filter using a modified Papanicolaou method.

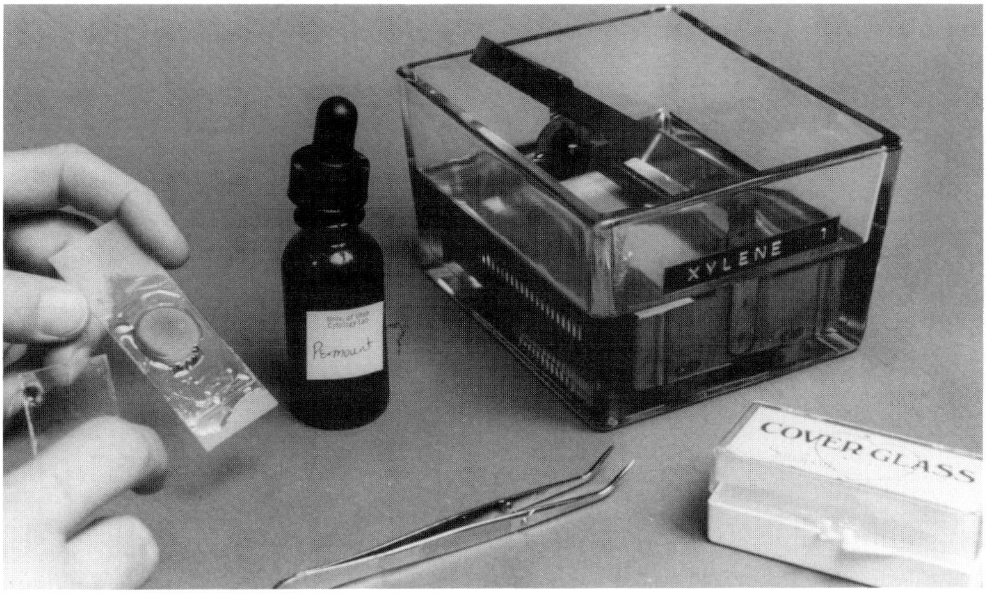

Figure 4.7. Coverslipping the filter.

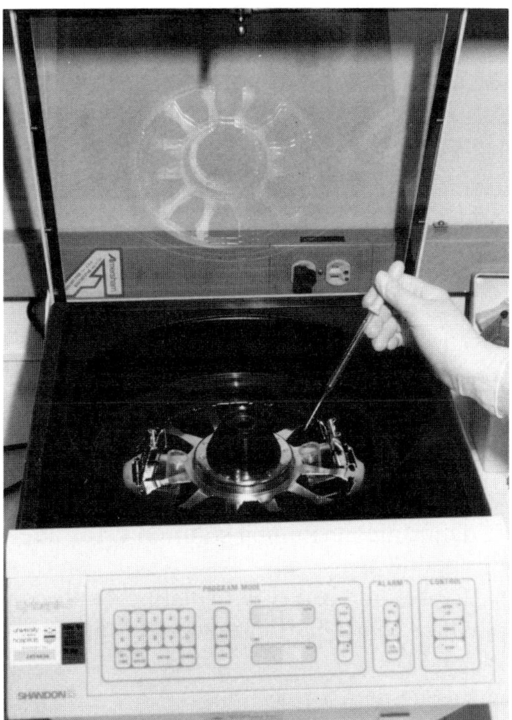

Figure 4.8. Shandon Cytospin and specimen chamber.

the method of choice for immunologic cell differentiation in CSF, which may allow equivocal morphologic findings to be clarified.

Cell Culture

The cell culture technique has been advocated for some cases involving brain tumors (22). Identification of glioma cells can be easily made in cell cultures because of their characteristic morphology and tendency to proliferate in vitro. Cell cultures are prepared by mixing 1 to 3 ml of CSF with 3 ml of a basic cultivating medium (Eagle's MEM) which has been supplemented with 20% fetal calf serum. The 4- to 6-ml mixture is then incubated at 37°C in Leighton tubes (17) with a coverslip being placed on top of the culture medium. The cells proliferate on the coverslip and can be harvested after a minimum of 3 days. The cells are fixed and stained on the coverslip. Permanent preparations are made by embedding the coverslip in Canadian balsam. This technique has been extensively utilized as a research

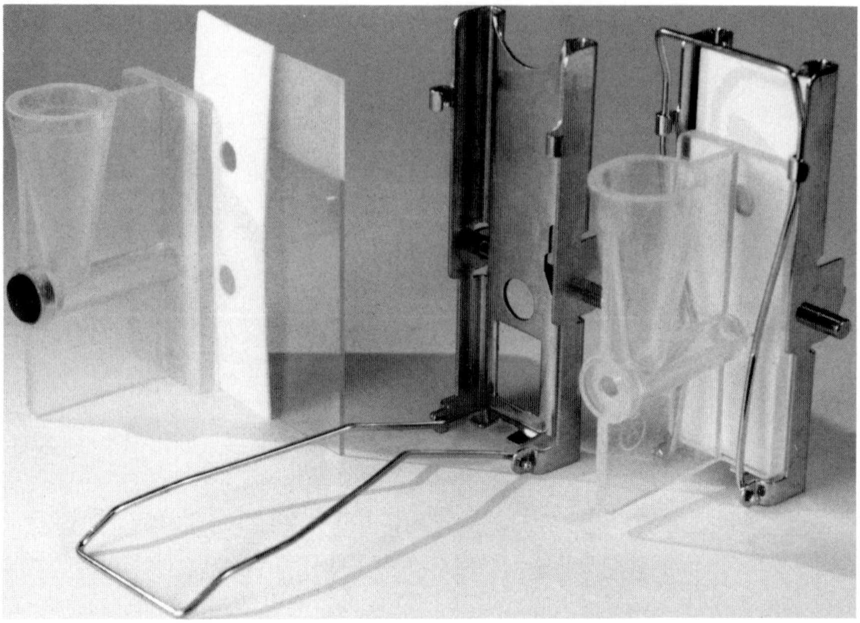

Figure 4.9. Specimen chamber, glass slide, paper filter, and alignment for cytocentrifugation.

tool but has not gained popularity in a clinical practice setting.

Staining

Selection of the staining method for CSF is usually based on the preference of the cytopathologist. The Papanicolaou stain is usually preferred by cytopathologists trained and practicing in the United States because of its demonstration of nuclear and cytoplasmic cellular detail (5, 6, 18, 29, 39, 42, 45, 46). Cytopathologists trained in Europe and those with a hematologic background typically prefer a variant of the Wright's stain (e.g., Diff-Quik [48]), especially for the identification of leukemic and lymphomatous cells (7, 13, 27, 41). An advantage of the Papanicolaou stain may be in facilitating recognition of CSF-lining cells and metastatic epithelial tumors (47), although more specific and sensitive immunohistochemical markers will be required to determine whether current assumptions are valid (5).

Wright Stain

Air-dried, cytocentrifuged CSF preparations can be stained with the commercially available Diff-Quik (Wright) stain. This stain is rapid, easy to perform, and provides good staining of the hematopoietic cells present (6).

The Diff-Quik (Harleco) procedure is as follows:

1. Dip slide in fixative solution *A* for five 1-second dips.
2. Drain slide on a paper towel.
3. Dip slide in staining solution *B* for five 1-second dips.
4. Drain slide on a paper towel.
5. Dip slide in staining solution *C* for five 1-second dips.
6. Rinse slide gently with distilled water and allow to air dry before coverslipping.

Diff-Quik fixative solution *A*: 1.8 mg/liter triarylmethane dye, 100% pure dye content in methyl alcohol.

Diff-Quik staining solution *B*: 1 g/liter

xanthene dye, 100% pure dye content buffer and sodium azide (0.01% as preservative).

Diff-Quik staining solution *C*: 1.25 g/liter thiazine dye mixture, 100% pure dye content (0.625 g/liter azure A and 0.625 g/liter methylene blue) and buffer.

Papanicolaou Stain

Alcohol-fixed slides are stained using a modified Papanicolaou technique. The following procedure is the one employed in our laboratory for the staining of all membrane filter preparations.

Procedure:

Step	Solution	Time (Interval)
1	Distilled H_2O	1 minute
2	Gill 1 hematoxylin	30 sec; agitate gently
3	Distilled H_2O	10 1-second dips
4	Distilled H_2O	10 1-second dips
5	Acid-H_2O (0.25% HCl)	10 1-second dips
6	Distilled H_2O	Five 1-second dips
7	Scott's tap H_2O	Five 1-second dips
8	Distilled H_2O	10 1-second dips
9	95% EtOH	10 1-second dips
10	95% EtOH	10 1-second dips
11	OG-6	1.5 minutes
12	95% EtOH	10 1-second dips
13	95% EtOH	10 1-second dips
14	EA-50	1.5 minutes
15	95% EtOH	10 1-second dips
16	95% EtOH	10 1-second dips
17	1-Propanol	10 1-second dips
18	1-Propanol	2 minutes
19	Xylene 1	1 minute (until clear)
20	Xylene 2	1 minute
21	Xylene 3	5 minutes

Solutions:

Gill 1 Hematoxylin (Lerner Laboratories)

OG-6 (Harleco)

EA-50 (Harleco)

Scott's tap H_2O: 40 g magnesium sulfate
8 g calcium carbonate
4 liters distilled water
(stir to mix solution)

Microscopic Interpretation

The microscopic examination of CSF should include a systematic and detailed assessment of the cellular and morphologic elements present on the slide regardless of the cell recovery and/or cytopreparatory method used. Because the cellular material is permanently fixed and stained, the slides can be periodically reviewed by several observers. This is ideal for developing CSF cytopathology laboratory quality control and assurance programs. The cytologist should initially determine the adequacy of the material on the slide, reporting whether the sample is satisfactory, unsatisfactory, or suboptimal (reasons or comments regarding unsatisfactory CSF specimens are listed in Table 4.5). The next goal for the microscopist is to determine whether the CSF sample contains normal or abnormal morphological elements.

Approach to the Microscopic Evaluation of CSF Cytology

The microscopic interpretation of CSF cytology specimens seems tedious and time consuming because of the hypocellularity of the specimens. The microscope should be in good working order and Köhler illumination should be achieved. Because of the hypocellularity and the amount of open space between cells it is important for the microscopist to allow his or her eyes to become accustomed to these small morphologic entities. A general rule of thumb is that the more specimens one examines, the easier and larger the images appear over time. Initially

Table 4.5.
Types of CSF Cytodiagnoses

I.	UNSATISFACTORY e.g., acellular specimen, contamination by fresh blood (traumatic tap) or by fungal or bacterial overgrowth, marked cellular degeneration, etc.	
II.	NEGATIVE (no malignant or blast cells identified).	
III.	INFECTIONS	
	Bacterial	
	Fungal	
		Candidiasis
		Cryptococcosis
		Blastomycosis
		Histoplasmosis
		Aspergillosis
		Acinetobacter calcoaceticus
	Viral	
		Cytomegalovirus
		Herpes simplex
IV.	INFLAMMATION/HEMORRHAGE	
	Acute (neutrophilic) inflammation	
	Chronic (lymphocytic) inflammation	
	Plasma cells (%)	
	Eosinophils (%)	
	Hemosiderin-laden macrophages present consistent with *prior* CNS bleeding	
	Multinucleated giant cells	
V.	DEGENERATION	
	Fat-laden macrophages present consistent with tissue damage	
	Cells of nucleus pulposus	
	Corpora amylacea	
VI.	ATYPIAS (suspicious for malignancy)	
	Atypical immature monocytes or myelocytes present suspicious for a myeloproliferating disorder.	
	Atypical lymphocytes present suspicious for a lymphoproliferative disorder	
	Atypical epithelial cells present suspicious for a carcinoma	
VII.	MALIGNANT NEOPLASIA	
	Primary	
		Astrocytoma
		Ependymoma
		Medulloblastoma
		Ganglioglioma
		Pinealoma
		Retinoblastoma
		Craniopharyngioma
		Chordoma
	Secondary	
		Leukemia
		Lymphoma
		Multiple myeloma
		Malignant histiocytosis
		Metastatic carcinoma (lung, GI, breast, prostate, renal cell, transitional cell, etc.)
		Seminoma
		Embryonal or germ cell
		Small-cell cancer
		Sarcoma

Table 4.6.
Comparison of Microscopic CSF Methods

Method	Volume Examination	Normal	Comments
Chamber count (hemocytometer)	3.2 mm^3	0–5 mononuclear cells/mm^3	
Cytocentrifugation	0.5 ml to 1.0 ml	?	300 times more concentrated than hemocytometer
Membrane filter	3 ml	0–5000 cells/ml	Most sensitive

one should try to identify the normal elements of the spinal fluid (i.e., lymphocytes and monocytes) and compare that population with the abnormal cells. One should concentrate on the nuclear staining intensity as well as the cell size in defining the cytologic categories. Lymphocytes typically have a darkly staining, coarse nuclear chromatin in comparison to the finely granular nuclear chromatin of monocytes. Another important distinction is the size of monocytes in comparison to neutrophils; the latter are approximately half the size of a normal monocyte.

After one feels comfortable regarding the staining qualities and has identified representative or reference normal cells, the next decision deals with the adequacy and preservation of the specimen. A comment should be made in the report regarding this aspect of the specimen (Table 4.5). In qualitative CSF cytopathology one must do a systematic screening of the entire microscopic field. Typically, cytologists or cytotechnologists start at one end of the slide or filter and systematically screen the specimen in a vertical or horizontal fashion. As one gains experience, samples that are hypercellular or show striking pleomorphism quickly become obvious. Therefore, we feel it is important initially for the microscopist to formally attempt to categorize the CSF as hypocellular, normocellular, or hypercellular (Table 4.6).

The separation of normal from abnormal CSF specimens is the next step (i.e., finding a second cell population) (Table 4.7). With experience one can readily recognize abnormal cells even using low power magnifications with Wright's or Papanicolaou stains, primarily due to the increased cell size and nuclear staining characteristics. Perhaps one of the most challenging areas deals with benign and neoplastic lymphoproliferative conditions. Table 4.8 reviews cell recognition aids we have found useful in our residency training, as well as the cytotechnology training program. Once one feels comfortable with recognition of these cell populations, distinguishing normal from neoplastic conditions becomes easier (33, 47).

A major challenge to the microscopic evaluation of CSF deals with the paucity of important or diagnostic cells. Table 4.9 describes an approach to the dilemma of the single malignant cell that we have found useful and that may be helpful in reducing the number of false-positive and

Table 4.7.
Common Types of Benign "Mononuclear" Cells Found in "Normal" CSF[a]

Hematopoietic/lymphoreticular cells
Neutrophils (rare)
Lymphocytes (small)
Monocytes
Histiocytes and macrophages
CNS "lining cells"; may include:
Leptomeningeal cells (pia-arachnoid mesothelial)
Choroid plexus cells
Ependymal cells
Benign glial cells
Chondrocytes

[a] From Schumann, G.B., and Colon, F.V. The Clinician's Guide to Diagnostic Cytology. Year Book, Chicago, pp. 236–250, 1982; used by permission.

Table 4.8.
CSF: Cell Recognition Aids

1. Lymphocytes:
   a. The most common cell type in the majority of specimens (excluding acute infections, etc.)
   b. Spend your first few moments at the microscope allowing your eyes to accommodate to these small blue round cells in a light background. With practice they can be recognized in Pap-stained material without using oil immersion objectives. Compare these cells for size and chromatin staining reference points. Then start scanning the slide and identify nonlymphocytic cell populations.
2. Reactive lymphocytes:
   a. Slightly larger than small lymphocytes in nuclear size.
   b. Slightly finer chromatin patterns than normal "resting" lymphocyte.
   c. Nucleolus present because finely granular chromatin is evenly dispersed.
3. Atypical lymphocytes:
   a. Still a recognizable lymphocyte, but larger than small lymphocyte, with irregular nuclear membrane outline (e.g., noses, indentations).
4. Blast:
   a. Nucleus two times the size of most reactive lymphocytes (exception: microblasts will be small).
   b. High nuclear to cytoplasmic (N/C) ratio.
   c. Only a very thin rim of cytoplasm around the nucleus (rare exception: microblastic type of leukemia). Myeloblasts typically have more cytoplasm than lymphoblasts.
5. Monocyte:
   a. Larger than a lymphocyte and larger than a neutrophil (PMN).
   b. Beware of mistaking a monocyte on edge for a PMN (e.g., band form).
   c. U-shaped nucleus, chromatin finer than lymphocyte.
   d. Occasionally E-shaped nucleus.
   e. Cytoplasm pale, much more abundant than in lymphocytes and granulocytes.
6. Reactive monocyte:
   a. Nucleus may be slightly larger and tends to round up, but the fine chromatin pattern remains.
   b. Nucleolus often present, and a few small chromocenters.
7. Atypical monocyte:
   a. A rarely used designation—would be difficult to distinguish from immature or reactive monocyte except perhaps for more nuclear irregularities and larger size.
8. Plasma cell:
   a. Eccentric nucleus, slightly larger than that of small lymphocyte.
   b. Characteristic nuclear chromatin pattern ("clock-face, spoke-wheel").
   c. Slightly more dense cytoplasm may be seen, compared to monocyte.
   d. Conspicuous "hof" (i.e., focal paranuclear cytoplasmic pallor).
9. Atypical plasma cell:
   a. Nucleus slightly larger but still with features reminiscent of the characteristic chromatin pattern and eccentric nuclear location in the cell.
   b. Nucleus shows indentations or irregularities in outline.
10. Neutrophil (polymorphonuclear leukocyte; PMN)
    a. Larger than resting lymphocyte; smaller than monocyte.
    b. Be sure you see the segmented nucleus clearly as you focus up and down. If you cannot, it is probably a monocyte nucleus on edge.
11. "Smudge cell":
    a. Smeared on slide to a varying degree. It may be a clue for the presence of leukemia or lymphoma cells if there are many on the slide, since these neoplastic cells are sometimes more fragile. However, it may also occur as an artifact (e.g., excessive centrifuge speed, pressing cells into the filter; degenerating cells).
12. Lining cells:
    a. May be seen in groups of polygonal or cuboidal cells in a strip, or can form gland-like rosettes.
    b. May look bizarre in chronic irritative conditions, and thus mimic malignancy.
    c. Nuclei resemble those of monocytes in chromatin pattern, but shape is more often round or elliptical.
    d. More often seen as bare nuclei or with more cytoplasm on one side than the other (as with columnar cells).
    e. If artificially stripped off (e.g., by needle aspiration) can be more spindle shaped.

Table 4.9.
The Dilemma of the Single Malignant Cell

a. First identify the normal small lymphocyte population to assess size and chromatin staining features. Then search for a distinct second cell population that has morphologic differences.
b. Keep in mind the usual criteria for malignancy you have learned before (e.g., high N/C ratio, large cells 2–3 times or more in size than normal lymphs, clumped chromatin, nuclear membrane irregularities), even though all such features are rarely present in a single cell, and you do not—in this instance—have the benefit of assessing cell-to-cell relationships in fragments for additional malignancy criteria.
c. Then determine whether you can find a spectrum of intermediate cell types between one or another normal cell component and the cell in question (i.e., is it at the extreme end of a reactive cell change, or truly a separate cell population?)
d. Note the company the cells in question are keeping (e.g., tumor diathesis, acute or chronic inflammation, giant cells of multinucleated type suggesting a granuloma)
e. Consider the clinical history; communicate with the clinician if you still have questions.
f. Compared with prior specimens, if available (e.g., a case of lymphoma treatment monitoring).
g. If there is still a question of reactive/atypical lymphs versus lymphoma/leukemia, recommend repeat examination with 10 ml of fluid submitted for marker studies.

false-negative CSF interpretations. It has been the authors' experience that well-stained and well-preserved cells make the interpretation relatively easy. Caution in the interpretation of technically unsatisfactory or suboptimal material is always warranted. For those unfamiliar with the Papanicolaou stain, dual staining of separate slides using both Pap and Wright's (Diff-Quik) stains provides a safe means of gaining the necessary experience. We particularly recommend that the Papanicolaou stain-trained cytologist become more familiar with the appearance of cells using the Wright's stains. While it is not necessary to employ both stains routinely, there are certain situations (e.g., leukemias) in which the ability to evaluate cellular features with both staining methods becomes important for proper diagnostic classification.

Figures 4.10 to 4.25 have been selected primarily to help the microscopist review the distinct morphologic features of these important cell populations. We also encourage the reader to seek other atlases and audiovisual aids available on this topic. Chapter 5 describes the importance of sequential evaluation of CSF cells in identifying cell profiles that are characteristic of certain disease processes, as well as for monitoring therapy (34, 46).

References

1. Andrews, J.M., and Schumann, G.B. Laboratory processing of cerebrospinal fluid specimens. Diagn. Cytopathol. 6:139–143, 1990.
2. Azzarelli, B., Mirkin, L.D., Goheen, M., et al. The leptomeningeal vein: A site of re-entry of leukemic cells into the systemic circulation. Cancer 54:1333–1343, 1984.
3. Barrett, D.L., and King, E.B. Comparison of cellular recovery rates and morphologic detail obtained using membrane filter and cytocentrifuge techniques. Acta Cytol. 20:174–180, 1976.
4. Beerman, W.F. Meningeal carcinomatosis. JAMA 58:1437–1439, 1912.
5. Bigner, S.H. Central nervous system. Chapter 18 in: Bibbo, M. (Ed.): Comprehensive Cytopathology. W.B. Saunders Co., Philadelphia, 1991, pp.478–479.
6. Bigner, S.H., and Johnston, W.W. Cytopathology of the Central Nervous System. New York, Masson Publishing, 1983.
7. Bigner, S.H., and Johnston, W.W. The cytopathology of cerebrospinal fluid. I. Non-neoplastic conditions, lymphoma and leukemia. Acta Cytol. 25:335–353, 1981.
8. Bigner, S.H., and Johnston, W.W. The cytopathology of cerebrospinal fluid. II. Metastatic cancer, meningeal carcinomatosis and primary central nervous system neoplasms. Acta Cytol. 25:461–479, 1981.
9. Bigner, S.H., and Johnston, W.W. The diagnostic challenge of tumors manifested initially by the shedding of cells into cerebrospinal fluid. Acta Cytol. 28:29–36, 1984.
10. Bots, G.T.A.M., Went, L.W., and Schaberg, A. Results of a sedimentation technique for cytology of cerebrospinal fluid. Acta Cytol. 8:234–241, 1962.

11. Choi, H.H., and Anderson, P.J. Diagnostic cytology of cerebrospinal fluid by the cytocentrifuge method. Am. J. Clin. Pathol. 72:931, 1979.
12. Chu, J-Y., and Hohenberger, J. Simple sedimentation method for cytology of cerebrospinal fluid. Am. J. Clin. Pathol. 74:471–472, 1980.
13. den Hartog Jager, W.A. Color Atlas of CSF Cytopathology. Philadelphia, J.B. Lippincott, 1980.
14. Drewinko, B., Sullivan, M., and Martin, T. Use of cytocentrifuge in the diagnosis of meningeal leukemia. Cancer 31:1331–1336, 1973.
15. Fishman, R.A. Cerebrospinal Fluid in Diseases of the Nervous System. W.B. Saunders, Philadelphia, pp. 175–186, 1980.
16. Glass, J.P., Melamed, M., Chernik, N., et al. Malignant cells in cerebrospinal fluid (CSF): The meaning of a positive CSF cytology. Neurology 29:1369–1376, 1979.
17. Gondos, B., and King, E. Cerebrospinal fluid cytology: Diagnostic accuracy and comparison of different techniques. Acta Cytol. 20:542–547, 1976.
18. Hajdu, S.I., and Hajdu, E.O. Cytopathology of Sarcomas and Other Nonepithelial Malignant Tumors. W.B. Saunders, Philadelphia, pp. 328–331, 1976.
19. Halhuizen, J.C., Bots, J.T.A.M., Schaberg, A., et al. Value of cerebrospinal fluid cytology for the diagnosis of malignancies in the central nervous system. J. Neurosurg. 48:747–753, 1978.
20. Hansen, H., Bender, R., and Shelton, B. The cytocentrifuge and cerebrospinal fluid cytology. Acta Cytol. 18:259–262, 1974.
21. Herndon, R.M., Brumback, R.A. The Cerebrospinal Fluid. Kluwer Academic Publishers, Boston, 1989.
22. Kajikawa, H., Ohta, T., Ohshiro, H., Harrado, K., Ishikawa, S., Vozume, T., Kodama, M., and Okoda, T. Cerebrospinal fluid cytology in patients with brain tumors: A simple method using the cell culture technique. Acta Cytol. 21:162–167, 1977.
23. Kemp, D., and Cox, B. Cytocentrifugation in the management of central nervous system leukemia. J. Pediatr. 81:992–994, 1972.
24. Kline, T.S. Cytological examination of the cerebrospinal fluid. Cancer 15:592–597, 1962.
25. Kokkoris, C.P. Leptomeningeal carcinomatosis. How does cancer reach the pia-arachnoid? Cancer 51:154–160, 1983.
26. Kölmel, H.W. A method for concentrating cerebrospinal fluid cells. Acta Cytol. 21:154–157, 1977.
27. Kölmel, H.W. Atlas of Cerebrospinal Fluid Cells. 2nd ed. Springer-Verlag, New York, 1977.
28. Komp, D.M., and Cox, B.J. Cytocentrifugation in the management of central nervous system leukemia. J. Pediatr. 81:992–994, 1972.
29. Koss, L.G. Diagnostic Cytology and Its Histopathologic Bases. J.B. Lippincott, Philadelphia, pp. 971–978, 1979.
30. Krantz, B.R., Thiel, E., Thierfelder, S. Immunocytochemical identification of meningeal leukemia and lymphoma: Poly-L-lysine-coated slides permit multimarker analysis, even with minute cerebrospinal fluid cell specimens. Blood 73:1942–1950, 1989.
31. Krentz, M.J., and Dyken, P.R. Cerebrospinal fluid cytomorphology sedimentation vs filtration. Arch. Neurol. 26:253–257, 1972.
32. Leif, R.C., Silverman, M.A., Bobbitt, D., and Ng, A. Centrifugal cytology: A new technique for cytodiagnosis. Lab Management 32–41, Sept. 1979.
33. Mathios, A.J., Nielsen, S.L., Barrett, D., et al. Cerebrospinal fluid cytomorphology identification of benign cells originating in the central nervous system. Acta Cytol. 21:403, 1977.
34. Mayer, J.R., and Watson, C.W. Cytologic monitoring of cerebrospinal fluid in the treatment of histiocytic lymphoma involving the central nervous system. Acta Cytol. 24:26–29, 1981.
35. McAlpine, L.L., and Ellsworth, B. A modified membrane filter technique for cytodiagnosis. Am. J. Clin. Pathol. 52:242–244, 1969.
36. McCormick, W.F., and Coleman, S.A. A membrane filter technique for cytology of spinal fluid. Am. J. Clin. Pathol. 38:191–197, 1962.
37. McGarry, P., Holmquist, N.D., and Carmel, S.A. A postmortem study of cerebrospinal fluid with histologic correlation. Acta Cytol. 13:48–52, 1969.
38. Meena, C.E., Olsen, W.H., and Yam, L.T. Light microscopic cytology of cerebrospinal fluid. Chapter 9 in: Herndon, R.M., and Brumback, R.A. (Eds.): The Cerebrospinal Fluid. Kluwer Academic Publishers, Boston, 1989, pp. 227–244.
39. Naib, Z.M. Exfoliative Cytopathology. Ed. 2. Little, Brown, Boston, pp. 443–456, 1976.
40. Naylor, B. Cytologic study of intracranial fluid. Acta Cytol. 5:198–202, 1961.
41. Oehmichen, M. Cerebrospinal Fluid Cytology: An Introduction and Atlas. W.B. Saunders, Philadelphia, 1978.
42. Papanicolaou, G.N. New procedure for staining vaginal smears. Science, 95(2469):438–439, 1942.
43. Reynaud, A.J., and King, E.B. A new filter for diagnostic cytology. Acta Cytol. 11:289–294, 1942.
44. Rich, J. A membrane filter technique for cerebrospinal fluid cytology. J. Neurosurg. 36:661–666, 1972.
45. Rosenthal, D.L. Cytology of the Central Nervous System. Monographs in Clinical Cytology. Ed. C.L. Weid, New York, S. Karger, 1984.
46. Schumann, G.B., and Colon, F.V. The Clinician's Guide to Diagnostic Cytology. Year Book, Chicago, pp. 236–250, 1982.
47. Schumann, G.B., and Crisman, L.G. Cerebrospinal fluid cytopathology. Clin. Lab. Med. 5:275–302, 1985.
48. Silverman, J.F., and Frable, W.J. The use of the Diff-Quik stain in the immediate interpretation of fine-needle aspiration biopsies. Diagn. Cytopathol. 6:366–369, 1990.

49. Spriggs, A.I. Malignant cells in cerebrospinal fluid. J. Clin. Pathol. 7:122–130, 1954.
50. Watson, P. A slide centrifuge: An apparatus for concentrating cells in suspension onto a microscope slide. J. Lab. Clin. Med. 68:494–501, 1966.
51. Whitmore, E.L., Hochberg, F., Wolfson, L., Royalty, J., and Taft, P.D. Quantitative cytocentrifugation in the evaluation of cerebrospinal fluid. Acta Cytol. 26:847-850, 1982.
52. Woodruff, K.H. Cerebrospinal fluid cytomorphology using cytocentrifugation. Am. J. Clin. Pathol. 60:621–627, 1973.

5 / Quantitative Approach to CSF Cytopathology

The purpose of this chapter on a quantitative approach to CSF cytopathology is to briefly review the rationale, describe the method and reporting of results, and use recently reported case situations to highlight some important advantages of this method. Skeptics of this approach may perceive the methodology and techniques to be time consuming and cumbersome, and to an extent this is true. At the time of this writing, however, the approach to be described below appears to us to be the most efficient one available to provide this type of information. It is likely that methods currently under active investigation will simplify this approach (see Chapter 10).

Rationale

As previously discussed (see Chapters 3 and 4), the medical laboratory examination of cerebrospinal fluid (CSF) may include biochemical determinations for glucose, protein, and enzymes; microbiologic studies for infectious agents; hematologic evaluations for inflammation and hematopoietic or lymphoproliferative disorders; and cytologic evaluations to identify epithelial malignancies. CSF specimens are routinely triaged to various laboratory disciplines based on clinical differential diagnosis (2, 14). Each laboratory discipline has a responsibility to ensure that clinicians receive proper instructions regarding specimen submission and reporting of results (2) (see Chapter 3).

Traditionally, laboratory analysis (in body fluid and "stat" laboratories) includes cell counts using a hemocytometer chamber count method for assessment of cellularity, and cell differentials for classifying mononuclear cells. (Chapter 4 reviews methods most cytopathology laboratories use in the course of qualitative approaches to CSF cytology.) Until recently, CSF cytology has been primarily utilized for detecting epithelial malignancies (4, 6, 27, 31), hematopoietic or lymphoproliferative disorders (5, 7, 13, 18, 23), opportunistic infections, and chronic inflammatory conditions (5, 13, 23). Within the last decade the clinical role of CSF cytology has expanded to include monitoring the course of metastatic disease and treatment response with serial or sequential cellular assessments (1, 21, 28). In this restricted setting it has become a high-priority test for oncologists, neurologists, and neurosurgeons in managing patients with neural system malignancies.

Frequently, CSF specimens with demonstrated normal cell counts (less than 5 mononuclear cells per mm^3) contain malignant cells (28, 32). Because of this observation, some investigators have advocated using cytocentrifugation (32) or membrane filter techniques (3, 4, 11, 14) as an alternative to the usual hemocytometer method to improve cell recovery. Chapter 4 reviews advantages and disadvantages of various cytopreparatory methods used for qualitative CSF cytology.

Collection of Specimens for Quantitative CSF Cytology

In the period from January 1, 1981, to December 30, 1986, 2563 (see Table 4.3) CSF specimens—including lumbar punctures,

Ommaya reservoir specimens, and ventricular taps—were analyzed by means of a previously reported semiquantitative microscopic approach using membrane filter preparations (28). Physicians were requested to submit 3 ml of unfixed CSF to the laboratory. Refrigeration was utilized to minimize cellular degeneration in any specimen delivered after laboratory working hours.

Cytopreparation

CSF specimens submitted to the laboratory were evaluated for volume and appearance. Each specimen was then mixed for 5 minutes using a test tube agitator. Specimens normal in color and character and of 3 ml or less were placed over a small-diameter (25-mm) Millipore membrane filter with a 5-μm pore size (Millipore Corporation, Bedford, MA). Any remaining specimen was refrigerated until the final microscopic assessment was completed. Additional preparations were made in cases suspicious for malignancy. A 1-ml aliquot was used in specimens obtained from cases with previous hypercellular counts (less than 5000 cells/ml). Specimens of abnormal color or character (i.e., bloody, milky, xanthochromic, or containing mucoid or other precipitate) were individually assessed for determination of aliquot and filter diameter size to be used. After cytopreparation using the modified membrane filter technique (see Chapter 4), the filters were fixed for 15 min in 95% ethyl alcohol and stained with a modified Papanicolaou method. Additional Wright's (Diff-Quik) cytocentrifuge slides were made on leukemic patients when necessary.

Microscopic Evaluation

The initial microscopic evaluation of CSF samples included a general overview of the slide to judge the cellularity, adequacy, and nature of the specimen (i.e., marked degeneration, blood contamination, or obvious malignancy). This rapid microscopic assessment was followed by a cell count and differential and by screening for abnormal cells, infectious agents, and other cellular elements.

Cell Differential

A microscopic examination of the CSF filter preparation under 400× magnification provided the 100-cell differential in a fashion similar to that in a peripheral blood smear. The cell differential should be taken from random areas of the filter to minimize cellular distribution problems. Lymphocytes, monocytes, neutrophils, lining cells (ependymal and/or choroid plexus cells), malignant cells, and others (plasma cells, hemosiderin-laden macrophages, chondrocytes, etc.) were recorded. Only intact (i.e., with cytoplasm) nucleated cells (excluding erythrocytes) were included in the cell differential.

Filter Count Method

In our laboratory, we have devised a formula to calculate the approximate cellularity of a CSF specimen using a membrane filter preparation. The counting area of the filter is established by viewing 20 random, medium-power (200× to 250×) fields (five fields per quadrant) (Fig. 5.1). Using this method, the overall cellularity of the specimen is assessed.

Because the area viewed varies with the type of microscope used, the percentage of area covered in 20 fields must be determined for each type of microscope employed in screening. For example, the area of an expanded (25-mm Millipore) filter is 283.38 mm^2; the viewed area of Zeiss 25× objective and 10× ocular lenses is 0.38 mm^2. Thus, for a Zeiss Standard Lab 16 microscope, a calculation factor of 32 was determined. The formulas for the calculation factor for 20 fields are:

Formula No. 1:

$$\frac{(0.38\ \text{mm}^2)\,(20)}{283.38\ \text{mm}^2} = 0.03$$

Formula No. 2:

$$1 - 0.03 = 0.97$$

Formula No. 3:

$$\frac{0.97}{0.03} = 32 = \text{calculation factor}$$

The cell-count formula is:

$$\frac{(\text{Calculation Factor})\,(x) + x}{\text{ml}}$$

$$= \text{Cells per ml of specimen}$$

where x = number of cells in 20 (medium-power or 25×) fields. For example, if 3 ml of CSF was prepared and screened at 250× magnification and 100 cells were counted in 20 fields, then the calculation factor = 32, x = 100 cells, and ml = 3, and the number of cells per ml is:

$$\frac{(32)\,(100\ \text{cells}) + 100\ \text{cells}}{3\ \text{ml}} = 1100$$

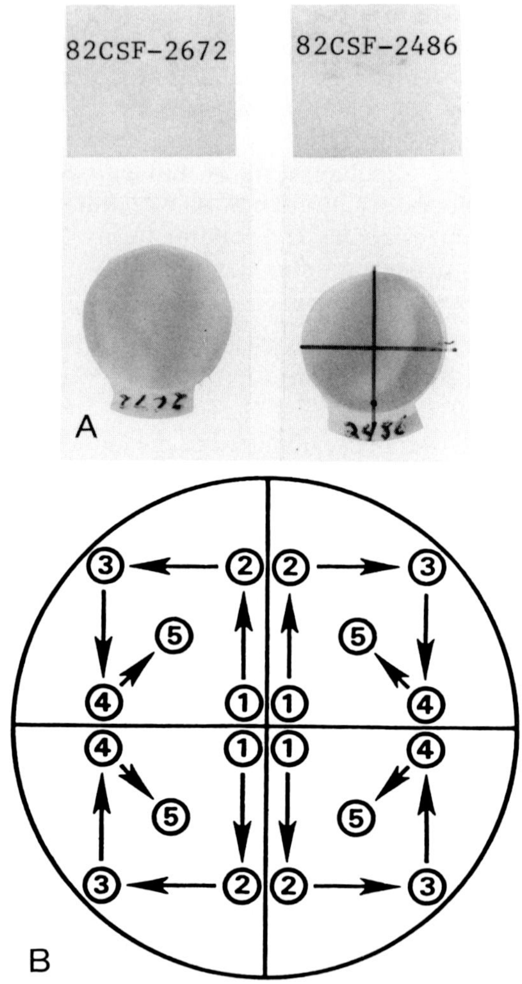

Figure 5.1. **A,** Small (25 mm) Millipore filter following staining and coverslipping (left); filter has been divided into quadrants (right). **B,** Quadrants illustrating the set number of medium-power field. Count the cells in the fields (labeled No. 1) in the immediate vicinity of the convergence of the lines. From the field labeled No. 1, count four fields (away from the horizontal line), and then count the cells in the fifth field (labeled No. 2). From the field labeled No. 2, count four fields (away from the vertical line), and then count the cells in the fifth field (labeled No. 3). From the field labeled No. 3, count four fields (toward the horizontal line), and then count the cells in the fifth field (labeled No. 4). From the field labeled No. 4, move toward the center of the quadrant (approximately two fields), and count the cells in the field. (From Schumann, G.B., and Grisman, L.G. Cerebrospinal fluid cytopathology. Clin. Lab. Med. 1985. Used by permission.)

Modified Correction Factors for Quantitative CSF

	Diameter		Area	
20×	= .93 mm	r = .465 mm	$(.465)^2$	= .68 mm^2
25×	= .7 mm	r = .35 mm	$(.35)^2$	= .38 mm^2
40×	= .44 mm	r = .22 mm	$(.22)^2$	= .15 mm^2
filter	= 15.4 mm	r = 7.7 mm	$(7.7)^2$	= 186.27 mm^2

Correction Factors (Area of Objective) (20) Divided into Total Area of Filter

$$20\times = .68\ mm^2 \times 20 = 13.6\ mm^2 \quad 186.27\ mm^2 = 13.7^*$$
$$25\times = .38\ mm^2 \times 20 = 7.6\ mm^2 \quad 186.27\ mm^2 \doteq 24.5^*$$
$$40\times = .15\ mm^2 \times 20 = 3\ mm^2 \quad 186.27\ mm^2 = 62.1^*$$

To adapt these corrections factors to the mathematically correct formula $\frac{(cf)(x) + x}{\#mls}$, we subtract one and have:

	cf
20×	(12.7) + x
25×	(23.5) + x
40×	(61.1) + x

Diagnostic Statement

The entire filter is screened under 250× magnification to detect rare malignant or atypical cells and infectious agents. The total microscopic examination is then summarized and reported.

Example 1 (Fig. 5.2):

Diagnosis: Hypercellular specimen with blastic cells present derived from a leukemic process. Cellular features consistent with acute lymphocytic leukemia (ALL).

Cell count: 6232 cells/ml

Cell differential:
- 56 lymphocytes (few atypical)
- 34 monocytes
- 2 neutrophils
- 8 blast cells

100 cells counted

Example 2:

Diagnosis: Malignant cells present derived from adenocarcinoma. Hemosiderin-laden macrophages present indicating prior bleeding.

Cell count: 2398 cells/ml

Cell differential:
- 17 lymphocytes
- 68 monocytes
- 5 lining cells
- 7 malignant cells
- 3 macrophages (occasional hemosiderin-laden)

100 cells counted

Benefits of Quantitative CSF Cytopathology

This new approach for CSF cytopathology was readily accepted by the technical staff

* It is easier to simply multiply *x* times the raw numbers above.

Table 5.1.
Abnormal CSF Interpretations Grouped by Cellularity[a]

	Atypical	Suspicious	Positive	Total
Normal cellularity (<5,000 cells/ml)	12 (13.2%)	3 (3.3%)	52 (57.1%)	67 (73.6%)
Hypercellular (>5,000 cells/ml)	5 (5.5%)	4 (4.4%)	15 (16.5%)	24 (26.4%)

[a] From Schumann, G.B., and Crissman, L.G. Semiquantitative approach to CSF cytopathology. Diagn. Cytopathol. 2:194–197, 1986.

in our laboratory. The complete cytologic examination required 15 to 20 minutes with most of the microscopic time involved with screening for malignant and blast cells. With experience we found the Papanicolaou (Pap) stain to be excellent in characterizing hematopoietic as well as epithelial cells. This may create a disadvantage for laboratories restricted to the use of Wright's stain. Because the Pap stain is a universal stain, most laboratories have experience with the method. Although more time is needed to perform the cell count and cell differential, the time required to summarize the microscopic findings and to establish the diagnostic or interpretative statement is decreased.

The medical acceptance of this semiquantitative protocol for CSF cytology has been increasing. The number of specimens has increased to approximately 500 specimens per year. Table 5.1 lists the abnormal CSF interpretations grouped by cellularity. As reported in Chapter 4, we have observed a higher percentage of malignant CSF results in hypocellular to normocellular specimens (57%) than in hypercellular specimens (16%). That is, the overall number of abnormal CSF cytologic interpretations was higher (74%) in normocellular specimens than in hypercellular specimens (26%), due to the preponderance of inflammatory rather than neoplastic conditions producing the latter.

In clinical practice, the identification of tumor cells is the major goal of the cytology laboratory (14). Barrett and King determined that the membrane filtration method provides maximum cell retrieval and minimum cellular distortion in hypocellular specimens and is the most reliable method (3). Recently, Whitmore et al. (32) have advocated a quantitative cytocentrifugation method over the standard hemocytometer method. Their study concluded that because of the large volume of CSF fluid used in cytocentrifugation, cells ($0.2/mm^3$) were found in 264 specimens that would have been considered devoid of cells by hemocytometry; six of these samples contained malignant cells (32). The differences in the normal cell count range obtained from the standard hemocytometer method versus the filter method are 0 to 5 cells/mm^3 versus 0 to 5000 cells/ml, respectively. Our results (Table 5.1) showed that 73.6% of the abnormal, noninfectious CSF diagnosed had normal cell counts, i.e., less than 5000 cells/ml. The designation of a CSF sample as hypercellular should be reported as an abnormality, and additional samples may be required to explain the increased cellularity.

The semiquantitative approach to CSF cytology described, therefore, combines a diagnostic statement, a cell differential, and a cell count. This becomes important in neoplastic conditions when serial or sequential specimens are compared following chemotherapeutic regimens. The necessity of monitoring the CSF has increased as the overall survival rates of patients with acute lymphocytic leukemia and diffuse histiocytic lymphoma, for example, have improved. These patients are more prone to develop CNS involvement and are frequently treated with intrathecal chemotherapy. Changes in cell counts and differentials may be useful in monitoring treatment response (11, 21, 29).

The following section of this chapter describes two previously reported cases that highlight the advantages of this quantitative approach to CSF cytology. While numerous examples could have been provided, these two cases were selected because comprehensive clinical information, histologic confirmation of diagnosis, and autopsy studies were available.

Cytodiagnosis and Monitoring of Acute Lymphocytic Leukemia and Eosinophilia in Cerebrospinal Fluid—A Case Report

The first case report describes a patient in whom CSF cytopathology was used to diagnose acute lymphocytic leukemia (ALL) (11). The patient initially presented with ALL and eosinophilia. Immunologic tumor markers were used to correctly classify the leukemia in CSF. This is a rare report describing the sequential, cytologic follow-up of ALL and the disappearance of malignant or blastic cells from the CSF in response to therapy (11).

Clinical Summary

A 22-year-old white male machinist from southern Utah presented to his local physician in April of 1984 with a 2-month history of myalgia, arthralgia, and low-grade fever. An erythematous rash and nonexudative pharyngitis were the only findings on physical examination. His peripheral white cell count was 51,000 cells/μl with 85% eosinophils. An iliac crest bone marrow aspirate was interpreted as normal except for increased eosinophils. The patient was given aspirin and prednisone for possible hypersensitivity to chronic streptococcal pharyngitis, but 1 week later he was admitted to the University of Utah Medical Center with increasing lethargy, apneic spells, deteriorating mental status, and unilateral inguinal adenopathy. No focal neurologic signs were detected, and his CSF was unremarkable at this first admission. His peripheral white cell count was 24,100 cells/μl, with 75% eosinophils and no immature cells. A bone marrow aspirate and biopsy were 100% cellular with diffuse replacement of normal marrow elements by common acute lymphoblastic leukemia antigen (CALLA)- and terminal deoxynucleotidyl transferase (Tdt)-positive lymphoblasts. B and T cell markers were negative. Chest x-ray and abdominal-pelvic computerized tomographic (CT) scans were normal. Clinically, it was felt the patient had a lymphoblastic lymphoma, and he was begun on the COMLA regimen (cytoxan, vincristine followed by methotrexate, with leucovorin rescue and cytosine arabinoside). Although a bone marrow aspirate done after three courses of chemotherapy showed no evidence of hypereosinophilia or residual malignancy, the CSF contained 22% eosinophils and rare immature lymphoid cells consistent with a leukemic process (see Fig. 5.4). CALLA, Tdt, and human T lymphocyte antigen (HTA) immunologic markers performed on the CSF lymphoblasts gave results identical to the lymphoblasts in the bone marrow aspirate studies.

The patient's bone marrow studies were reinterpreted as aleukemic acute lymphocytic leukemia with an isolated CNS relapse. He then began reinduction chemotherapy with vincristine, prednisone, and Adriamycin with twice-weekly intrathecal methotrexate to continue until the CSF cleared, followed by craniospinal axis irradiation (2400 rad to the cranium, 1400 rad to the spinal cord) with oral maintenance therapy of 6-mercaptopurine and methotrexate. The CSF was cytologically evaluated at twice-weekly intervals. The CSF was negative after 4 weeks of intrathecal methotrexate, but by the time the irradiation therapy had been completed 3 weeks later the CSF was again positive for lymphoblasts. Intrathecal methotrexate was resumed, and an Ommaya reservoir was placed. Seven months after the first CNS relapse the patient was readmitted with anorexia, somnolence, flat affect, and stumbling. Neurologic examination showed a rapid decay of mental functioning and frontal release signs. No adenopathy was noted, and all laboratory tests on blood and CSF were normal.

While hospitalized, the patient developed tonic-clonic seizures controlled with dilantin and phenobarbital. Antibiotic therapy was started when a head CT scan showed a diffuse white matter process and two masses thought to be abscesses, the larger in the left frontotemporal cortex adjacent to the anterior horn of the left lateral ventricle. An electroencephalogram showed diffuse slowing. CSF cytology showed no evidence of acute inflammation or leukemia. The patient deteriorated and died 16 months after diagnosis.

Postmortem examination revealed no evidence of residual leukemia. The brain showed severe necrotizing leukoencephalopathy in areas corresponding to the masses identified on CT, attributed to irradiation and intrathecal methotrexate; there was no microscopic evidence for infection, and brain cultures were negative.

Materials and Methods

A total of 19 CSF specimens were obtained over 8 months (Table 5.2). CSF examination consisted of a 3-ml volume of CSF processed by vacuum filtration through a small Millipore filter (25-mm diameter, 5-μm pore size) (Millipore, Bedford, MA). The filter was fixed with 95% ethanol and stained with a modified Papanicolaou stain. The slides were then screened for small, reactive, and atypical lymphocytes, reactive and normal monocytes, neutrophils, eosinophils, macrophages, lining cells, and parenchymal elements. A total cell count (cells/ml) and a 100-cell differential count were determined for each sample.

Standard immunoperoxidase staining methods were used for the CALLA and HTA marker studies, which were performed on air-dried, acetone-fixed material. CALLA antibody was provided by Becton-Dickinson Immunocytometry Systems (Mountain View, CA), and HTA antibody was provided by Hybritech (San Diego, CA). The Tdt antibody was from Pharmacia P-L Biochemicals (Piscataway, NJ), and the test was performed using standard indirect immunofluorescence methods.

Results

In the CSF, small lymphocytes were small cells with smudged, dense chromatin. Reactive and atypical lymphocytes had dense chromatin and larger or irregular nuclear contours, respectively. Normal mature monocytes had an eccentric bean-shaped nucleus with fine chromatin and slightly more cytoplasm than normal small lymphocytes. Reactive monocytes were characterized by a larger nucleus than normal with a single prominent nucleolus. Lymphoblasts were characteristically larger than normal small lymphocytes and had high nuclear/cytoplasmic (N/C) ratios (Fig. 5.2). The lymphoblast nuclear membrane was usually regular, although convolutions were variably present; chromatin was slightly hyperchromatic with a single prominent nucleolus, and only a thin rim of cytoplasm was visible. Immunologic cell surface markers indicated a null-cell ALL.

Differential counts of CSF samples from the time of the patient's relapse are summarized in Table 5.2. Initial CSF cell counts showed a markedly hypercellular fluid containing rare lymphoblasts, with high total

Table 5.2.
Cytologic CSF Flow Sheet for a Patient with ALL and Eosinophilia

Date (1985)	Cell count (cells/ml)	Blasts	Cell Differential: Monocytes	Lymphocytes	Neutrophils	Eosinophils	Other	Cytodiagnosis[a]	Comments
1/10	160,000	Rare	20	58	Rare	22		ALL	
1/17	64,680	Rare	32	14	11	43		ALL	CALLA+; Tdt+; HTA−
1/21	21,665	Rare	46	36	1	16	One "lining cell"	ALL	
1/24	26,565		9	14	77	Rare		NBCI	Diluted by fresh blood
1/28	5,764	Rare	59	31	Rare			ALL	
1/31	25,080		32	4	54	10	Rare "lining cells"	NBCI	Diluted by fresh blood
2/5	4,092	Rare	40	4	55	1		ALL	Diluted by fresh blood
2/7	1,425		20	73	7	Rare		NBCI	
3/4	20,944			7	93			NBCI	
3/18	154		16	5				NBCI	
4/29	924	Rare	72	27 (few atypical)			One plasma cell	ALL	
5/13	1,287	Rare	52	48				ALL	
5/15	9,702	Rare	3	6			44 "lining cells"; 47 parenchymal elements	ALL	
5/25	11,154		40 (rare; react)	41 (rare; atypical)	19		Rare macrophages	NBCI	Diluted by fresh blood
6/3	14,569		49 (few; react)	41 (few atypical)	8		Rare macrophages	NBCI	Diluted by fresh blood
6/18	14,569		29	20	3		48 hemosiderin macrophages	NBCI	Diluted by fresh blood
8/5	1,023		50	46	Rare		One "lining cell"; 3 hemosiderin macrophages	NBCI	
8/23	7,810		44	6	50			NBCI	Diluted by fresh blood
8/26	10,560		76	24	Rare			NBCI	

[a] NBCI, no blast cells identified.

cell counts persisting at a lower but still elevated level through the first 3 weeks of treatment with i.v. and intrathecal chemotherapy. Lymphoblasts were identified after six courses of intrathecal chemotherapy in specimens that were normocellular. By the time radiation therapy was completed, malignant cells that were morphologically identical to the lymphoblasts in the initial CSF had reappeared in specimens with normal to mildly elevated cell counts. There did not appear to be a relationship between cell count and number of lymphoblasts. That is, blasts were never numerous even in hypercellular specimens. CSF cell counts steadily decreased during the initial stages of therapy except when the specimen was contaminated by blood. Because this patient never exhibited blasts in his peripheral blood smears, blasts found in CSF samples diluted by fresh blood were considered to be a significant indicator of CNS disease.

Hypereosinophilia was an additional feature followed in early CSF specimens. The eosinophils (Fig. 5.3) were mature cells with characteristic bilobed nuclei; no immature cells from the myeloid series were present. As the CSF total cell counts fell the number of eosinophils also fell, and eosinophilia did not reappear at the time of CNS relapse.

Discussion

Cytopathologists who examine CSF are chiefly concerned with identifying malignant cells. Approximately 30% of patients who die of cancer have CNS involvement at the time of autopsy (5). If no CNS prophylaxis is given to patients with ALL, 60% will have CNS relapse (5). Twenty percent of leukemic adults achieving complete bone marrow remission will have CNS involvement (30), and the incidence of CNS relapse has increased due to prolonged survival with radiation and chemotherapy. Finding malignant cells in the CSF generally indicates that immediate treatment to the craniospinal axis is necessary. Sequential CSF studies are needed to monitor the efficacy of therapy and to assist the clinician in making management decisions. CSF involvement is not always manifested by signs or symptoms; two-thirds to three-quarters of patients with autopsy-proven CNS involvement with metastatic disease had no clinically detectable signs or symptoms (5); therefore, cytologic examination of CSF may be the only method for accurately determining a patient's true status. Multiple CSF examinations increase the detection rate of malignant cells from 45% on one examination to 80% on multiple examinations (1, 24).

The utility of cytologic monitoring of the CSF has recently been described by several investigators for benign and malignant histiocytic proliferations; the characteristic morphology of the histiocytes was used to identify atypical and malignant cells in multiple patient samples (16, 21). A similar method for comparing morphologically malignant cells in serial samples was applied in this case of an adult male with acute lymphoblastic leukemia, null-cell type, who had achieved a bone marrow remission but suffered an isolated CNS relapse.

Clinical decisions affecting the duration of intrathecal chemotherapy were based on whether blasts were identified in each specimen. CSF was removed at each lumbar puncture used to inject methotrexate and was cytologically examined. Prompt specimen preparation, screening, and reporting are essential to this type of evaluation to optimize the implementation of treatment decisions based on the CSF data. An-Foraker has listed proper sampling, preparation, and cell interpretation as critical factors in cytodiagnostic accuracy in studying CSF for the presence of malignancy (1).

In 1983, Casper et al. (9) reported a series of patients in whom morphology and the cell marker Tdt were used to differentiate pleocytosis from malignancy in a sequential series of samples. The use of cell surface markers and cytochemistry is now a well-established method of identifying cell origin and is usually considered an adjunct to light microscopy. However, the markers were used in this case not to identify malignant cells but rather to type the cells to give an indication of prognosis and to specify appropriate treatment. We believe that the use of such costly techniques on a routine basis for each specimen is usually unnecessary, and we reserve them for initial studies and when the morphology of the malignant cells appears to be altered. Whenever a new malignancy is suspected, marker studies are appropriate. Once the malignant cells have been identified, subsequent specimens can be morphologically compared with slides from the initial fluid sample. This more limited use of marker studies will also reduce delays in reporting, since marker studies generally take at least several hours to complete and interpret.

The clinical significance of eosinophils associated with ALL is unknown. Few cases of ALL with eosinophilia in the CSF have been reported (8, 10, 34). One case demonstrated peripheral blood as well as CSF eosinophilia (8). The eosinophil count in one case, as in our own case, decreased with intrathecal chemotherapy (8).

We believe the monitoring of sequential CSF specimens from patients with acute leukemia by cell morphology may prove advantageous as a rapid means of assessing the patient's condition accurately, and can provide the clinician with information useful in determining treatment decisions and assessing prognosis (11).

Cytodiagnosis and Monitoring of Hodgkin's Disease in Cerebrospinal Fluid—A Case Report

Malignant cells may be shed into the CSF when tumor reaches the ventricular system or subarachnoid space. Central nervous system (CNS) involvement is infrequent with Hodgkin's disease (HD), involvement of the epidural space occurring far more often than the involvement of the intracranial cavity (12, 25, 29).

We report here a patient with involvement of the base of the skull and penetration of the dura by nodular sclerosing HD. Reed-Sternberg cells were identified in the CSF, and sequential cytologic examinations proved useful in evaluating the efficacy of therapy (29).

Clinical Presentation

A 22-year-old woman developed left cervical lymphadenopathy in October of 1978. Biopsy revealed nodular sclerosing HD, and subsequent staging procedures established that disease was restricted to the left neck and mediastinum (stage IIA). The patient was treated with extended-field radiotherapy. A recurrence was detected in a high left-sided cervical node in May of 1979. Five monthly cycles of chemotherapy (MOPP) and regional radiation were administered. Therapy was complicated by radiation pneumonitis and pericarditis.

In August of 1980, the patient developed diplopia. She was referred to the University of Utah Medical Center where she was discovered to have a left 6th cranial nerve palsy and bilateral, firm, posterior cervical adenopathy. Within a month, she developed bilateral 6th nerve palsies and a right 12th nerve paresis. Computerized tomography (CT) of the brain demonstrated a 1.5×2 cm enhancing mass in the posterior fossa just above the foramen magnum. The initial CSF cytologic examination, using a membrane filtration method, demonstrated a cell count of 10,170 cells/ml (normal is less than 5,000) composed of eosinophils, lymphocytes, and atypical mononuclear cells. CSF examination 4 days later demonstrated a rare Reed-Sternberg cell and atypical mononuclear cells, confirming the clinical diagnosis of intracerebral HD involving the brain stem. Whole-brain radiation, radiotherapy to the neck nodes, systemic combination chemotherapy, and intrathecal chemotherapy (cytosine arabinoside) were administered. Sequential CSF cytologic examinations were used to monitor the efficacy of therapy. The cranial nerve palsies improved rapidly following initial therapy. Six monthly treatments with Adriamycin, bis-chloroethyl nitrosourea (BCNU), vinblastine, and dimethyl-triazeno-imidazole carboxamide were administered. The patient did well until March 1981, when she developed interstitial pneumonitis and died of respiratory failure. At autopsy there was no evidence of residual HD in the CNS or systemically. The interstitial pneumonia was compatible with that reported in other patients treated with BCNU.

Materials and Methods

CSF examination consisted of a 3-ml volume of CSF processed by vacuum filtration through a Millipore filter (25-mm diameter, 5-μm pore size) (Millipore, Bedford, MA). The filter was fixed with 95% ethanol and stained with a modified Papanicolaou stain. A total cell count (cells/ml) and a 100-cell differential count were determined for each sample. A total of 14 CSF specimens were obtained over 5 months.

Cytologic Findings

Initial CSF total cell counts ranged from 3,000 to 10,000 cells/ml (normal total amount less than 5,000 cells/ml). Reed-Sternberg (R-S) cells were rare but atypical mononuclear cells (mononuclear variant of R-S cells) were far more common and represented 3 to 10% of the cells counted in the first four samples examined prior to intrathecal chemotherapy. Eosinophils (Fig. 5.4) were present in the initial samples (up to 8% of the cells counted). Three days after the initiation of intrathecal chemotherapy the cell count had diminished to less than 1,000 cells/ml, and remained so through the rest of the clinical course. Reactive monocytes and lymphocytes (Fig. 5.5) and so-called "lining cells" (Fig. 5.6) continued to be seen but eosinophils, R-S cells (Fig. 5.7), and atypical mononuclear cells had disappeared.

Discussion

HD rarely involves the cranial cavity (17). However, like non-Hodgkin's lymphomas, it may enter the cranial cavity by several routes (15, 19, 22, 33). Nasopharyngeal and high cervical lymph node involvement may lead to intracranial spread by penetration of the thin lamellar bone at the base of the skull or by extension through various foramina and fissures (such as the sphenomaxillary and orbital fissures) (33). Involvement of the sixth cranial nerve is the most common clinical manifestation, but other cranial nerves may also be affected (15, 19, 27, 33). The tumor is most commonly extradural (33), but when it penetrates the thin bone at the base of the skull it can present in the pituitary fossa and sella turcica (19, 33). Penetration of the meninges, as in the case reported here, may result in shedding of malignant cells into the CSF. The tumor may also extend along Virchow-Robin spaces into the brain parenchyma (20).

Billingham et al. (7) have described three types of malignant cells in serous effusions and CSF from patients with HD: the classic R-S cell, the mononuclear R-S cell, and the lacunar cell. In our case, we noted the first two types together with eosinophils and lymphocytes. Because of the relative paucity of cells in the CSF, cytocentrifugation (12) or membrane filters have been employed for cytologic examination. We have found vacuum filtration through a small (25-mm) Millipore membrane filter to be superior to these techniques, confirming the report of Barrett and King (3).

Cytologic examination of CSF has previously proven valuable in the diagnosis and staging of non-Hodgkin's lymphoma (21, 26). This case report demonstrates the value of serially monitoring the CSF cytology in HD. Others (12, 25, 29) have also demonstrated the detection of R-S cells of patients with intracranial involvement by HD in the CSF. In addition to the identification of R-S cells in the CSF, our case also illustrates the serial cytology profile of HD when the CNS involvement is successfully treated (29).

In conclusion, maximum cell retrieval, localization of cells, and preservation of cell morphology are the advantages of using this membrane filter technique. By employing a 25-mm diameter filter instead of a 47-mm diameter filter, microscopic evaluation time is also shortened without loss in total number of cells retrieved. CSF cytopathology remains an important test in the differential diagnosis of CNS diseases (1, 4, 13, 23, 27), and its potential value in monitoring certain nervous system diseases in serial fashion may be underutilized.

References

1. An-Foraker, S. Cytodiagnosis of malignant lesions in cerebrospinal fluid. Acta Cytol. 29:286–290, 1984.
2. Andrews, J.M., and Schumann, G.B. Laboratory processing of cerebrospinal fluid specimens. Diagn. Cytopathol. 6:139–143, 1990.
3. Barrett, D.L., and King, E.B. Comparison of cellular recovery rates and morphologic detail obtained using membrane filter and cytocentrifuge techniques. Acta Cytol. 20:174–180, 1976.
4. Bigner, S.H., and Johnston, W.W. Cytopathology of the Central Nervous System. Masson, New York, 1983.
5. Bigner, S.H., and Johnston, W.W. The cytopathology of cerebrospinal fluid. I. Non-neoplastic conditions, lymphoma and leukemia. Acta Cytol. 25:335–353, 1981.
6. Bigner, S.H., and Johnston, W.W. The cytopathology of cerebrospinal fluid. II. Metastatic cancer, meningeal carcinomatosis and primary central nervous system neoplasms. Acta Cytol. 25:461–479, 1981.
7. Billingham, M.E., Rawlinson, D.G., Berry, P.F., and Kempson, R.L. The cytodiagnosis of malignant lymphomas and Hodgkin's disease in cerebrospinal, pleural and ascitic fluids. Acta Cytol. 19:547–556, 1975.
8. Budka, H., Guseo, A., Jellinger, K., et al. Intermittent meningitic reaction with severe basophilia and eosinophilia in CNS leukaemia. J. Neurol. Sci. 28:459–463, 1976.
9. Casper, J.T., Lauer, S.J., Kirchner, P.A., et al. Evaluation of cerebrospinal fluid mononuclear cells obtained from children with acute lymphocytic leukemia: advantages of combining cytomorphology and terminal deoxynucleotidyl transferase. Am. J. Clin. Pathol. 80:666–670, 1983.
10. Catovsky, D., Bernasconi, C., Verdonck, P.J., et al. The association of eosinophilia with lymphoblastic leukaemia or lymphoma: a study of seven patients. Br. J. Haematol. 45:523–534, 1980.
11. Coleman, A., and Schumann, G.B. Cytodiagnosis and monitoring of acute lymphocytic leukemia and eosinophilia in cerebrospinal fluid. Diagn. Cytopathol. 3:330–334, 1987.
12. Cuttner, J., Meyer, R., and Huang, Y.P. Intracerebral involvement in Hodgkin's disease. A report of 6 cases and review of the literature. Cancer 43:1497–1506, 1979.
13. den Hartog Jager, W.A. Color Atlas of CSF Cytopathology. J.B. Lippincott, Philadelphia, 1980.
14. Fishman, R.A. Cerebrospinal Fluid in Diseases of the Nervous System. W.B. Saunders, Philadelphia, 175–186, 1980.
15. Griffin, J.W., Thompson, R.W., Mitchinson, M.J., et al. Lymphomatous leptomeningitis. Am. J. Med. 51:200–208, 1971.
16. Hamilton, S.R., Supta, P.K., Marshall, M.E., et al. Cerebrospinal fluid cytology in histiocytic proliferative disorders. Acta Cytol. 26:22–28, 1982.
17. Kaplan, H.S. Hodgkin's Disease. Harvard University Press, Cambridge, MA, 1972.
18. Kölmel HW. Atlas of Cerebrospinal Fluid Cells. 2nd ed. Springer-Verlag, New York, 1977.
19. Lascelles, G., and Burston, J. Hodgkin's disease presenting with symptoms of cranial nerve involvement. Arch. Neurol. 7:359–364, 1962.
20. Marshall, G., Roessmann, U., and Noort, S.V.D. Invasive Hodgkin's disease of brain. Report of two new cases and review of American and European literature with clinical pathologic correlations. Cancer 22:621–630, 1968.
21. Mayer, J.R., and Watson, C.W. Cytologic monitoring of cerebrospinal fluid in the treatment of histiocytic lymphoma involving the central nervous system. Acta Cytol. 24:26–29, 1981.
22. Morrell, R.M. Cranial neuropathy in advanced Hodgkin's disease. Dis. Nerv. Syst. 19:261–263, 1958.

23. Oehmichen, M. Cerebrospinal Fluid Cytology. An Introduction and Atlas. W.B. Saunders, Philadelphia, 1976.
24. Olson, M.E., Chernik, N.L., and Posner, J.B. Infiltration of the leptomeninges by systemic cancer: a clinical and pathologic study. Arch. Neurol. 30:122–137, 1974.
25. Orlowski, E.P., Hansen, R.M., Anderson, T., Hanson, G.A., Kun, L.E., and Pisciotta, A.V. Hodgkin's disease with leptomeningeal involvement. Report of a case with long survival. Cancer 53:1883–1885, 1984.
26. Rawlinson, D.G., et al. Cytology of the cerebrospinal fluid in patients with Hodgkin's disease or malignant lymphoma. Acta Neuropathol. 69 (suppl):187–191, 1975.
27. Rosenthal, D.L. Cytology of the Central Nervous System. Karger, New York, 1984. (Weid, C.L., ed.: Monographs in clinical cytology.)
28. Schumann, G.B., and Crisman, L.G. Semiquantitative approach to CSF cytopathology. Diagn. Cytopathol. 2:194–197, 1986.
29. Shenoy, U.A., Kushner, J.P., and Schumann, G.B. Cytologic diagnosis and monitoring of Hodgkin's disease in cerebrospinal fluid. Diagn. Cytopathol. 3:323–325, 1987.
30. Stewart, D.J., Keating, M.J., McCredie, K.B., et al. Natural history of central nervous system acute leukemia in adults. Cancer 47:184–196, 1981.
31. Wertlake, P.T., Markovits, B.A., and Stellar, S. Cytologic evaluation of cerebrospinal fluid with clinical and histologic correlation. Acta Cytol. 16:224–239, 1972.
32. Whitmore, E.L., Hochberg, F., Wolfson, L., Royalty, J., and Taft, P.D. Quantitative cytocentrifugation in the evaluation of cerebrospinal fluid. Acta Cytol. 26:845–850, 1982.
33. Woltman, H.W. Malignant tumors of nasopharynx with involvement of nervous system. Arch. Neurol. Psychiatr. 8:412–429, 1922.
34. Youniou, P., Andrieu, J.M., and Cassussus, P.H. Leucemie algue lymphoblastique accompagnee d'une eosinophille sanguine et meningee. Nouv. Presse. Med. 8:527, 1979.

6 / Cytologic Methods Applied to Neural Tissue Biopsies and Aspirates—General Aspects

Developments discussed in Chapter 1 and in several recent articles and reviews now result in an increasing proportion of neurosurgical specimens received by surgical pathologists being obtained by means of stereotactic surgery. The vast majority of such surgeries are performed for the management of cerebral neoplasms (1, 5, 6, 12, 18–21, 29, 33, 37b). Virtually any intracranial site is now within reach of this technology, and the spectrum of applications of such methods will likely be expanded by technological developments currently being explored (3, 4, 20, 23, 38, 39, 42).

Studies of glial neoplasms comparing histologic data with lesion margins as demonstrated by neuroimaging methods demonstrate reasonably good correlation, particularly with magnetic resonance imaging (MRI) methods (10, 24, 25). Such studies do, however, note that isolated tumor cells may extend beyond the MRI-defined lesion boundary (especially in recurrent tumors) (16) and indicate that the combination of smear and routine histologic techniques in the delineation of tumor margins are complementary (10).

Suggested indications and contraindications for stereotactic neurosurgical biopsy are summarized in Tables 6.1 and 6.2 (6, 20).

CNS lesions caudal to the foramen magnum may be subject to many of the same neuroimaging methods for localization, but anatomic factors preclude the required degree of stereotactic frame-to-target stability, and open biopsy remains the procedure of choice for these sites as well as for certain intracranial lesions (see Table 6.2).

Accuracy of Diagnosis

Few would challenge the rationale, whenever feasible, to obtain histologic confirmation of a diagnosis when the literature suggests the accuracy of clinical, presurgical diagnoses to be only in the range of 74 to 86% (8, 14). The accuracy of frozen-section diagnosis (excluding cases deferred to permanent sections, which vary from 0.5 to 10% of all cases in published series) for all specimens (neural and non-neural) in general surgical pathology departments, based on concordance between frozen-section and the final histologic diagnosis, is generally claimed to be in the range of 96.5 to 99% (22). The accuracy rate of intraoperative diagnoses based on stereotactic neurosurgical biopsies, using frozen-section and/or cytologic and permanent paraffin-embedded section methods combined, is estimated to be in the range of 82 to 97% in several published reports (6, 7, 9, 11, 30, 31, 35, 37, 40, 41).

The interpretation of such results must be considered with some caution. The stereotactic biopsy fragment is typically less than 2.0 mm^3 in maximum size. Not all studies indicate whether diagnosis was based on single or multiple stereotactic biopsy samples. Also not universally stated is whether results were based on frozen section alone, cytologic techniques alone, or some combination of these with or without the results of permanent sections included.

Colbassani et al. (9) note that two or more stereotactic biopsies were required to obtain an intraoperative diagnosis in 39% of their cases, using frozen sections only. A single specimen was diagnostic in only 67% of their cases. On the other hand, Silverman et al. (37), using smear techniques in the diagnosis of CNS biopsies, reported a sensitivity of 90.7%, a specificity of 100%, a positive predictive value of 100%, and efficacy of the test of 91%, with 34 cases yielding a false-negative result in three cases. In a separate

Table 6.1.
Indications for Stereotactic Neurosurgical Biopsy, Past and Present[a]

Surgery for psychiatric disorders
Surgery for parkinsonism
Surgery for pain syndromes (e.g., hypophysectomy)
Local delivery of chemotherapeutic agents
Local delivery of radiation therapy
Depth electrodes for diagnosis and localization of epileptic foci
Third ventriculostomy
Tissue grafts to brain
Procedures related to neoplasia/mass lesions
Diagnosis of histologic type and grade (e.g., for planning of definitive therapy)
Verification of resection margins
Diagnosis of tumor recurrence versus radionecrosis
Biopsy and/or treatment of cystic lesions
Biopsy of deep and/or small lesions where open biopsy either is contraindicated (e.g., certain intrinsic brain stem lesions) or is associated with greater operative risk (e.g., motor cortex)
Evacuation of intratumoral hematoma
Biopsy of focal lesions of uncertain nature
Neoplasia versus inflammatory versus vascular versus demyelinating disease (e.g., biopsy of cerebral mass not responding to anti-toxoplasmosis therapy in AIDS patient, to rule out primary CNS lymphoma)
Verification of clinically suspected herpes simplex encephalitis prior to treatment
Diagnosis of diffuse lesions of uncertain etiology when other tests are negative (e.g., Canavan's disease; Alexander's disease; certain pre-senile dementias)

[a] Sources: Chandrasoma and Apuzzo (6), Gildenberg (15), Hirschfeld (20).

Table 6.2.
Potential Problems/Contraindications Regarding Stereotactic Biopsy[a]

Potential problems
Less control of hemorrhage than with open biopsy
Potential for cerebral edema
Small sample size and associated increased chance for non-representative sample
Needle may displace, rather than penetrate, a firm lesion.
Increased risk of hemorrhage in patients with significant cerebral atrophy
Implantation of tumor along biopsy needle path (32)
Potential contraindications
Superficially situated lesion in which an immediate attempt at total or subtotal removal is likely to follow biopsy
Poorly controlled systemic and/or intracranial hypertension
Poorly controlled coagulopathies
Suspected vascular lesions
Diagnosis has already been established by other means
Patient is so ill no treatment is justified

[a] Sources: Chandrasoma and Apuzzo (6), Hirschfeld (20).

study of fine-needle aspiration (FNA) results in a pediatric population, Silverman et al. (35) also reported a sensitivity of 90.6%, a specificity of 100%, a positive predictive value of 100%, a negative predictive value of 94.7%, and efficiency of the test 96.5% (in a total of 135 biopsies from varying sites in 123 children). More relevant to our area of concern, however, is that their sensitivity of FNA biopsies in CNS sites alone was only 57.1% and that of four false-negative diagnoses in the entire study, three involved FNA biopsies of the CNS (in a total of eight CNS cases). Ferracini et al. (11) reported an accuracy rate of 89% in stereotactic biopsies in cerebral tumors, and Adams et al. (2) an accuracy rate of 93.6%, using only smear techniques.

Guarda (17) has compared intraoperative cytology and frozen-section methods in a variety of tissues, including neurosurgical specimens, indicating an error rate for the two methods of 1.6 and 0.8%, respectively, but also indicating this difference was largely a consequence of inexperience with cytologic methods at the outset of the study. He mentions a preference for cytologic methods over frozen-section techniques for brain specimens by the end of his study.

Less information is available concerning the accuracy of FNA in orbital tumors (see Tumors of the Eye and Orbit in Chapter 7), although some studies report accuracy rates exceeding 90%. Krohel et al. (27) studied 34 cases by simultaneous FNA (performed under direct visualization of the mass) and conventional open biopsy. They reported an accuracy rate for FNA alone of only 47% (i.e., good cytologic-histopathologic correlation in 16 cases; an inaccurate or misleading cytologic diagnoses in seven cases; and nondiagnostic FNA material in 11 cases, the latter consisting of nonspecific fibrosis or blood, or no tissue). Glasgow and Layfield (15a) have recently reported a more favorable experience with FNA of orbital and periorbital masses, achieving a specific diagnosis in 13 of 18 cases (72%).

In summary, it is our belief that the potential for misinterpretation of CNS and orbital intraoperative biopsy material remains substantial, certainly for some entities more than others, even with the combined advantages of frozen-section and cytologic methods. Such factors as sampling error, inexperience of the examiner, overlapping morphologic features seen in several types of primary and secondary CNS neoplasms and in non-neoplastic lesions, the varying degree of glial and/or inflammatory reaction seen around certain neoplastic and non-neoplastic lesions, varying degrees of lesion heterogeneity, varying host response capabilities, the spectrum of paraneoplastic syndromes that occur in neural tissues, and effects of therapy can, alone or in combination, make accurate diagnoses difficult or impossible under certain circumstances. In some lesions it will be found that the diagnosis is more dependent on architectural (i.e., frozen section) features, and in others on cytologic (i.e., smear/imprint) features.

These issues are dealt with further in the sections on the specific entities to which they may apply, as well as in the chapter on pitfalls (Chapter 9) and the chapter on future trends (Chapter 10).

Techniques

The method of making cytologic preparations will vary with the nature of the biopsy, tissue consistency, and examiner preference (Fig. 6.1). Flushing the biopsy needle into a container (e.g., with physiological saline, fixative, etc.) after the tissue sample is removed can potentially increase the yield for cytologic studies by means of smears, cytocentrifuge, membrane filter preparations, or cell block methods. The choice of methods and stains also depends on the amount of tissue retrieved and the clinical differential diagnosis. Material to be utilized for smear techniques may be incised by scalpel from a portion of each tissue fragment received and placed on one or more slides (Fig. 6.2). Making touch preparations (imprints), rolling the specimen on a slide, or scraping the surface of the specimen by scalpel and then transferring the retrieved material from the scalpel to the glass slide (Fig. 6.2**A**) are all methods applicable to more fibrous tissue that does not smear well. With sparse samples of tissues that smear poorly, however, we tend to apply such techniques sparingly to minimize mechanical trauma to the fragment(s), and expect that the frozen section will usually provide the greater diagnostic yield in such circumstances. In specimens of softer consistency and/or with a more discohesive cell population suitable

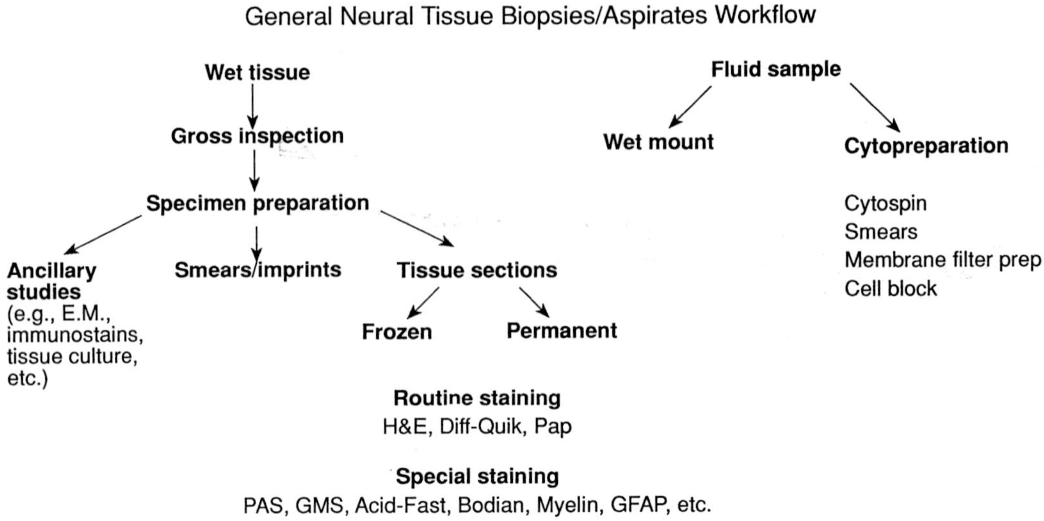

Figure 6.1. General neural tissue biopsies/aspirates workflow.

for smears, the smear may be made by a variety of means. These include combined crush (squash) preparations produced by pressing the specimen between two slides (Fig. 6.2**B**), generally followed by a pull-apart technique (Fig. 6.2**C**) to distribute the tissue over a larger surface area of each slide. Applying a mild pressure gradient during the pull-apart will provide both thicker and thinner areas of the smear for study (Fig. 6.2**D**). With very limited material, we immediately fix most smears by immersion in alcohol to minimize air drying artifacts, and select one or two slides for prompt hematoxylin and eosin staining to determine the presence or absence of diagnostic material in the biopsy and/or provide an immediate diagnosis (see Appendix). Figure 6.3 reveals the amount of material that is examined with smear techniques in comparison to a paraffin section. Figure 6.4 illustrates smear patterns commonly observed with various brain tumors.

We also prepare one or two air-dried smears for Diff-Quik staining (see Appendix) in the event an unexpected lymphoproliferative lesion is encountered. The extra smears can also be subsequently utilized for selected special stains. We prefer to do marker studies on frozen or paraffin-embedded material, however, to exploit the serial slide-to-slide consistency of tissue sampling that is so helpful in the interpretation of a panel of immunostains. Preparing additional air-dried sections and cutting additional unstained permanent sections for possible later special study are also options for conserving tissue, as described by Scheithauer (34). It is important to screen the entire smear at low power prior to the selection of fields for scrutiny at higher magnification.

Immediate decisions the pathologist must make include determining whether the material received is adequate for diagnostic purposes and is sufficient in amount for anticipated ancillary studies that may be required for a diagnosis precise enough to allow the necessary therapeutic decisions; whether the process is non-neoplastic or neoplastic; and, if neoplastic, whether it is benign or malignant, primary or secondary, and of a histologic type prone to vague infiltrating margins or narrow, well-demarcated margins.

Specimens obtained from non-neoplastic neurologic disorders usually are either the result of diagnostic uncertainty (see Chapter

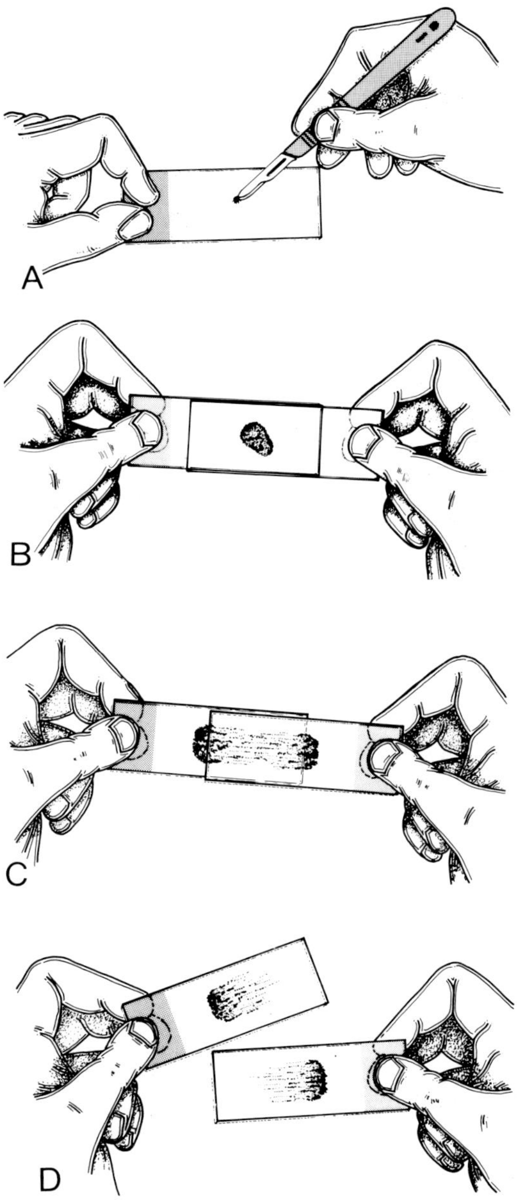

Figure 6.2. A–D, Smear (squash and pull apart) preparatory method for brain tissue.

8) or are taken as elective procedures for diagnostic or special study purposes. The protocol for specimen handling will vary with the clinical differential diagnosis and planned procedures, and requires careful preoperative coordination with all investigative team members to optimize the information obtainable from the specimen.

Needle aspirates of liquid cyst contents are processed in a manner similar to those utilized for CSF (see Chapters 3 and 4), with the exception that a wet mount is examined immediately to determine the presence or absence of cholesterol crystals and parakeratotic or anucleate squamous cells (e.g., seen in cysts within craniopharyngiomas, epidermoid and dermoid cysts, teratomas with a squamous cystic component), cholesterol crystals alone (e.g., any of the above plus colloid cysts, xanthogranulomas of the choroid plexus), parasites, or other abnormalities that may provide a preview of diagnostic possibilities.

Diagnostic neurosurgical material suitable for both cytologic and histologic study may also be obtained by means of the Cavitron ultrasonic surgical aspirator, despite the mechanical forces to which the tissue is subjected by this procedure; such aspirates should not be discarded on the assumption that the tissue is too pulverized to be useful (13, 28, 36).

Artifacts

In addition to the usual artifacts that may be encountered in smears and aspirates, which include many of the elements outlined as artifacts in CSF preparations (see Table 3.7), any of the soft tissue or neural elements encountered en route to the target tissue may be found in the specimen (see Chapter 2).

We also concur with Chandrasoma and Apuzzo (6) that it is important not to confuse slide contamination by bone dust from the skull drill hole with true calcification intrinsic to the biopsied tissue. This error should be avoidable by insisting that a characteristic tissue reaction or cellular whorl surrounds the calcification for it to be interpreted as intrinsic (see Table 7.8 for lesions associated with CNS calcification).

Although not an artifact in the usual sense, diagnostic problems may occur when biopsies are obtained from tissue sites previously sampled by FNA (37a), reemphasizing the need for close communication between diagnostic and therapeutic team members.

Summary

Major advantages of frozen-section material are familiarity to the pathologist, and superiority to cytologic methods in evaluating tissue architecture and cellularity. Disadvantages include relatively poor cytologic detail and introduction of freezing artifacts (neither of which are completely reversed by post-fixation of frozen tissue, and which can also compromise subsequent ultrastructural or routine histological study). Further, the inevitable loss of tissue from the facing of the specimen block in the cryostat, and increasing difficulty of interpretation (as well as decreasing relevance of the advantages listed above) as the specimen diminishes in size, are to be considered.

Cytologic techniques provide superior cytologic detail (sufficient in many cases for diagnosis without ancillary techniques) and provide the advantage of tissue conservation. The latter is especially important for very small stereotactic biopsy specimens in which one may wish to prioritize a potential list of ancillary technique applications (e.g., pituitary adenomas). Further, cytologic methods may allow a confident diagnostic impression to be salvaged from a specimen that would, by frozen section alone, be nondiagnostic (26) and may provide a three-dimensional image of certain tissue structures that can be useful (e.g., glomeruloid vascular proliferations, meningothelial whorls).

It follows that, assuming tissue is adequate in amount, we recommend both frozen-section and cytologic methods be used simultaneously. The additional time required for both methods to be used is insignificant, and the combined advantages of both can be helpful in formulating a diagnostic impression. In addition, experience so gained is invaluable when a subsequent specimen from another patient is very small, and cytologic methods may be the only sensible initial approach. We, in agreement with other workers (17, 26) see these methods (i.e., frozen section and cytologic) not as being in competition with one another but rather as complementary of one another in the overall efforts of the pathologist to achieve the maximum possible accuracy, particularly when confronted with the smaller samples now being received in the intraoperative consultation setting with increasing frequency. Kim et al. (26), in examining a variety of tissues, clearly demonstrate a significant reduction in both false-negative and false-positive diagnoses when using these methods in combination, compared to the use of either frozen-section or cytologic methods alone.

References

1. Abernathy, C.D., Camacho, A., and Kelly, P.J. Stereotaxic suboccipital transcerebellar biopsy of pontine mass lesions. J. Neurosurg. 70:195–200, 1989.
2. Adams, J.H., Graham, D.I., and Doyle, D. Brain Biopsy. The Smear Technique for Neurosurgical Biopsies. J.B. Lippincott Co., Philadelphia, 1981.
3. Berger, M.S. Ultrasound-guided stereotaxic biopsy using a new apparatus. J. Neurosurg. 65:550–554, 1986.
4. Bullard, D.E., and Makachinas, T.T. Measurement of tissue impedance in conjunction with computed tomography-guided stereotaxic biopsies. J. Neurol. Neurosurg. Psychiatry 50:43–51, 1987.
4a. Cappabianca, P., Spaziante, R., Caputi, F., Pettinato, G., Del Basso De Caro, M., Carrabs, G., and de Divitiis, E. Accuracy of the analysis of multiple small fragments of glial tumors obtained by stereotactic biopsy. Acta Cytol. 35:505–511, 1991.
5. Carapella, C.M., Mastrostefano, R., Raus, L., and

Riccio, A. Methodology of stereotactic biopsy. J. Neurol. Sci. 33:5–10, 1989.

6. Chandrasoma, P.T., and Apuzzo, M.L.J. Stereotactic Brain Biopsy. Igaku-Shoin, New York, 1989.
7. Chandrasoma, P.T., Smith, M.M., and Apuzzo, M.L.J. Stereotactic biopsy in the diagnosis of brain masses: comparison of results of biopsy and resected surgical specimen. Neurosurgery 24: 160–165, 1989.
8. Choksey, M.S., Valentine, A., Shawdon, H., Freer, C.E.L., and Lindsay, K.W. Computed tomography in the diagnosis of malignant brain tumours: do all patients require biopsy? J. Neurol. Neurosurg. Psychiatry 52:821–825, 1989.
9. Colbassani, H.J., Nishio, S., Sweeney, K.M., Bakay, R.A.E., and Takei, Y. CT-assisted stereotactic brain biopsy: value of intraoperative frozen section diagnosis. J. Neurol. Neurosurg. Psychiatry 51:332–341, 1988.
10. Daumas-Duport, C., Scheithauer, B.W., and Kelly, P.J. A histologic and cytologic method for the spatial definition of gliomas. Mayo Clin. Proc. 62:435–449, 1987.
11. Ferracini, R., Poletti, V., Manetto, V., Frank-Ricci, R., and Del Borrello, E. Smear biopsy for on-the-spot diagnosis in stereotactic surgery of CNS tumors. Experience of 101 cases. Ital. J. Neurol. Sci. 8:347–349, 1987.
12. Finizio, F.S., Frank, F., Ricci, R., and Ruggiero, G. Contribution of stereotactic techniques to the diagnosis and treatment of cerebral tumors in childhood. J. Neuroradiol. 15:353–371, 1988.
13. Finley, J.L., Silverman, J.F., and Dickens, M.A. Immunocytochemical evaluation of central nervous system tumors obtained by the Cavitron ultrasonic surgical aspirator. Diagn. Cytopathol. 6:308–312, 1990.
14. Friedman, W.A., Sceats, D.J., Nestok, B.R., and Ballinger, W.E. Jr. The incidence of unexpected pathological findings in an image-guided biopsy series: a review of 100 consecutive cases. Neurosurgery 25:180–184, 1989.
15. Gildenberg, P.L. The article reviewed. Oncology 3:37–40, 1989.
15a. Glasgow, B.J., and Layfield, L.J. Fine-needle aspiration biopsy of orbital and periorbital masses. Diagn. Cytopathol. 7:132–141, 1991.
16. Greene, G.M., Hitchon, P.W., Schelper, R.L., Yuh, W., and Dyste, G.N. Diagnostic yield in CT-guided stereotactic biopsy of gliomas. J. Neurosurg. 71:494–497, 1989.
17. Guarda, L.A. Intraoperative cytologic diagnosis. Evaluation of 370 consecutive intraoperative cytologies. Diagn. Cytol. 6:235–242, 1990.
18. Guthrie, B.L., Steinberg, G.K., and Adler, J.K. Posterior fossa stereotaxic biopsy using the Brown-Roberts-Wells stereotaxic system. J. Neurosurg. 70:649–652, 1989.
19. Hashimoto, N., and Kikuchi, H. Transsphenoidal approach to infrasellar tumors involving the cavernous sinus. J. Neurosurg. 73:513–517, 1990.
20. Hirschfeld, A. Stereotactic techniques in the management of cerebral neoplasms. Oncology 3:25–32, 1989.
21. Hood, T.W., Gebarski, S.S., McKeever, P.E., and Venes, J.L. Stereotaxic biopsy of intrinsic lesions of the brain stem. J. Neurosurg. 65:172–176, 1986.
22. Howanitz, P.J., Hoffman, G.G., and Zarbo, R.J. The accuracy of frozen-section diagnoses in 34 hospitals. Arch. Pathol. Lab. Med. 114:355–359, 1990.
23. Jenny, A.B., Biondetti, P.R., Layton, B., and Knapp, R.H. The computer and stereotactic surgery in neurological surgery. Comput. Med. Imaging and Graphics. 12:75–83, 1988.
24. Kelly, P.J., Daumas-Duport, C., Kispert, D.B., Kall, B.A., Scheithauer, B.W., and Illig, J.J. Imaging-based stereotaxic serial biopsies in untreated intracranial glial neoplasms. J. Neurosurg. 66:865–874, 1987.
25. Kelly, P.J., Daumas-Duport, C., Scheithauer, B.W., Kall, B.A., and Kispert, D.B. Stereotaxic histologic correlations of computed tomography—and magnetic resonance imaging—defined abnormalities in patients with glial neoplasms. Mayo Clin. Proc. 62:450–459, 1987.
26. Kim, K., Phillips, E.R., and Paolino, M. Intraoperative imprint cytology: its significance as a diagnostic adjunct. Diagn. Cytopathol. 6:304–307, 1990.
26a. Kontozoglou, T.E., and Cramer, H.M. The advantages of intraoperative cytology. Analysis of 215 smears and review of the literature. Acta Cytol. 35:154–164, 1991.
27. Krohel, G.B., Tobin, D.R., and Chavis, R.M. Inaccuracy of fine needle aspiration biopsy. Ophthalmology 92:666–670, 1985.
27a. Mair, S., Lash, R.H., Suskin, D., and Mendelsohn, G. Intraoperative surgical specimen evaluation: frozen section analysis, cytologic examination, or both? A comparative study of 206 cases. Am. J. Clin. Pathol. 96:8–14, 1991.
28. Malhotra, V., Malik, R., Gondal, R., Beohar, P.C., and Parkash, B. Evaluation of histological appearance of tissues removed by Cavitron ultrasonic surgical aspirator (CUSA). Acta Neurochir. (Wien) 81:132–134, 1986.
29. Mathisen, J.R., Giunta, F., Marini, G., and Backlund, E.O. Transcerebellar biopsy in the posterior fossa: 12 years experience. Surg. Neurol. 28: 100–104, 1987.
30. Mennel, H.D., Rossberg, C., Lorenz, H., Schneider, H., and Hellwig, D. Reliability of simple cytological methods in brain tumour biopsy diagnosis. Neurochirurgia 32:129–134, 1989.
31. Mouriquand, C., Benabid, A.L., and Breyton, M.

Stereotaxic cytology of brain tumors. Review of an eight-year experience. Acta Cytol. 31:756–764, 1987.
32. Rosenfeld, J.V., Murphy, M.A., and Chow, C.W. Implantation metastases of pineoblastoma after stereotactic biopsy. Case report. J. Neurosurg. 73:287–290, 1990.
33. Sahni, K.S., Ghatak, N.R., Gulati, A.N., Leshner, R.T., Alberico, A., and Young, H.F. CT-guided stereotactic biopsies of lesions in the medulla and a case of Leigh's disease. Appl. Neurophysiol. 50:203–209, 1987.
34. Scheithauer, B.W. Central nervous system and pituitary. Chapter 8 in: Silva, E.G., and Kraemer, B.B. (Eds.): Intraoperative Pathologic Diagnosis. Frozen Section and Other Techniques. Williams & Wilkins, Baltimore, 1987, pp. 167–219.
34a. Sidawy, M.K., and Silverberg, S.G. Intraoperative cytology. Back to the future? Am. J. Clin. Pathol. 96:1–3, 1991.
35. Silverman, J.F., Gurley, A.M., Holbrook, C.T., and Joshi, V.V. Pediatric fine-needle aspiration biopsy. Am. J. Clin. Pathol. 95:653–659, 1991.
36. Silverman, J.F., Jones, F.D., Unverferth, M., and Berns, L. Cytopathology of neoplasms of the central nervous system in specimens obtained by the Cavitron ultrasonic surgical aspirator. Acta Cytol. 33:576–582, 1989.
37. Silverman, J.F., Timmons, R.L., Leonard, J.R. III, Hardy, I.M., Harris, L.S., O'Brien, K., and Norris, H.T. Cytologic results of fine-needle aspiration biopsies of the central nervous system. Cancer 58:1117–1121, 1986.
37a. Tabbara, S.O., Frierson, H.F. Jr., and Fechner, R.E. Diagnostic problems in tissues previously sampled by fine-needle aspiration. Am. J. Clin. Pathol. 96:76–80, 1991.
37b. Taratuto, A.L., Sevlever, G., and Piccardo, P. Clues and pitfalls in stereotactic biopsy of the central nervous system. Arch. Pathol. Lab. Med. 115:596–602, 1991.
38. Thomas, D.G.T., Dairs, C.H., Ingram, S., Olney, J.S., Bydder, G.M., and Young, I.R. Stereotaxic biopsy of the brain under MR imaging control. Am. J. Neuroradiol. 7:161–163, 1986.
39. Uematsu, S., Erozan, Y.S., Gupta, P.K., Kumar, A.A.J., McArthur, J., and Rosenbaum, A.E. Intraoperative CT-guided serial microbiopsy of brain lesions and concomitant use of CT air and angiographic studies. Stereotactic Funct. Neurosurg. 52:250–261, 1989.
40. Wilden, J.N., and Kelly, P.J. CT computerized stereotactic biopsy for low density CT lesions presenting with epilepsy. J. Neurol. Neurosurg. Psychiatry 50:1302–1305, 1987.
41. Willems, J.G.M.S., and Alva-Willems, J.M. Accuracy of cytologic diagnosis of central nervous system neoplasms in stereotactic biopsies. Acta Cytol. 28:243–249, 1984.
42. Young, R.F. Application of robotics to stereotactic neurosurgery. Neurol. Res. 9:123–128, 1987.

7 / Neoplasia and Related Disorders

The goals of this chapter are to briefly review the cytohistologic features of well-defined neural neoplasms and to summarize morphologic observations based on wet tissue smears, imprint methods, aspirates, and/or the appearance of exfoliated cells in the CSF for tumors to which such methods have been applied. Selected morphologic and behavioral features of tumors that may be useful from the standpoint of differential diagnosis (e.g., tumors containing melanin, patterns of spread of primary neural tumors, etc.) are tabulated.

Theories of oncogenesis; incidence statistics; age and topographic distribution; and immunohistochemical, ultrastructural, and other specialized features of such tumors not directly related to cytohistologic observations by routine methods are not within the scope of this review, but are widely available in standard references. The recently published text by the late Drs. Russell and Rubinstein is, in our opinion, unsurpassed in the field of neuro-oncology and has been an important source of much of the information included in this chapter (194). The text by Burger et al. (26) deserves the wide use it enjoys among surgical pathologists as a current and practical guide to both neoplastic and non-neoplastic disorders of the nervous system. We also have found the monograph by Franks (57) to be useful for the number and quality of its color illustrations of CNS tumors, which encompass not only routine histologic preparations but also frozen section and smear preparations. The monographs on CNS cytopathology by Rosenthal (188) and by Bigner and Johnston (14), in particular, are among those we regard as essential to those interested in enhancing their skills in this area.

Fundamentals that apply to cytology in general should be kept in mind when reviewing published material in neuropathological disorders. Cells from the same lesion will differ in appearance depending on whether they are examined using imprint techniques, smear or crush preparations, or aspiration techniques, which subject cells to more or less mechanical force. Smears may emphasize tumor components that tend to be either unapparent or less prominent in routine histologic descriptions of certain tumor types (e.g., fibrillary processes in hemangioblastomas). The presence or absence of spontaneously exfoliated cells within CSF undoubtedly depends on a variety of factors (e.g., whether the neoplastic cells are sequestered in neural parenchyma or have broached anatomic barriers to gain access to the subarachnoid space; whether or not the tumor cells are cohesive and are able to survive and/or proliferate within the CSF environment). As with exfoliated cells in other body fluids, surface tension forces will often result in a round configuration of the cell, with obscuration of previously apparent cytoplasmic processes or other more characteristic native cell shapes. Spinal fluid also represents a hostile environment for many cell types, leading to degenerative changes that tend to blur distinctions between normal, reactive, and neoplastic cells. Such changes include, but are not limited to, alterations in nuclear and cytoplasmic volume and chromatin appearance, and the presence of bare nuclei. These issues and potential diagnostic pitfalls have been discussed in detail elsewhere (60). We favor an approach that is based on a thorough foundation in differential diagnostic possibilities given the clinical setting and morphologic appearance, comparison of sections from previous tumors in the same patient whenever possible, and application of

Table 7.1.
Neoplasia and Related Disorders

I Tumors of Neuroglial Cells
  A. Diffuse astrocytomas
    1. Astrocytoma
      a. Fibrillary
      b. Protoplasmic
      c. Gemistocytic
      d. Giant cell
    2. Anaplastic astrocytoma
    3. Glioblastoma multiforme
  B. Special variants of astrocytomas
    1. Protoplasmic astrocytoma
    2. Pilocytic astrocytoma
    3. Astroblastoma
    4. Polar spongioblastoma
    5. Pleomorphic xanthoastrocytoma
    6. Gliomatosis cerebri
    7. Mixed gliomas
  C. Oligodendroglial tumors
    1. Oligodendroglioma
    2. Anaplastic (malignant) oligodendroglioma
  D. Ependymal tumors
    1. Ependymoma
    2. Myxopapillary ependymoma
    3. Tanycytic ependymoma
    4. Subependymoma
    5. Anaplastic (malignant) ependymoma
  E. Glial heterotopias and ectopic tumors
II Tumors of Neuronal Cells
  A. Primitive neuronal and/or glial precursor cell tumors (embryonal neoplasms, primitive neuroectodermal tumors [PNETs])
    1. Medulloblastoma
    2. Central neuroblastoma
    3. Ependymoblastoma
    4. Medulloepithelioma
    5. Neurocytoma
  B. Neuronal tumors with more mature ganglion cell components
    1. Gangliocytoma/ganglioglioma
    2. Uncommon variants
      a. Desmoplastic infantile gangliocytoma
      b. Intrasellar endocrinologically active gangliocytoma
      c. Dysplastic gangliocytoma of the cerebellum (Lhermitte-Duclos disease)
      d. Hypothalamic neuronal hamartoma
    3. Neuronal ectopias and ectopic tumors
III Meningiomas and Other Tumors of Meningeal Origin
  A. Common histologic types of meningioma
    1. Meningotheliomatous
    2. Fibrous
    3. Transitional
  B. Uncommon variants of meningioma
    1. Microcystic (humid) meningioma
    2. Myxomatous (myxoid) meningioma
    3. Xanthomatous meningioma
    4. Lipoblastic (lipomatous) meningioma
    5. Granular meningioma
    6. Secretory meningioma
    7. Papillary meningioma
    8. Other (chordoid, etc.)
  C. Malignant meningiomas
  D. Angiomatous and angioblastic meningiomas, and dural hemangiopericytomas
  E. Ectopic meningiomas
  F. Miscellaneous meningeal tumors
    1. Primary meningeal melanoma
    2. Other meningeal tumors
IV Hemangioblastoma and Other Primary Neuraxis Tumors with a Prominent Vascular Component
  A. Hemangioblastoma (capillary hemangioblastoma)
  B. Other primary neuraxis tumors with a prominent vascular component
V Craniopharyngioma
VI Choroid plexus tumors
  A. Xanthogranuloma
  B. Papilloma
  C. Carcinoma
VII Pineal body tumors
  A. Pineoblastoma
  B. Pineocytoma
VIII Germ Cell Tumors
  A. Germinoma
  B. Embryonal carcinoma
  C. Endodermal sinus tumor (yolk sac tumor)
  D. Choriocarcinoma
  E. Teratoma
  F. Mixed germ cell tumor
IX Lipoma
X Pituitary Tumors
  A. Pituitary adenoma
  B. Tumors of the neurohypophysis
    1. Astrocytoma
    2. Granular cell tumor
  C. Other sellar area mass lesions
XI Peripheral Nervous System Tumors
  A. Tumors of the nerve sheath elements
    1. Schwannoma
    2. Neurofibroma
    3. Malignant peripheral nerve sheath tumor
    4. Other primary peripheral nerve sheath tumors
  B. Tumors of peripheral neuronal and neuroendocrine elements

Table 7.1.—*Continued*

1. Peripheral neuroblastoma
2. Peripheral neuroepithelioma
3. Ganglioneuroblastoma and ganglioneuroma
4. Pheochromocytoma and paraganglioma
5. Carcinoid tumor

XII Neuroectodermal Dysplasias (phakomatoses, neurocutaneous syndromes)

XIII Cytologic Components of Benign Cystic Lesions of the CNS

XIV Patterns of Spread of Primary CNS and PNS Tumors

XV Secondary Tumors of the Nervous System

XVI Lymphoma, Leukemia and Related Disorders
- A. Primary cerebral lymphomas
- B. Secondary non-Hodgkin's lymphoma of the nervous system
- C. Hodgkin's disease
- D. Multiple myeloma and related disorders
- E. Histiocytosis X
- F. Leukemia
- G. The problem of blast-like cells in the CSF

XVII Tumors of the Eye and Orbit
- A. Nevi and melanomas
- B. Retinoblastoma
- C. Ocular medulloepithelioma (dictyoma)
- D. Glial and other miscellaneous tumors

XVIII Radiation and/or Chemotherapeutic Effects on CNS Tumors and Adjacent Tissues
- A. Effects on neural tumors
- B. Effects on adjacent neural tissues

XIX Paraneoplastic Syndromes (Remote effects of cancer on the nervous system)

ancillary methods in case of doubt concerning non-neoplastic versus neoplastic, or specific type of neoplasm. Enthusiasm concerning the advantages provided by cytologic methods as applied to neuropathology, particularly during this era of its expanding use, should be balanced by a respect for the number of neuropathological problems that morphology alone, no matter how elegant or esthetically pleasing the preparation, simply cannot solve. Morphologic approaches, nonetheless, play a key role in directing and prioritizing the ancillary studies that may be required to precisely define a given tumor type within the limits of currently available knowledge.

The topics reviewed in this chapter are outlined in Table 7.1. In the sections on tumor cytology, references following the heading "Cytology" include illustrations of the tumor category under discussion.

Tumors of Neuroglial Cells

Diffuse Astrocytoma

Discussion of the cytologic appearance of astrocytomas requires a background in classification schemes. A classification currently in common use separates astrocytomas into diffuse types (based on a tendency for infiltration of neoplastic cells well beyond the grossly evident limits of the neoplasm) and special types that, on the basis of morphology or tendency toward a less infiltrative (i.e., better demarcated) interface with adjacent normal neural tissue and/or more favorable biologic behavior, warrant separation from the other group (26). A three-tiered grading system (27, 148) (see Table 7.2) has now replaced the four-tiered system of Kernohan in our institution and many others. It applies to the diffuse astrocytomas but is not applicable to the special types of astrocytomas or other pure or mixed glial neoplasms (e.g., oligodendrogliomas, ependymomas, gangliogliomas) with comparable prognostic accuracy. For example, the presence of prominent cellularity, pleomorphism, and a certain pattern of necrosis in a diffuse astrocytoma is virtually synonymous with gliobiastoma multiforme and implies a uniformly poor prognosis. However, it is not unusual for the same findings in an oligodendroglioma or a ganglioglioma to correlate poorly with survival

Table 7.2.
Grading of Diffuse Astrocytomas

Astrocytoma	
	Mildly increased cellularity
	Mild pleomorphism and cytologic atypia
	Few or no mitotic figures
Anaplastic Astrocytoma	
	Moderate to marked cellularity
	Moderate to marked pleomorphism and atypia with or without giant cells
	Mitoses not unusual and may be prominent
	Vascular endothelial proliferation may be present
	No necrosis
Glioblastoma Multiforme	
	Features of anaplastic astrocytoma plus:
	One or more foci of necrosis, with or without pseudopalisading or "serpiginous" outline
	High cellularity
	Mitoses often, but not invariably, prominent
	Vascular and endothelial proliferation commonly prominent

statistics. Clearly, for some tumor types morphologic features alone—such as cellularity, necrosis, or the presence of bizarre cells—may provide limited insight to future clinical behavior. Serial biopsy studies of recurrent tumors may also demonstrate progressively increasing anaplasia and/or conversion to another dominant cell line. Finally, heterogeneity of tumor grade (and dominant cell type), while not exclusive to gliomas, is a common feature (25, 173). Since the highest tumor grade determines both prognosis and treatment decisions, and sampling by small-biopsy methods may yield a falsely lower grade (or even miss tumor if the mass is deep and/or small or if the interface between tumor and non-neoplastic tissue is abrupt), treatment decisions in such circumstances should appropriately include consideration of clinical and radiologic, as well as pathologic, information.

Astrocytoma

Diffuse astrocytomas contain one, and often more than one, of the following cell types:

1. *Fibrillary astrocytoma.* The nuclei closely resemble those of normal astrocytes, with only a moderate increase in size, angularity, and/or pleomorphism (Fig. 7.1**A** and **B**). They tend to be unevenly dispersed in the neuropil. Cell bodies may vary considerably in size and shape, and the cytoplasm is usually less conspicuous in neoplastic than in the often associated reactive astrocytes. The background is an exaggerated fine fibrillary one compared with normal neuropil, and mitoses are rarely seen. Perivascular pseudorosettes are often present. Rare perivascular cuffs of small lymphocytes may occur but are seldom prominent. Microcysts are frequent but may be difficult to appreciate on frozen sections and smears. Calcifications may be present, especially in relation to capillary walls. Infiltration of pre-existing white matter tracts may impart a bipolar (pilocytic) appearance to cells, which should not be confused with the adult and juvenile types of pilocytic astrocytomas described under special variants below.
2. *Protoplasmic astrocytoma.* Considered in the diffuse astrocytoma category when admixed with one or more other cell types (fibrillary, gemistocytic, or giant-cell), as is commonly the case, this tumor is considered a special variant when in pure form. The nuclei differ in no important respect from the other types of astrocytomas included in this category. However, the cytoplasmic features are characterized by a more stellate outline to the cell, sparse and often vacuolated cytoplasm, and a paucity of processes (i.e., sparse fibrillarity of the background). The cell distribution is often more uniform than in other forms of astrocytoma, although this is not constant. Microcystic change is common. Endothelial proliferation may occur without other evidence of malignancy, particularly in pure forms of protoplasmic astrocytoma, and does not connote malignant behavior in such circumstances.

3. *Gemistocytic astrocytoma.* This cell type is generally admixed with other astrocytoma cell types and only rarely occurs as a virtually pure population. The gemistocytic astrocytoma cell is a large cell, in the range of 25 μm diameter, with the parakaryon consisting of eosinophilic, homogeneous hyalin material (Fig. 7.1**C**). Glial filaments tend to aggregate preferentially just beneath the cell membrane (Fig. 7.1**D**). Short, coarse, fibrillary processes are present and nuclei are often eccentrically placed, with binucleation or multinucleation present. Coarse chromatin and a more prominent nucleolus are often present in this cell type, compared with other low-grade astrocytoma cell types. The neuropil background is often less tightly packed with fibrillar processes, but those present may be more coarse than in classical fibrillary astrocytomas. Perivascular pseudorosettes (referred to by some as perivascular radial collars, to distinguish them from the more orderly perivascular pseudorosette of ependymomas) are common, and there is a much higher percentage of conversion (about 80%) of pure forms of gemistocytic astrocytoma to glioblastoma. Perivascular lymphocytic infiltrates are more common in this variant than in other low-grade diffuse astrocytoma types.
4. *(Subependymal) giant cell astrocytoma.* Variably sized (but often large) fusiform or pyramidal cells are present, with prominent hyalin eosinophilic cytoplasm and short, stubby processes (Fig. 7.4**E**). Some cells resemble gemistocytic astrocytes (with eccentric nuclei, etc.). Others are more strap-shaped, reminiscent of strap cells in rhabdomyoblastoma but devoid of cross-striations. Yet others resemble ganglion cells, particularly with regard to nuclear features, but are of glial origin. Finally, some cells are bizarre in appearance and difficult to classify as neuronal or glial in type. Perivascular pseudorosettes are common. Vessels are usually thin-walled, and mitoses rare or absent. Nucleoli may be prominent, but chromatin coarseness and distribution are quite variable, often having bland characteristics. This tumor type is characteristically seen in the first and second decades in subependymal locations in patients with tuberous sclerosis. Similar cells may occur, however, in a background of glioblastoma multiforme. Thus, it is the cytologic company such cells keep, rather than the giant cells, to which one's attention should be directed for the proper classification of the giant cell-containing tumors.

   Giant cells of glial, neuronal, or uncertain lineage, reminiscent of those seen in the giant-cell astrocytoma group, may be seen in several situations. They may have single or multiple nuclei and can be difficult to categorize even with immunohistochemical and ultrastructural study. Conditions in which giant cells may form a prominent morphologic feature are summarized in Table 7.3.

While it is generally appreciated that astrocytomas frequently exhibit microcystic or grossly evident cystic change, perhaps less generally appreciated is the spectrum of other tumors and related conditions in which cysts may be prominent (Table 7.4).

Table 7.3.
Conditions in Which Prominent Giant Cells May Occur

Astrocytomas (e.g., pilocytic astrocytoma; subependymal giant cell astrocytoma; glioblastoma multiforme)
Capillary hemangioblastoma
Germ cell tumors
Gliosarcoma (and primary CNS sarcoma)
Malignant peripheral nerve sheath tumor
Medulloblastoma
Meningioma
Pheochromocytoma and extra-adrenal paraganglioma
Primary cerebral lymphoma
Post-radiation therapy

Table 7.4.
Neoplasms and Related Conditions in Which Cystic Change May Be Prominent

Astrocytoma (all types, including unusual variants such as pleomorphic xanthoastrocytoma, angioglioma, etc.)
Craniopharyngioma
Ganglion cell tumors and variants (including desmoplastic infantile ganglioglioma), both central and peripheral types
Hemangioblastoma
Meningioma
Neuroblastoma
Neurofibroma
Pineocytoma
Schwannoma
Teratoma
Ependymoma (particularly in spinal areas)
Vascular malformations
Oligodendroglioma

Cytology of Well-Differentiated, Diffuse Astrocytomas (1, 28, 39, 50, 57, 88, 119, 155, 164, 188) (Fig. 7.1A to D). In general, smears of well-differentiated fibrillary astrocytomas reveal mildly increased cellularity, mild pleomorphism, and a tendency for nuclei to appear "bare" on a finely fibrillar, neuropil-like background. The degree of fibrillary change in the background, as well as the prominence of the parakaryon cytoplasm, will vary with the astrocyte cell component included in the tumor, as described above. Some types exhibit long, fine fibrillary processes. Cell borders are indistinct, except for the gemistocytic and some giant-cell variants. There is generally minimal deviation in nuclear shape, contour, and chromatin content compared to normal astrocytes. The fibrillary background is typically more delicate in gliomas than in smooth muscle or fibroblastic spindle cell tumors. Adjectives used to describe the glial fibrils include "thready," "delicate," and "interlacing." In most examples in the literature, nuclear chromatin is fine and evenly distributed, and nucleoli are small or inconspicuous. Careful comparison with normal white or gray matter is often necessary to appreciate the mild degree of pleomorphism present. The latter should be distinguished from the smudging and distortion of nuclei that may be seen in any smear preparation, but particularly when excessive pressure has been applied. Most well-differentiated astrocytomas smear easily, although this is variable and more fibrillary forms may smear poorly. Smears often demonstrate a more prominent population of small, round nuclei slightly larger than lymphocytes, the source of which may include oligodendrocytes and/or protoplasmic astrocytes. The occurrence of large numbers of the latter nuclei would raise the question of a mixed oligo-astrocytoma (see below). The tendency of many astrocytomas to form perivascular pseudorosettes may, on smear preparations, be reflected in a pseudopapillary appearance due to the firm adherence of tumor cells to branching blood vessels. This appearance, so reminiscent of ependymomas, is well illustrated by Adams et al. (1). The smear appearance, as described in this chapter, is primarily based on H&E preparations. If Papanicolaou-stained smears are used, cytoplasmic components that are eosinophilic will almost invariably stain varying shades of blue-green, and cytoplasmic detail will often be less well appreciated. In our experience in CNS tissue samples other than lymphoproliferative disorders, Diff-Quik stained smears are far less helpful and are discussed primarily in the context of lymphomas and leukemias.

Gemistocytic astrocytomas tend to demonstrate a greater range of nuclear pleomorphism and more prominent paranucleolar eosinophilic cytoplasm from which profuse short, pointed extensions terminate in fine fibrillary processes within a distance, generally, of one to two cell diameters from the soma. Subependymal giant-cell astrocytomas, in the single example illustrated by Franks (57), smeared poorly, with cohesive aggregates of large, bizarre cells easily confused with a ganglioglioma or glioblastoma on smear; the example illustrated by Adams et al. (1) appears to have smeared easily, with individual cells well displayed.

Well-differentiated astrocytomas do not tend to exfoliate spontaneously into spinal fluid. Most examples of exfoliated cells in the literature consist either of aspirated cyst contents from cystic astrocytomas or of examinations of the spinal fluid in the immediate postoperative period, neither of which is comparable to other situations in which tumor cells spontaneously exfoliate into CSF. Examples we have seen were interpreted as tumor cells based on comparison with histologic sections and/or smears, with no additional descriptive features that would be helpful, and often with superimposed degenerative change. The cytoplasm of such cells is sometimes described as "wispy" or trailing off one aspect of the cell more than another, probably reflecting recent avulsion from the neuropil by the aspirating needle or as a consequence of the preceding surgical procedure.

Anaplastic Astrocytoma

This type of diffuse astrocytic tumor is defined by both architectural (i.e., more marked cellularity) and cytologic (i.e., more pronounced nuclear pleomorphism, hyperchromatism, coarseness and irregularity of chromatin, nucleolar prominence, etc.) features in varying combinations (see Table 7.2). One or more of the cell types described under astrocytoma, above, may be present, but necrosis must be absent (Fig. 7.1**E** and **F**).

Cytology of Diffuse Anaplastic Astrocytoma (1, 10, 14, 28, 39, 57, 164, 188) (Fig. 7.1E and F). Smears are more cellular, with the nuclear features described above. Mitoses, increased prominence of vascular structures, and endothelial proliferation may be seen (see Glioblastoma). Anaplastic astrocytomas with a prominent fibrillary background may, in smears, be virtually indistinguishable from some spindle-cell sarcomas that have relatively limited nuclear pleomorphism, particularly on Diff-Quik stains. Intimate admixture with neuropil in infiltrating margins of the tumor in astrocytomas, compared with the more abrupt interface between tumor and neuropil seen in sarcomas, may be a helpful distinguishing feature.

Glioblastoma Multiforme

This tumor, frequently referred to herein only by the term "glioblastoma," is defined by the features noted for anaplastic astrocytoma (Table 7.2), most of all of which are often in exaggerated form. In addition, there must be the superimposition of necrosis, required for the diagnosis (Fig. 7.2**A**). Since the necrosis may be sparsely distributed within the tumor it may or may not be present in small biopsies, giving a false impression of a lower-grade tumor. Mitoses vary in prominence even with cytologically poorly differentiated examples. To any of the cell types described above in the astrocytoma and anaplastic astrocytoma categories may be added small cells with hyperchromatic nuclei and sparse cytoplasm that are not, in isolation, clearly identifiable as astrocytic (and probably represent the more poorly differentiated component of the tumor); bizarre, giant single or multiple nucleated cell forms (Fig. 7.2**C**) that exceed the pleomorphism of most subependymal giant-cell astrocytomas; and a variety of intermediate forms. Oligodendroglial nuclei may be admixed to varying degrees. There also may be a considerable variation in cellular appearance in different portions of the tumor and an admixture of hemorrhagic changes, vascular and endothelial proliferation (Fig. 7.2**B**), and varying degrees of lymphoplasmacytic infiltrates and even acute inflammatory cell infiltrates, the latter more frequent in the vicinity of large areas of necrosis. With poorly differentiated examples, ancillary techniques (GFAP staining, etc.) may be necessary for definitive diagnosis. Rare variants can pose especially difficult diagnostic problems. These include tumors exhibiting prominent populations of granular cells (resembling granular cell tumors of Schwann cell origin); cells with extensive cytoplasmic vacuolization due to lipid globules; and tumor cells with epithelial appearance (Figs. 7.3**A** and **B**) arranged in solid cellular trabeculae, nests, or forming cribriform, pseudoacinar, and papillary structures. These epithelial features are particularly likely to be misinterpreted as metastatic carcinoma, and the latter impression may be enhanced—rather than contradicted—by immunohistochemical stains that can reveal keratin positivity in some of the epithelial-like cells (194). Glioblastomas are most frequently associated with a background of more clearly identifiable astrocytoma elements, but may arise from oligodendrogliomas.

Vascular and endothelial hyperplasia (Fig. 7.2**B**) is so characteristically present in glioblastomas, and is so frequently emphasized (with necrosis) as a component of the morphologic diagnosis, that it is useful to recall other situations in which this finding may appear. While this vascular change is most consistent and most well-developed in glioblastomas, it can be surprisingly prominent in some of the other tumors listed in Table 7.5. The plump endothelial cells in areas of vascular proliferation may occasionally demonstrate mitotic figures as well as bulbous cellular aggregates with convoluted or "glomeruloid" formations. The presence of this finding in ependymomas, oligodendrogliomas, and pilocytic astrocytomas does not correlate well with clinical behavior (i.e., does not necessarily imply malignant behavior).

Table 7.5.
Conditions in Which Vascular and Endothelial Hyperplasia May Be Prominently Demonstrated

Anaplastic (malignant) ependymoma
Astrocytoma (cerebellar pilocytic, astroblastoma, brain stem astrocytoma, protoplasmic astrocytoma, glioblastoma multiforme)
Medulloblastoma
Oligodendroglioma
Secondary carcinoma (renal cell carcinoma, oat cell carcinoma)
Primary and secondary sarcomas
Surrounding abscesses and infarctions (typically to mild degree)

Cytology of Glioblastoma Multiforme (1, 14, 39, 50, 57, 88, 104, 106, 119, 155, 164, 188) (Fig. 7.2C, D, E, and F; Fig. 7.3A and B). Given the remarkable degree of cytologic heterogeneity in anaplastic astrocytomas and glioblastomas, it is not surprising that descriptions of such tumors by smears, imprints, and exfoliative cytology techniques are also quite varied from case to case. Helpful features include pleomorphism and/or prominence of primitive-appearing anaplastic cells with nuclear features of malignancy including coarse, irregularly distributed chromatin and prominent nucleoli, as well as variation in nuclear size, shape, and regularity. Multinucleation can be seen in some tumors but is absent in others. Similarly, the amount of cytoplasm will vary depending on the dominant cell component. Necrosis, based on the presence of cell ghosts, basophilic nuclear fragments, and/or eosinophilic granular debris, is necessary for the diagnosis of glioblastoma but may prove difficult to distinguish from fibrin and/or other crushed neuropil components on smears, and should be confirmed in frozen or permanent sections if there is any doubt. Astrocytic fibrillary processes are often but not invariably prominent in the background. The degree of inflammatory cell infiltration in glioblastomas, as noted above, may be a diagnostic pitfall if the zone surrounding a large necrotic area is sampled in a small biopsy, since either chronic or acute inflammatory cells may dominate such zones. Neuroimaging studies may not be able to distinguish between necrotic tumor and brain abscess, and consultation with the surgeon to determine the feasibility of sampling tissue from areas of the non-necrotic periphery of the lesion is warranted to search for evidence of neoplasia.

The vascular and endothelial proliferation produces a fairly characteristic smear appearance, with thick-walled vessels containing large numbers of predominantly parallel-oriented endothelial cells, and often an impression of an excess number of nuclei present for the caliber of the vessel. Cohesive groups of endothelial-like spindle cells, resembling syncytial groups, may form irregular knots or outpouchings along the course of the vessel. These are not, however, associated with sheets of cells and individual cells in the immediate vicinity, the latter being more characteristic of an epithelial tumor.

We have seen two examples of the epithelioid variant of glioblastoma that provided diagnostic difficulty not only on frozen section but also on smears. Smears and aspirates tend to select the more discohesive epithelial cells in such variants, leaving the more typical fibrillary astrocytic stroma behind. This results in a very skewed population of epithelial-like cells on the smear, virtually to the exclusion of admixed tumor astrocytic components (Fig. 7.3**A** and **B**). An erroneous preliminary diagnosis of metastatic carcinoma may be rendered under such circumstances. We recommend that this variant be kept in mind in such cases and that the surgeon be advised that the differential diagnosis would include a primary glioma of this type, deferring to permanent sections to make the distinction with greater certainty. This may spare the patient an unnecessary search for occult extraneural primary tumor site. The differential diagnosis also includes the rare occurrence of metastasis to an existing primary glioma by a nonneural primary tumor (see Table 7.17).

Reports of the cytologic appearance of exfoliated cells from glioblastomas in cerebrospinal fluid vary from primitive forms indistinguishable from leukemia blasts to others that encompass much of the spectrum of cell types described above (Fig. 7.2**F**). Descriptive emphasis is on atypical nuclear features and prominent, variably staining cytoplasm that is more irregular than spherical in outline, and asymmetrically distributed.

Descriptions of tumor cell nucleoli range from unapparent to prominent. Neoplastic cells are often accompanied by inflammatory cells in both primary and secondary CNS malignancies. There is no consistency in available reports with regard to the prevalence of single cells versus cell clusters. Multinucleated forms have been described. General features emphasized as helpful in the distinction between glioblastoma and metastatic carcinoma cells include the greater tendency of cells from carcinoma to be encountered as tightly cohesive fragments or as solitary round cells with round rather than irregular or angular nuclei, and nucleoli that are often more prominent than those seen in many glioblastomas. The cell membrane is also generally better defined in epithelial than in glial cells. Morphology has proved far less reliable than a panel of markers in such situations (see Chapter 10).

Preferential aggregation of neoplastic cells in certain locations (e.g., subpial, subependymal, perivascular, and/or perineuronal) may occur in gliomas of various types (Fig. 7.3**C**, **D**, **E**, and **F**). This tendency may be helpful in distinguishing neoplasia from reactive gliosis (see Chapter 8 for more complete discussion of Scherer's secondary structures) (200).

Special Variants of Astrocytoma

Protoplasmic Astrocytoma

This cell type is described above, and in pure form (i.e., without admixture of fibrillar, gemistocytic, or giant-cell morphology) is usually a superficially situated neoplasm in the cerebrum, and is often cystic.

Pilocytic Astrocytoma

In the adult type bipolar astrocytes—typically with minimal nuclear pleomorphism—are associated with a profuse fibrillary background of intersecting glial cell processes. As opposed to the juvenile variant, perivascular pseudorosettes are infrequent, and there is little or no tendency to form microcysts or grossly evident cysts. A few stellate or gemistocytic astrocytes may be admixed. Adult-type pilocytic astrocytomas are relatively rare, are more prone to occur in older patients, and undergo anaplastic change in a significant percentage of cases.

The more common juvenile type of pilocytic astrocytoma is, as the name implies, prone to occur in children and is most commonly encountered in the cerebellum or in the floor of the third ventricle (Fig. 7.4**A** and **B**). It may rarely occur in the cerebral hemispheres. Fibrous astrocytic elements tend to form perivascular pseudorosettes or may form longitudinal sheaths along blood vessels. The astrocytic component may also include prominent protoplasmic astrocytes, which have a more stellate appearance and more sparse fibrillar processes. Nuclei tend to be similar in both the pilocytic (or bipolar) and the protoplasmic elements. There is a marked tendency for the development of microcystic change and grossly evident cysts; the contained material, often eosinophilic by H&E, may stain metachromatically with the Diff-Quik stain. Rosenthal fibers are also a very common and useful diagnostic feature, but may be seen in several other situations (see Table 7.6) (71). Rosenthal fibers are typically brightly eosinophilic, hyalin to glassy-appearing ovoid, elongate, or carrot-shaped, irregularly outlined structures within astrocyte processes. They have a very characteristic light microscopic appearance (Fig. 7.4**C** and **D**). The ovoid Rosenthal fiber aggregates are sometimes also described as "cytoid bodies."

Cytology of Pilocytic Astrocytomas (1, 57) (Fig. 7.4B, C, and D). Smear preparations have emphasized the bipolar appearance of astrocytes with elongate processes, and the frequent presence of Rosenthal fibers. Nuclei tend to be typical of low-grade astrocytomas (see above), with minimal pleomorphism, bland chromatin, and inconspicuous nucleoli. We are not aware of descriptions of exfoliated pilocytic astrocytoma cells in the CSF.

Table 7.6.
Conditions Associated with Rosenthal Fiber Formation

Pilocytic astrocytoma (particularly in cerebellum and optic nerve)
Other low-grade astrocytomas (generally not as prominent as in the pilocytic group)
Malignant oligodendroglioma
Alexander's disease
Associated with longstanding, intense fibrillary gliosis in several situations such as:
a. Around syringomyelic cavities
b. Around cystic tumors (especially craniopharyngioma and capillary hemangioblastoma) or slowly growing solid tumors
c. Around multiple sclerosis plaques
d. Around a wide variety of benign cysts (pineal, colloid, parasitic, etc.)
Within glial tissue in ovarian teratomas.

Astroblastoma

This tumor is rare in pure form; it is most often seen as a minor component of one of the more common low- or high-grade astrocytoma types. It is very vascular, often with hyalinization of vessel walls and prominent, uniform perivascular pseudorosettes. The astroblastoma cell processes abutting vascular walls tend to be more broad or blunt, as opposed to the fine fibrillary processes seen in most of the previously described astrocytomas or those seen in ependymomas (see below). The nuclei are oval, slightly irregular or notched in outline at times, and with a more coarse chromatin than is typically seen in ependymoma cells. Cellular atypia is variable: it is usually mild but may be marked. Multinucleated cells may occur. Mitoses vary from few to moderate. Vascular endothelial proliferation is not typical. The cells between perivascular pseudorosettes are rather discohesive and separate easily on smears and in routine paraffin sections, giving a pseudopapillary appearance to the lesion. Hence the tendency for astroblastomas to be confused with papillary ependymomas.

Cytology of Astroblastoma (57, 88). Smears produce appearances reminiscent of ependymomas, but with more discohesive cells. The differential diagnosis from ependymoma and oligodendroglioma, in particular, may be problematic.

Polar Spongioblastoma

This rare tumor is composed of thin, delicate cells of uni- or bipolar shape, with small, dark, oval nuclei. The main distinguishing feature is the architecture rather than the cytology, with nuclei aligned in parallel rows (palisading) separated by delicate glial fibrils (Fig. 7.4**F**). This palisading appearance dominates extensive portions of the lesion. Similar but usually less prominent palisading may be seen in several other tumors, including cerebral neuroblastoma, schwannoma, and oligodendroglioma, but such tumors typically have nearby areas in which the architecture is more characteristic of the basic tumor type and have differing nuclear characteristics (described below with each individual tumor) (165).

Pleomorphic Xanthoastrocytoma

This is an important tumor to recognize for several reasons. Its xanthomatous features and desmoplastic background (the latter related to its typical superficial location with infiltration of leptomeninges) calls to mind soft tissue tumors of mesodermal origin, benign or malignant, which may also arise from dura and/or leptomeninges. The variable presence of a bizarre, pleomorphic cell component with hyperchromatic nuclei, frequently multinucleated and of giant size, together with the presence of mitotic figures can readily be confused with the cellular components of a sarcoma or glioblastoma. Occurrence in the first 3 decades of life, a prominent cystic component in most cases, superficial location (in temporal, parietal, or frontal lobe), local leptomeningeal invasion but with sparing of dura and bone, presence of a dissection plane of demarcation from underlying brain, occasional presence of perivascular lymphocytic infiltrates, and absence of necrosis are all useful features in avoiding errors in interpretation. With few exceptions, the prognosis of pleomorphic xanthoastrocytoma is far more favorable than the tumors with which it is most likely to be confused, and tumors with these features should have appropriate ancillary techniques applied for precision in diagnosis. The potential for error based on interpretation of a small sample by smear alone is obvious but is unlikely to occur in view of the superficial location of most of these lesions. Such locations typically encourage a more extensive debulking procedure via open biopsy or an attempt at complete extirpation by the surgeon. Several recent sources of information and illustrations of this unusual lesion and its differential diagnosis are available (97, 100, 231). CNS lesions in which xanthomatous change may be prominent are listed in Table 7.7.

Cytology of Pleomorphic Xanthoastrocytoma. An illustration of the appearance of this tumor on a smear preparation is provided by Franks (57), in which the smear closely resembles that of a malignant glial tumor.

Gliomatosis Cerebri

This should be considered an architectural, rather than cytological, tumor category. It

Table 7.7.
CNS Lesions in Which Xanthomatous Cells May Be Prominent

Hemangioblastoma
Histiocytosis X
Malignant gliomas (several types, most prominently pleomorphic xanthoastrocytoma)
Sarcomas
Schwannoma
Secondary carcinoma (renal cell carcinoma; adrenal carcinoma)
Choroid plexus xanthogranuloma

refers to a diffusely infiltrating form of glioma that may involve large areas of brain, even extending into posterior fossa and spinal cord tissues, with or without obvious diffuse expansion or formation of one or more grossly apparently mass lesions. The majority of tumors with this architectural feature have been composed of elongate, poorly differentiated neoplastic cells with a tendency toward astrocytic differentiation in areas. Foci of architectural features consistent with Scherer's secondary structures (200) are common (see Chapter 8 for more detailed discussion of Scherer's secondary structures) (Fig. 7.3**C**, **D**, **E**, and **F**). Foci of typical glioblastoma may occur. The clinical course may suggest a pre-senile dementia or other degenerative disease (201), rather than a neoplasm, since mass lesions may not be apparent on neuroimaging studies. If brain tissue is obtained antemortem, it may be for the purpose of histologically confirming a clinical impression of untreatable dementia. Careful attention to even subtle degrees of nuclear atypia and/or the presence of Scherer's secondary structures will reduce the possibility of an erroneous histologic diagnosis in such settings.

Cytology of Gliomatosis Cerebri. Miller et al. (137) described the CSF cytology in a case of gliomatosis cerebri in which all the cells were small (10 to 15 μm in diameter), with round to oval nuclei, coarse chromatin clumping, inconspicuous nucleoli, and scant red cytoplasm (Papanicolaou stain). Although the cells were felt to be atypical, they were considered insufficient for the diagnosis of malignancy (many of the abnormal cells being degenerated). Similar cells were subsequently documented at autopsy, as well as a spectrum of larger and multinucleated cells and frequent mitoses in tissue sections.

Mixed Gliomas

This category of tumors is arbitrarily discussed in the context of the astrocytic tumors, since the glial component is most often exclusively or preponderantly astrocytic. Cases have been described in which mixtures of oligodendroglia and/or ependymal elements occurred. Russell and Rubinstein (194) categorize this group of neoplasms in the following manner: mixed gliomas consist of a diffuse blend of different neoplastic glial cell types, or—alternatively—close juxtaposition of two or more larger areas of distinct glial tumor types. In addition, glial and non-glial neoplastic cells may be admixed. In gangliogliomas, for example, neoplastic neuronal and glial cell lines appear in varying combinations (Fig. 7.8**A** and **B**). A nearly pure population of ganglion cells would be termed a gangliocytoma, but the glial component is often conspicuous or nearly obscures the ganglion cell component in many cases (termed gangliogliomas). Mixed gliomas and mesodermal neoplastic elements may also occur. These may be in the form of gliosarcomas, with a malignant transformation of fibroblastic or endothelial elements within the stroma of a glioblastoma (149). Alternatively, a sarcoglioma may occur, defined as a malignant transformation of a glial element at the margin of an infiltrating malignant meningioma or sarcoma. A third category would be an angioglioma, in which there are mixed capillary hemangioblastoma and glioma components.

Cytology of Mixed Gliomas, Gangliogliomas, and Gliosarcomas (14, 57, 88). Gliosarcomas, the most frequently encountered of the mixed glial and sarcomatous variety of tumor, should be diagnosed primarily on tissue sections rather than smears, and generally require ancillary techniques. Many anaplastic gliomas may have a prominent spindle cell component, related to either vascular endothelial proliferation and/or spread to the leptomeninges. The latter type of spread may stimulate a significant fibroblastic response. Further, as noted above, glial cells may become quite spindle-shaped and bipolar, mimicking spindle cell tumors of non-glial origin.

The cytology of gangliogliomas is discussed under Tumors of Neuronal Cells below (Fig. 7.8**A** and **B**).

The mixed gliomas (most commonly a mixture of astrocytoma and oligodendroglioma cells) may be suspected in small biopsies if the biopsies are multiple and differ from one another in predominant cell type. A preliminary diagnosis of primary glial tumor with an estimate of grade, and deferral of final diagnosis to permanent sections may be most appropriate for such cases.

Oligodendroglial Tumors

Oligodendroglioma

As with normal oligodendrocytes, neoplastic oligodendrocytes often display a marked tendency toward a "fried-egg" appearance in which the nucleus is completely surrounded by a clear zone as a consequence of cell swelling, associated with delayed fixation (Fig. 7.5**A**, **B**, and **C**). This tendency is minimal or absent in promptly fixed biopsy material, in frozen sections, and in smear preparations (Fig. 7.5**D** and **E**). The common variety of oligodendroglioma is moderately cellular, with sheets of cells having nuclei in the range of 1.5 to 3 times the size of normal oligodendrocyte nuclei, and with a dispersed fine to mildly coarse chromatin pattern. They often appear as bare nuclei in a background of a mildly fibrillar neuropil. Cytoplasmic eosinophilia varies from minimal to prominent, the latter predominantly in more anaplastic oligodendrogliomas (see below). Nuclei are round, with variable tendency toward more elongate or even fusiform profiles. Nucleolar prominence is variable but usually not conspicuous. Oligodendrogliomas have a pronounced tendency (in about 90% of cases) to demonstrate calcification and also have a prominent tendency to form Scherer's secondary structures (200). This is especially true with regard to the perineuronal satellitosis and is not just limited to subpial, subependymal, or perivascular increased neoplastic cell concentrations (see Gliosis versus Glioma in Chapter 8 and Fig. 7.3**C**, **D**, **E**, and **F**). Uncommon architectural patterns include nuclear palisading resembling a polar spongioblastoma, prominent perivascular pseudorosettes, cytoplasmic mucinous change (including PAS-positivity) with or without microcystic foci, and a signet ring appearance. Intracytoplasmic crystals are a rarely described finding in oligodendrogliomas (178). Calcification is often initially related to vascular structures, but calcific foci may coalesce to become quite large. While calcifications within tumors as well as in non-neoplastic brain tissue are very characteristic of oligodendrogliomas, it should be emphasized that they are common in a variety of situations, summarized in Table 7.8 (13a, 26, 58, 194, 220b).

A plexiform capillary network is often present in more cellular, central portions of classical oligodendrogliomas and is a helpful clue since this pattern is unlikely to occur in other glial tumors. However, similar types of delicate angular branching networks of capillaries are seen in other types of tumors, including hemangioblastomas, and in nonneural tumors such as liposarcomas. Diagnosis is rendered more difficult in cases in which there is a mixed astrocytoma and oligodendroglioma component (mixed glioma), or in which there exists a prominent reactive fibrillary background unlike the classical form generally illustrated in textbooks. This can also make it difficult or impossible to distinguish the oligodendroglioma from an astrocytoma, but most oligodendrogliomas have a more uniform round nuclear population compared with the more angular or elliptical nuclei of many of the astrocytomas. GFAP positivity is also present in some oligodendrogliomas in which conspicuous evidence of a significant astrocyte component is absent in routine H&E sections, a potential diagnostic pitfall (21, 194).

Table 7.8.
CNS Calcifications

Calcifications in Normal Brain
- Pineal body
- Choroid plexus
- Leptomeninges and dura mater
- Around and/or within vascular walls in lentiform nucleus, hippocampus, dentate nucleus, and striate cortex

Non-Neoplastic Calcifications
- In basal ganglia associated with disturbed calcium or phosphorus metabolism:
  - a. Hypoparathyroidism
  - b. Pseudohyperparathyroidism
  - c. Albright's hereditary osteodystrophy
  - d. Familial forms
  - e. Associated with neural degenerative syndromes (e.g., Cockayne syndrome, mitochondrial myoencephalopathies, juvenile form of Canavan's disease, Down's syndrome)
- In association with pre-existing tissue injury such as:
  - a. Radiation therapy
  - b. Chemotherapy
  - c. AIDS with CNS involvement
  - d. Necrosis (e.g., perinatal injury, infectious granulomas)
  - e. Ischemic or hemorrhagic lesions
  - f. Various congenital malformations and neuroectodermal dysplasias (i.e., phakomatoses)
  - g. Glial scars
  - h. Disseminated necrotizing leukoencephalopathy

CNS/PNS Mass Lesions
- Arteriovenous malformations
- Astrocytomas (including glioblastoma)
- Calcifying pseudoneoplasm of the neural axis (13a)
- Choroid plexus papilloma
- Ganglioglioma
- Ganglioneuroblastoma
- Ganglioneuroma
- Germinoma
- Meningioma
- Neuroblastoma, medulloblastoma, and related tumors
- Neurocytoma
- Oligodendroglioma
- Pineocytoma
- Polar spongioblastoma
- Pituitary adenoma
- Secondary tumors (metastatic carcinoma or sarcoma)
- Subependymoma and ependymoma
- Associated with radionecrosis
- Craniopharyngioma

Bone Formation May Occur In:
- Craniopharyngioma
- Choroid plexus papilloma
- Ependymoma
- Ganglioglioma
- Lipoma
- Medulloepithelioma
- Meningioma
- Oligodendroglioma
- Normal leptomeninges and dura mater
- Vascular malformations

Anaplastic (Malignant) Oligodendroglioma

There is considerable controversy concerning the histologic criteria that may be used to separate the common, relatively benign oligodendrogliomas from those with more aggressive or malignant clinical behavior. Our own correlation of histology and clinical course in approximately 30 oligodendrogliomas is consistent with the conclusions of Russell and Rubinstein (194). Briefly, there is no single histologic criterion that dependably distinguishes the more benign from the malignant group, but the more developed are certain atypical features (e.g., high cellularity, high mitotic index, cytologic atypia, pleomorphism, poorly defined cytoplasmic outlines, extensive necrosis and/or endothelial and vascular proliferation) the more likely is the clinical behavior to be aggressive. To be distinguished are the common mixed gliomas in which the astrocytic, rather than the oligodendrocytic, component is demonstrating changes in the direction of a glioblastoma. Burger et al. (26) also point out that oligodendroglioma cells with more prominent glassy fibrillar, eosinophilic cytoplasm (resembling small gemistocytes) and Rosenthal fiber-like aggregates may occur more commonly in atypical oligodendrogliomas.

Cytology of Oligodendroglioma and Anaplastic Oligodendroglioma (1, 10, 14, 28, 39, 88, 155, 188) (Fig. 7.5D and E). Cytologic features of typical benign oligodendrogliomas include regular round nuclei with powdery to mildly coarse chromatin, small to inconspicuous nucleoli, and an indistinct wispy cytoplasm causing a general appearance, particularly on smears, of naked nuclei on a nondescript eosinophilic background. Smears taken from the infiltrating margin are likely to demonstrate a confusing array of admixed reactive astrocytes. Vessels may demonstrate the angular branching of fine capillaries that reflect the "chicken-wire" vascular pattern often seen in histologic sections, but there is much less tendency for tumor cells to adhere to vessels in smear preparations of oligodendrogliomas compared to astrocytomas (1). In cells with more prominent cytoplasm the nucleus is often eccentrically placed. Cytoplasmic processes, when present, tend to be short. The background in some oligodendrogliomas is more fibrillar, increasing the opportunity for confusion with an astrocytoma, but the roundness of the nuclei (compared with the more angular nuclei of many astrocytomas) is helpful. Paranuclear halos, as noted above, are usually not evident in rapidly fixed tissue (e.g., in frozen sections or smear preparations). Burger et al. (26) suggest that, in many instances, it may not be possible using techniques available for intraoperative consultation to be more specific than "well-differentiated infiltrating glioma" on the preliminary diagnosis. Other tumors readily confused with oligodendrogliomas on the basis of morphology alone include pituitary adenoma, pineocytoma, and particularly neurocytoma (see discussion of neurocytoma below). In our experience, nucleoli have been more prominent in pituitary adenomas than in the low-grade oligodendrogliomas with which they are most likely to be confused.

Malignant oligodendrogliomas demonstrate a greater degree of pleomorphism, more coarse chromatin, prominent nucleoli, and often a more conspicuous paranuclear eosinophilic cytoplasm as well as a greater fibrillar component. Permanent sections will often be necessary to distinguish it from other high-grade gliomas as well as from secondary tumors.

Ependymal Tumors

Ependymoma

Normal ependymal cells demonstrate certain structural characteristics that may persist to varying degrees in neoplastic ependymal cells, including cilia formation with blepharoplasts, glial fibril proliferation, tubules with "true" (i.e., Flexner-Wintersteiner) rosette formation (Fig. 7.6**A** and **B**), and/or a papillary architecture reminiscent of choroid plexus. The most common ependymoma variant demonstrates a neuropil-like, finely fibrillar background upon which are loosely grouped aggregates of cellular zones. The cells contain bland round to ovoid nuclei with finely granular chromatin and inconspicuous or small dark nucleoli. In the center of the fibrillar areas blood vessels are often present, completing the perivascular pseudorosette pattern (Fig. 7.6**A**). The fibrillar zone consists of elongate, tapering fibrillary process of the neoplastic ependymal cells forming the perivascular pseudorosette, without an expanded footplate on the vessel (as is seen in the astroblastoma, for example). True rosettes with tubules (Fig. 7.6**B**), as well as light microscopically visible cilia and blepharoplasts, are much less commonly encountered and may even be absent. Papillary variants are rare and must be distinguished from choroid plexus papillomas, astroblastomas, infrequent papillary metastatic lesions, and papillary meningiomas. The latter are unlikely to cause confusion not only because of cytologic differences but also because of the neuropil background in ependymomas, which is not apparent in meningiomas. Ependymomas may have cytologic and architectural features other than those that are classic and readily recognized,

Table 7.9.
Rosettes, Fleurettes, and Tumors in Which They Occur

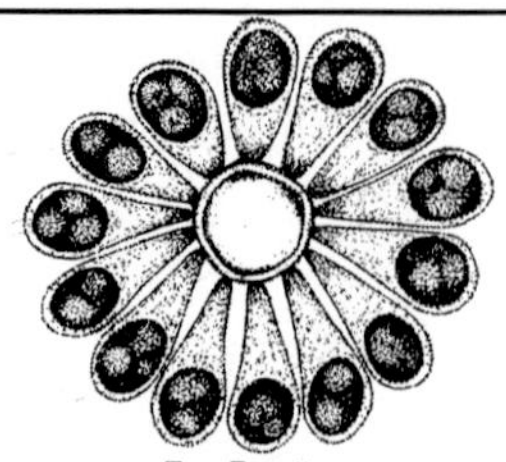 True Rosette (Flexner-Wintersteiner) Cell processes surround a membrane-bound lumen	True rosette (Flexner-Wintersteiner) Ependymoblastoma Ependymoma Malignant pineocytoma Olfactory neuroblastoma (esthesioneuroblastoma) Peripheral neuroepithelioma Pineoblastoma with retinoblastic differentiation Retinoblastoma (and retinal dysplasia) Subependymoma
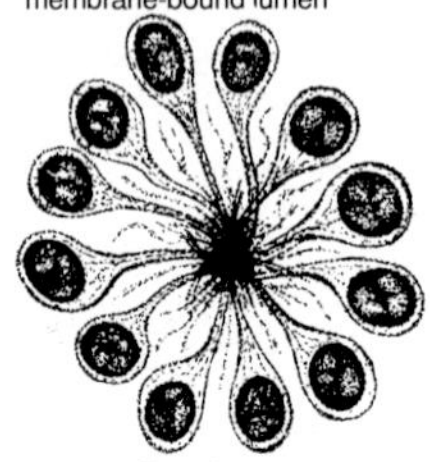 Pseudorosette (Homer Wright) with central tangle of fibrillary processes	Pseudorosette (Homer Wright) Ganglioneuroblastoma Medulloblastoma Medulloepithelioma Neuroblastoma Neurocytoma Olfactory neuroblastoma (esthesioneuroblastoma) Peripheral neuroepithelioma Pineoblastoma Pineocytoma Retinoblastoma Undifferentiated small-cell carcinoma (oat cell carcinoma)
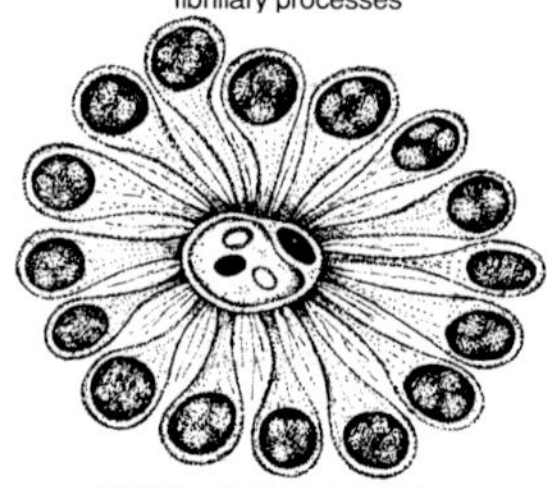 Perivascular Pseudorosette Cell processes (e.g., filamentous, broad, with or without terminal expansions, etc.) surround a central vessel	Perivascular pseudorosette Astroblastoma Astrocytoma (several types, including low- and high-grade astrocytomas, and subependymal giant-cell astrocytomas) Ependymoma Medulloblastoma Neurocytoma Oligodendroglioma Pineocytoma Pituitary adenoma Sarcoma (primary or metastatic) Subependymoma Retinoblastoma
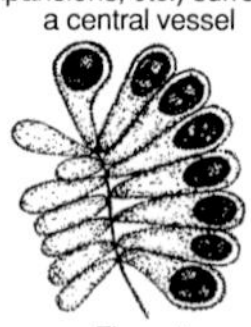 Fleurette Broad cytoplasmic processes of aligned cells traverse a fenestrated membrane	Fleurette Pineoblastoma with retinoblastic differentiation Pineocytoma Retinoblastoma Retinocytoma

increasing the potential for misinterpretation. These latter include myxopapillary and tanycytic forms (see below), a papillary variant (see Choroid Plexus Papillomas) and clear-cell variants in which the perinuclear halo resembles that seen in oligodendrocytes. Distinction of the latter from a mixed glioma may require ancillary studies. Since several types of tumors may have rosettes of one type or another as an architectural feature, these are summarized in Table 7.9.

Myxopapillary Ependymoma

This common variant of ependymoma is almost exclusively found in the lower spinal canal. Architecturally, this variant demonstrates a centrally positioned vessel surrounded by hyalinized, acellular material surfaced by cuboidal or low columnar tumor cells with nuclear characteristics similar to those described for the ependymoma (Fig. 7.6**F**). Fibrous tissue varies in prominence. Tumor cells may also line spaces or tubules, and cystic change is common. At times, the architecture is dominated by pools of mucin-like material (positive with PAS, mucicarmine, and Alcian blue stains), with relatively sparse cellularity consisting of stellate cells (i.e., resembling chordomas) (1). Fibrinoid change may occur.

Tanycytic Ependymoma

While it has been speculated that tanycyte-like cells play a role in the genesis of astroblastoma (194), their possible importance as a source for more highly fibrillated ependymomas that architecturally and cytologically closely mimic fibrillary astrocytomas (including the presence of prominent GFAP positivity) has been suggested more frequently in recent years (26, 59). The distinction of tanycytic ependymoma from a well-differentiated fibrillary astrocytoma by light microscopy depends on its more fascicular architecture, as well as evidence of ependymal differentiation in adjacent portions of the tumor. The latter features would include nuclear differences between typical ependymomas and astrocytomas, with ependymal nuclei generally being more round to oval rather than angular, and containing a larger amount of dense chromatin than is seen in most low-grade astrocytomas. More reliable, however, are architectural features consistent with ependymoma elsewhere in the tumor, which provide a clue to its true origin. True rosettes (Flexner-Wintersteiner type) are seldom present in this variant. The importance of this differential diagnosis is that an erroneous diagnosis of astrocytoma (particularly in spinal sites, where this problem is more likely to arise) could possibly influence the surgeon to be less vigorous in attempting to locate a plane of dissection in an effort to completely extirpate the lesion grossly, since, in an astrocytoma as opposed to ependymoma, a plane of dissection is very unlikely to be found.

Subependymoma

Most of these tumors are incidental findings in the fourth or lateral ventricle, but they may become large enough or be situated strategically enough to produce obstructive symptoms (e.g., hydrocephalus). The histologic pattern is that of a low-grade fibrillary astrocytoma, within which are unevenly distributed, small aggregates of bland-appearing polygonal ependymal cells. The latter may or may not form true rosettes or perivascular pseudorosettes. Cellularity is low except in the focal ependymal cell aggregates, where it is moderately cellular. Some examples contain areas merging into more classic ependymoma patterns. Larger tumors may contain cysts, hemorrhages, and/or calcifications. Their similarity to the smaller benign, reactive ependymal granulations is well described in the literature.

Anaplastic (Malignant) Ependymoma

The ependymomas described above are generally slow growing, fairly well circumscribed tumors more analogous to the special variants of astrocytomas than to the diffuse astrocytoma group, although there are exceptions to this rule (particularly in children). There are also rare ependymomas (usually intracranial in location) that demonstrate anaplastic changes, including cellular and nuclear pleomorphism, nuclear hyperchromasia, marked increase in cellularity, a high mitotic index, and vascular and endothelial proliferation. They may occasionally demonstrate such poor differentiation as to resemble the primitive cells in medulloblastomas, on the one hand, or sufficient pleomorphism to resemble a glioblastoma on the other hand. The original cell type can be determined in such circumstances only by persistence of a well-differentiated ependymoma pattern in another portion of the lesion or by evidence of a gradual cytomorphologic evolution toward an increased anaplasia in cases of serial biopsies of recurrent tumors. In analogy with the atypical oligodendroglioma, however, the presence of such histologic features simply increases the statistical chance that the clinical course in that patient will be a more rapidly progressive one, but is not as reliable a prognostic guide as are similar changes in diffuse astrocytomas (66, 184). The distinction between malignant ependymoma and ependymoblastoma is important in this regard and is discussed in detail by Rubinstein and co-workers (138, 190).

Cytology of Ependymal Tumors (1, 10, 14, 28, 39, 50, 57, 76, 88, 106, 155, 164, 188) (Fig. 7.6C, D, and E). The low-grade ependymoma nuclei in smears appear round to oval and may show columnar orientation, perivascular pseudorosettes, or true rosettes in fortuitous biopsies. In smear preparations they generally form cohesive cell clusters with few single cells, but highly cellular examples (probably comparable to the anaplastic ependymoma noted above but not designated as such in all published cases) may be more discohesive. In the latter group there is also greater nuclear pleomorphism, although the chromatin pattern is most often uniform and finely granular. Nucleoli are variable, being absent in some cases and conspicuous in others. The prominence of astroglial elements may complicate the diagnosis, especially in subependymomas. Frozen sections are particularly helpful in the latter, since the low-power appearance is architecturally virtually diagnostic. Eccentrically placed nuclei are often present in the cells. Rare mention is made of nuclear grooves and folds.

Smears of myxopapillary ependymomas emphasize the papillary pattern and the presence of mucin clumps between the tumor cells and the central vessels (1, 57). The mucin accumulates beneath the basement membrane on which the cells rest and is unevenly distributed along the vessel. The smear appearance of mucin clumps surrounded by tumor cells, particularly under low-power magnification, is reminiscent of smears of adenoid cystic carcinoma and may also stain metachromatically with toluidine blue or similar stains.

The only smear preparation of a subependymoma with which we are familiar is that by Adams et al. (1), which emphasizes the fibrillar stroma and thick aggregates of cells due to the difficulty with which this tumor smears.

The more anaplastic group of malignant ependymomas may be indistinguishable from medulloblastomas or other related neoplasms (see below). The differential diagnosis of primary cauda equina tumors includes not only ependymomas, schwannomas, and astrocytomas but also paragangliomas, which may have perivascular pseudorosettes similar to those described above. Many cauda equina paragangliomas will have a ganglionic component, which may be helpful in distinguishing it from the other common tumors in this location, but gangliogliomas must also be kept in mind as a rare tumor in spinal (as opposed to intracranial) locations.

Glial Heterotopias and Ectopic Tumors

Neuronal and glial elements, alone or in varying combinations, may occur in a variety of ectopic sites and are presumably the source of neoplasms that occasionally occur in unexpected locations. Those relevant to glial tissue have been categorized by Russell and Rubinstein (194) as follows:

Leptomeningeal heterotopias (177) are generally microscopic in size and are composed of fibrillary astrocytes with or without other glial components such as ependyma; intracranial and intraspinal meningeal gliomas may arise from such a source. Extracranial gliomas and hamartomas (153) most commonly occur at the bridge of the nose and less often in the nasopharynx, orbit, or other sites. Extraspinal sacral gliomas are usually ependymal in nature, especially the myxopapillary ependymoma variant; astrocytomas may also occur in this latter location. Clinically, the latter may be mistaken for a "pilonidal cyst." Intra-abdominal gliomas have been reported in a number of sites: ependymal tumors have been described in the ovary and broad ligament, and astrocytomas have been described as arising in the uterine endometrium (234). Gliomatosis peritonei (72, 224) are implants of benign-appearing astrocytic tissue on the peritoneum. They arise as a result of seeding from a mature solid or cystic ovarian teratoma and are not to be confused histologically with peritoneal carcinomatosis or sarcomatosis.

Tumors of Neuronal Cells

Primitive Neuronal and/or Glial Precursor Cell Tumors: Embryonal Neoplasms, Primitive Neuroectodermal Tumors (PNETs)

Medulloblastoma

This is the prototype of the highly cellular, small blue cell tumors of the nervous system, the cytology of which is typically dominated by a round to angular, hyperchromatic cell population (Fig. 7.7**A** and **B**). At times the nuclei are more elongate and are frequently described as being carrot-shaped. Nuclei are hyperchromatic with a high nuclear-to-cytoplasmic ratio and a frequent tendency to demonstrate nuclear molding. The cytology is virtually identical to that of the small-cell undifferentiated carcinoma of pulmonary origin (oat cell carcinoma) as well as to several other poorly differentiated small-cell tumors (i.e., retinoblastoma, pineoblastoma, ependymoblastoma, neuroblastoma, and others) (Fig. 7.7**C**, **D**, and **E**) and rare benign conditions (see Retinoblastoma section of this chapter and Fig. 7.7**F**). Distinction between these various tumors is made not by the most poorly differentiated portions but by areas that may also be present in the tumor demonstrating differentiation toward true rosettes, pseudorosettes, ganglion cells, or other features that would allow more accurate categorization. The cytoplasm in most examples is sparse, ill-defined, and "wispy." Mitotic figures and zones of necrosis and hemorrhage are common, and leptomeningeal spread often results in seeding throughout the neuraxis with or without a local desmoplastic response (the latter is more common in adults). Although an extended discussion of the many controversial aspects of this group of neoplasms is beyond the scope of this book, these issues are important and are worth reviewing in the literature (26, 37, 183, 185, 192-194). The term medulloblastoma is restricted to the form of primitive precursor-cell tumor that arises in the cerebellum in which the poorly differentiated cell is often virtually the exclusive element. It also refers to similarly located tumors in which the more primitive population is admixed with cells demonstrating varying degrees of differentiation toward neuronal (e.g., Homer Wright rosette; immature or rarely mature ganglion cells) or glial forms (typically astrocytic with or without perivascular pseudorosettes). The amount of intervening neuropil appears to be more a consequence of the intensity of infiltration of adjacent brain parenchyma than to be related to intrinsic processes of tumor cells; the latter are sparse in most examples. Architectural patterns include sheets of cells, a more lobular arrangement, and areas of streaming of cells in indian-file fashion. The latter may occur intrinsic to the tumor but is also often seen in areas where leptomeningeal invasion has provoked a desmoplastic response. The spread of tumor cells into adjacent brain may demonstrate a sawtooth pattern, and subpial linear aggregation over extended distances may occur. Papillary configurations are rarely seen. Complex examples with other cellular components traditionally receive special designations. Examples of the latter include the medullomyoblastoma (with a skeletal muscle component that usually resembles rhabdomyoblasts) and the melanotic medulloblastoma (with a prominent component of tumor cells resembling the medulloblastoma, but also producing melanin).

Central Neuroblastoma

The neuroblastoma has many features in common with the medulloblastoma, but differentiation is, by definition, only along neuronal lines if and when it is present. Clues to differentiation along neuronal lines are the same as noted for medulloblastomas, and in both instances differentiation may be further confirmed by ancillary ultrastructural and/or immunochemical studies. Homer Wright rosettes are more often present, and better developed, in central neuroblastomas than in medulloblastomas. Mitoses are common, as are desmoplastic areas.

Ependymoblastoma

Cytologically very similar to the medulloblastoma, this tumor is, by light microscopy and routine stains, distinguished by its propensity to also form true ependymal rosettes (Flexner-Wintersteiner), the central lumen surrounded by a few or several layers of neoplastic cells.

Medulloepithelioma

This tumor, unlike the group of poorly differentiated tumors noted above, has an architecture characterized by papillary and tubular profiles surfaced by ribbons of primitive cells of columnar to cuboidal shape. Nuclei contain coarse chromatin and variable, but occasionally multiple, nucleoli. The cell ribbons may vary from one to several cell layers thick. The pseudostratification of nuclei resembles primitive medullary epithelium of the embryonic neural tube. Mitoses are readily found. Approximately half of the reported examples of this rare tumor have displayed differentiation along one or more of the following lines: neuronal, astrocytic, oligodendroglial, and ependymal. The mesenchymal stroma may be delicate or prominent, with one reported example exhibiting areas of cartilaginous, osseous, and striated muscle metaplasia (194).

Cytology of Medulloblastoma and Related Tumors (1, 14, 28, 39, 50, 57, 76, 88, 104, 106, 155, 164, 181b, 188, 198) (Fig. 7.7A, B, C, D, and E). Smears and imprints of this group of primitive neuronal and/or glial precursor cell tumors demonstrate hypercellularity, round to angular nuclei, hyperchromatism, granular chromatin where it is discernible, and nucleoli that vary from inconspicuous to prominent. Mitotic figures, necrosis, and, occasionally, poorly differentiated rosettes are described in several reports. The cells are discohesive, but this diagnosis, both in smears and cerebral spinal fluid, should include fragments of three or more cells as a criterion, owing to the ease with which lymphoproliferative disorders could otherwise be erroneously diagnosed. Ancillary studies may be necessary for confirmation of suspected cell origin.

In addition to the tumors listed above, metastatic small-cell tumors of pulmonary origin and small-cell glioblastomas would be indistinguishable by cytology alone, particularly in the absence of more differentiated elements. The smear background may demonstrate some sparse, delicate fibrillary processes, but stroma is generally not prominent except in areas of more pronounced glial or neuronal differentiation or in desmoplastic forms that include leptomeningeal elements.

A potential diagnostic pitfall, particularly

considering the cerebellar location of the medulloblastoma, is confusion of tumor cells with normal granular cells. In addition to the anaplasia already noted for the medulloblastoma, the regularity of the granule cell neuronal nuclei, the targetoid nuclear appearance that persists in a substantial percentage of the granule cell population, and the admixture of other normal cerebellar cortex constituents (i.e., Purkinje cells) are helpful clues in the distinction (see Chapter 2).

Cerebrospinal fluid cytology demonstrates cytologic features essentially as described above on smears, with a somewhat greater tendency for the cells to have a round configuration. Again, it is important to demonstrate fragments as well as individual cells. Nuclear molding is a frequent and helpful feature (Fig. 7.7**C**). CSF cytology is useful as an aid to pretreatment staging of medulloblastomas and to monitoring for tumor recurrence (40).

(Central) Neurocytoma

This infrequent tumor is typically located in or near the septum pellucidum and foramen of Monro region in young adults and is most often misinterpreted as an oligodendroglioma because of its considerable cytologic similarity to the latter (Fig. 7.5**F**). The nuclei are small and round with small nucleoli and contain a delicate, speckled chromatin pattern giving a "salt-and-pepper" appearance reminiscent of carcinoid tumor cells. This feature is better appreciated on imprints and smears than in routine paraffin sections and also resembles the chromatin pattern in normal pineocytes (see Chapter 2), but without the prominent nuclear membrane irregularities of the latter. Perinuclear clear halos and foci of calcification, as well as a delicate vasculature, are all oligodendroglial-like features that encourage misinterpretation. Mitoses are rare or absent. Aside from the age group and topographic features, one should also question the diagnosis of oligodendroglioma if either of the following characteristics of a neurocytoma is noted. First, prominent cell streaming (resembling indian-file configurations) may occur on a delicate neuropil-like background. In addition, perivascular pseudorosettes occur, reminiscent of cellular ependymomas. Less often, pseudorosettes of the Homer Wright type are encountered. Markers for neuronal antigens and ultrastructural study (to demonstrate neurosecretory granules and synapses) may be necessary to confirm the diagnosis.

This tumor can be differentiated from the neuroblastoma by the light microscopy appearance and by the ultrastructural evidence of more mature neuronal tissue and well-formed synaptic junctions. It can be regarded as a tumor intermediate in differentiation between the primitive group of neuronal tumors noted above and the more mature ganglion cell tumors discussed below (74, 174, 222).

Cytology of Neurocytomas (9, 26). Smears and imprints of neurocytomas reveal markedly uniform nuclei with a salt-and-pepper chromatin pattern, delicate nucleoli, rare mitoses, and occasional perinuclear halos. The cytoplasm is inconspicuous and may be a helpful differential feature if carcinoid tumor is considered, since carcinoid tumors often demonstrate much more obvious cytoplasm on both H&E and Diff-Quik smears (155) (Fig. 7.14**D** and **E**). Photographs of imprints of this rare tumor are provided by Burger et al. (26, p. 326) and Barbosa et al. (9). In the absence of rosettes the illustrations in the literature, including paraffin sections of such lesions, indicate that distinction from oligodendroglioma would probably not be possible without the ancillary techniques noted above.

Neuronal Tumors with More Mature Ganglion Cell Components

Gangliocytoma/Ganglioglioma

Diagnosis of this group of tumors requires (*a*) identification of ganglion cells distinct from ganglion-like cells that are of glial origin (e.g., as in subependymal giant-cell astrocytomas or giant-cell glioblastomas) and (*b*) identification of neoplastic ganglion cells as distinct from normal neurons infiltrated and surrounded by neoplastic glial cells (194). The relative proportions of neoplastic ganglion cells and a neoplastic glial element vary (Fig. 7.8**A** and **B**), and tumors with an essential absence of the latter are designated gangliocytoma. Features helpful in differentiating neoplastic ganglion cells from entrapped normal neurons include the tendency of the former to occur in atypical locations (e.g., white matter), to occur in irregular groups, and to demonstrate excessive pleomorphism (i.e., increased variation in size, shape, orientation, and branching of processes; bizarre forms; and multinucleation) (227). Application of all of these criteria is important, since ectopic gray matter or rare binucleate ganglion cells may be an incidental finding in otherwise normal brain, and some glial and even metastatic neoplasms can mimic a neuronal appearance rather closely. Other features helpful in the diagnosis of this tumor category include the frequent presence of calcification, a tendency to become cystic, a more prominent fibrous tissue component than is present in many gliomas, and the frequent presence of perivascular lymphocytic infiltrates. There is a tendency for this tumor to occur in the temporal lobe in young adults. Distribution in the neuraxis is widespread, however; our most recent case was situated in the cerebellum of a female in her fourth decade.

Russell and Rubinstein (194) cite evidence to suggest that, while the perivascular round cell infiltrates can be lymphocytic, some of these small cells may be primitive ganglion cell precursors analogous to those seen in cerebral neuroblastomas. Gangliogliomas also provide another example of a glial-type neoplasm to which the three-tiered grading system—so useful in diffuse astrocytomas—does not reliably apply. That is, histologically bland neoplasms may recur, and features suggestive of an aggressive nature (e.g., high cellularity, local leptomeningeal invasion, necrosis, etc.) do not correlate well with subsequent prognosis (89, 90).

It is important to recognize ganglion cells as such in these tumors, since misidentification can lead to an erroneous diagnosis of sarcoma, glioblastoma, or other pleomorphic and more aggressive lesions. Rare examples demonstrate melanin-containing cells (87, 227).

Cytology of Ganglioglioma (57, 88, 121) (Fig. 7.8B). The cytologic appearance of a cerebral ganglioglioma has been reported by Loesel (121). The biphasic cell population consisted of occasionally multinucleated and somewhat bizarre-appearing neurons admixed with glial-like cells with round to ovoid nuclei on a fibrillar background. As noted above, ganglion cells may be very infrequent in some examples, in which case the cytologic preparations will be indistinguishable from an astrocytoma. The glial component may also vary in grade, with rare examples demonstrating evolution to a glioblastoma.

Uncommon Variants

Desmoplastic Infantile Gangliocytoma. This tumor usually occurs in the first few months of life, and is typically situated superficially in the cerebral hemisphere (frontal or parietal lobe). It invades leptomeninges with resultant desmoplasia, usually has a cystic component, and has a more favorable course than, for example, the usual diffuse astrocytomas. They typically demonstrate neoplastic astrocytes that stain with GFAP, admixed with cells with immunohistochemical staining characteristics of neurons. The latter may be difficult in some cases to distinguish as neurons on routine H&E stained sections, however. In some examples, more obvious mature ganglion cells are distinguishable. Thus, the cytologic components include fibroblastic elements, pleomorphic cells with features of astrocytes (i.e., GFAP positive), and other cells, either similar in appearance to the more fibrillar component or with more obvious mature ganglion cell cytoplasmic and nuclear morphology, which are positive with neuronal stains (150).

Intrasellar Endocrinologically Active Gangliocytoma. This term refers to the presence of nodules of distinct neurons in the adenohypophysis. Such neurons may demonstrate markers for one or another hypothalamic releasing factor (e.g., usually growth hormone releasing hormone) and are often in the company of a pituitary adenoma with corresponding hormonal production (e.g., growth hormone) and the associated clinical syndrome (e.g., acromegaly). This lesion is referred to by Okazaki and Scheithauer (166) as an adenohypophyseal neuronal choristoma. (A choristoma is a mass of tissue histologically normal for an organ or part of the body other than the site at which it is located; also called aberrant rest and heterotopic tissue.)

Dysplastic Gangliocytoma of the Cerebellum (Lhermitte-Duclos Disease). This, together with the preceding condition and a few other neural lesions, can be regarded as straddling the gray zone between unequivocal neoplasia, malformations, and hamartomas. (A hamartoma is a benign tumor-like nodule composed of an overgrowth of mature cells and tissues that normally occur in the affected part, but often with one element predominating.) A typical case demonstrates a focal loss of normal cerebellar architecture. Such zones are largely occupied by a neuronal-type cell population intermediate in size between granular neurons and Purkinje cells but with immunohistochemical properties of both of these neuronal types (194). Folia so involved are often abnormally thickened and present as slowly expanding mass lesions. Normal-appearing granular and Purkinje cells in and near such zones are reduced in number or absent, accompanied by reduced white matter and an outer (corresponding to molecular) cortical layer with a large component of radially oriented myelinated nerve fibers (41, 135). Reactive gliosis is variable. Padberg et al. (169) have recently established a link between Lhermitte-Duclos disease and Cowden disease and suggest that this disorder should be grouped with the phakomatoses (see Neuroectodermal Dysplasias later in this chapter).

Hypothalamic Neuronal Hamartoma. Slowly expanding cellular aggregates falling within the broad definition of hamartoma (see above) include this lesion. As with the intrasellar gangliocytoma described above, it may have hormonally active neurons and be associated with a pituitary adenoma of corresponding type. Cellular components can include neurons exhibiting an unusual degree of variation in size, shape, and polarity; myelinated axons; and glial cells (astrocytes and oligodendrocytes), often with an associated fibrillary astrocytic gliosis.

Neuronal Ectopias and Ectopic Tumors

Neuronal ectopias (i.e., gray matter) occur in white matter, near spinal ependyma, and occasionally in the meninges, particularly in some of the neuroectodermal dysplasias (e.g., neurofibromatosis, tuberous sclerosis, and Sturge-Weber disease). As already described under Glial Heterotopias, they may be accompanied by glial elements. The melanotic neuroectodermal tumor of infancy is an example of an unusual location of neuronal tumor elements in which neuroblast-like cells in small aggregates are admixed with melanin pigment-containing cuboidal to columnar cells, the latter in rows or gland-like clefts, with a fine neuropil background. This tumor is most commonly located in the maxilla, and is also referred to as a melanotic progonoma or retinal anlage tumor. More mature-appearing neuronal elements have been reported in one case, and malignant examples rarely occur. In addition, gangliocytic differentiation (to be dis-

Table 7.10.
Tumors in Which a Prominent Ganglion Cell Component May Occur

Gangliocytoma
Gangliocytic paraganglioma
Ganglioglioma
Ganglioneuroblastoma
Ganglioneuroma
Gangliorhabdomyosarcoma
Lipoma
Medulloblastoma
Nasal glioma
Neuroblastoma
Pheochromocytoma
Pineoblastoma
Pineocytoma

tinguished from entrapped normal ganglion cells) may occur with varying frequency in several neoplasms (Table 7.10).

Meningiomas and Other Tumors of Meningeal Origin

Meningiomas are an architecturally and cytologically heterogeneous group of tumors that can mimic, particularly in their less common variants, a wide variety of neural and non-neural tumors. We recommend review of the more detailed discussions of these tumors in the general references provided following Chapter 1, and particularly in the texts by Russell and Rubinstein and by Burger et al., and in the monograph by Kepes (26, 99, 194). Thick-walled hyalinized vessels and variable, but often prominent, connective tissue elements are common accompanying features of many of the following tumor types.

Common Histologic Types of Meningioma

Meningotheliomatous (Syncytial, Meningothelial, Endotheliomatous) Meningioma

The typical cell has a nucleus that is moderately large, round to elliptical, and often with a varying degree of nuclear membrane infolding or nuclear pseudoinclusions (cytoplasmic spurs), as described in Chapter 2 under Normal Pia-arachnoid Cells (Fig. 7.8**C**, **D**, and **E**). Excessive reliance on this nuclear feature to the exclusion of other tumor characteristics is to be avoided, however, due to the wide variety of tumors in which nuclear pseudoinclusions may be prominent (e.g., papillary carcinoma of the thyroid, bronchioloalveolar carcinoma, poorly differentiated carcinoma, malignant melanoma, Hurthle cell carcinoma, hepatocellular carcinoma). Rarely, true nuclear inclusions occur (194). The chromatin is fine, and a small nucleolus is often visible. There is a moderate amount of cytoplasm, but cell membranes are not well defined due to their interdigitating folds, best appreciated at the ultrastructural level. Fibrovascular connective tissue trabeculae tend to separate tumor cells into ill-defined lobules of varying size.

Fibrous (Fibroblastic) Meningioma

The dominant cell type is spindle shaped and occurs in interlacing bundles with a more loosely packed, fibrillar background than in syncytial forms. Nuclear palisading, reminiscent of Antoni type A areas of schwannomas, may be present.

Transitional Meningioma

As the name implies, this tumor exhibits features of both the syncytial and fibrous forms and has two additional distinctive structures. The first is the formation of whorls, the tumor cells forming circular, tightly wrapped aggregates (reminiscent of squamous pearls) around each other or around small vessels, collagen fibers, or other structures (Figs. 7.8**F** and 7.9**A**). The second distinctive feature is the presence of the psammoma body, generally formed by central mineralization of whorls with calcium apatite and iron (Fig. 7.9**B**).

The separation of histologic subtypes

noted above is useful for descriptive purposes, so long as it is understood that in practice one commonly encounters lesions that demonstrate features of more than one type in varying proportions. Tumors in which psammoma bodies dominate the architecture are often referred to as psammomatous meningiomas and are most often encountered in the mid to upper spinal canal of middle-aged or elderly females. Although generally best developed in meningiomas (among the primary intracranial tumors), similar whorls may occur in arachnoid cell aggregates in normal leptomeninges (see Chapter 2), in schwannomas, and occasionally in secondary tumors of the nervous system (e.g., squamous cell carcinoma, melanoma).

Uncommon Variants of Meningioma

Microcystic (Humid) Meningioma

This type contains cells with vacuolated or clear cytoplasm, but with distinct cell membranes, occasionally with stellate processes reminiscent of an astrocytoma. Varying glycogen or fat positivity has been described, from none to florid. Potential diagnostic errors to which this pattern could lead would be consideration of metastatic renal cell carcinoma, capillary hemangioblastoma, and microcystic astrocytoma, among others. One example with nuclear palisading mimicking a schwannoma has been described (194).

Myxomatous (Myxoid) Meningioma

Although similar to the humid type on H&E sections, this variant displays prominent neutral and acid mucopolysaccharides within the small cystic spaces present. Cysts may coalesce to form larger pools of myxoid material.

Xanthomatous Meningioma

Foam cells (with a "ground-glass" cytoplasm due to numerous small vacuoles) containing neutral fats or fatty acids may constitute a smaller population within more typical syncytial, fibroblastic, or angiomatous meningiomas, for example, but in this tumor type xanthomatous cells dominate the histologic pattern (Fig. 7.9**C** and **D**).

Lipoblastic (Lipomatous) Meningioma

This form is characterized by prominent areas of adipose metaplasia of meningothelial cells, with a (usually) single larger fat droplet resembling normal, mature adipose tissue, as a prominent component within an otherwise common variety of meningioma. This may give the cells a signet-ring appearance. It is regarded as a form of benign metaplasia and is to be distinguished from liposarcoma, metastatic mucinous carcinoma, and chordoma (116).

Granular Meningioma

The tumor cell in this form is similar in morphology to that described under Granular Cell Tumors of the Neurohypophysis later in this chapter.

Secretory Meningioma

This form is characterized by prominence of PAS-positive, eosinophilic, hyalin ovoid inclusions in syncytial meningioma cells. The droplets appear to be composed of basic proteins and are within intracytoplasmic lumina, consistent with a form of glandular metaplasia. The potential for confusion with certain epithelial metastatic tumors is apparent.

Papillary Meningioma

Papillary meningiomas, more common in children and often demonstrating aggressive clinical growth characteristics, are a histologic variant in which pseudopapillary formations are prone to occur as a result of partial separation of blood-vessel-oriented tumor cells during tissue processing (26), leading to "papillary" aggregates, often surrounding a central vessel or fibrillar aggregate. This pattern may occur in tumors that cytologically otherwise resemble one of the more common histologic varieties of meningioma (syncytial, etc.), although other histologic stigmata that can be correlated with a more aggressive growth characteristic are often present (see Malignant Meningiomas, below).

Other Rare Variants of Meningioma

A form of meningioma resembling a chordoma (chordoid meningioma) and rare examples with conspicuous bizarre cells and/or lymphoplasmacytic infiltrates (including lymphoid follicle formation) have been described. Pleomorphism and the presence of bizarre cells without other histologic evidence of malignancy in meningiomas do not necessarily indicate a more ominous clinical course (e.g., analogous to schwannomas, subependymal giant cell astrocytomas, etc.) (see Fig. 7.9**E** to **H**).

Meningiomas may also occur in unexpected intracranial locations, such as within cerebral ventricles. Intraventricular meningiomas are believed to arise from leptomeningeal elements in association with choroid plexus and are typically in the left lateral ventricle trigone region. Their histology does not differ from that of meningiomas in more typical locations, except for a relative preponderance of fibrous meningiomas. This can pose a difficult diagnostic problem, since both smear preparations and frozen sections may closely resemble fibrillary astrocytomas (1).

In addition to the lipoblastic meningiomas noted above, other metaplastic features in meningiomas may include the presence of bone, cartilage, and melanin.

Malignant Meningiomas

Histologic features that, in association with one of the other histologic types of meningioma noted above, are suspicious for an increased likelihood of aggressive or malignant clinical behavior include high cellularity, prominent nucleoli, high mitotic index, tumor cell necrosis, invasion of adjacent normal brain parenchyma, cellular atypia, multinucleation, hyperchromasia, and the presence of sheets of neoplastic cells uninterrupted by whorls or connective tissue (see Fig. 7.9**E** to **H**) (26, 194). Penetration by direct extension into adjacent bone or even temporalis muscle, while complicating attempts at total surgical extirpation, is not necessarily associated with "true" malignant characteristics (such as cerebral parenchymatous invasion or extraneural metastases). Such tumors are often referred to as "atypical meningiomas" if some, but not all, criteria for malignancy are present.

Angiomatous and Angioblastic Meningiomas, and Dural Hemangiopericytomas

We presently concur with the opinion expressed by Burger et al. (26) on this controversial topic. That is, the term angiomatous meningioma may be reasonably applied to meningiomas of one or another of the above histologic types in which an unusual prominence of vascularity prompts comment. The other tumor type often included under this heading is analogous in virtually every manner to the tumor described elsewhere in the body as a hemangiopericytoma, and its occasional origin from dura would not seem to justify the additional designation of angioblastic meningioma. This remains a controversial area, however, and for a more thorough discussion and description of unusual cases combining histologic features of both tumor groups, the reader is referred to Burger et al. (26, pp. 107-112) and Russell and Rubinstein (194, pp. 473-479).

Ectopic Meningiomas

Meningiomas may occur in a variety of ectopic sites, including skull bones, the glabellar area, orbit, middle ear, pterygopalatine fossa, nasal cavity, paranasal sinuses, oral cavity, parotid gland, bifurcation of the common carotid artery, skin (scalp, face, and paravertebral region), mediastinum, pleura, lung, brachial plexus, adrenal gland, and even a finger (55, 194).

Cytology of Meningiomas and Dural Hemangiopericytomas (1, 10, 14, 26, 28, 39, 50, 57, 68, 76, 88, 106, 151, 152, 155, 182a, 188, 220a) (Figs. 7.8C through 7.9H). Franks (57) demonstrates smear preparations of several meningioma varieties, including syncytial, fibroblastic, transitional, myxoid, and psammomatous types. Several meningioma types smear easily, with syncytial types demonstrating cells primarily in clusters and sheets and with abundant, fairly well defined, and filmy cytoplasm and round to ovoid nuclei, with the nuclear characteristics already described above and demonstrated in Chapter 2. That is, nuclei have delicate chromatin that is evenly distributed, a small to inconspicuous nucleolus, and often a few small chromocenters. The cells sometimes have a more polygonal appearance. Fibroblastic meningiomas demonstrate spindle cells with nuclear characteristics similar to these, and the transitional forms are more likely to demonstrate whorls and psammoma bodies. In smear preparations, insisting that psammoma bodies be surrounded by at least a few meningothelial cells will avoid the pitfall of confusing psammoma bodies with, for example, contaminants such as bone dust or talc crystals. Several of the uncommon variants have not been described in cytologic preparations. The smear background in meningiomas is typically clean, but the degree of collagen present may sometimes mimic astrocytic gliosis. Hemosiderin-laden macrophages are sometimes present, especially in the more vascular tumors, and mast cells and mononuclear chronic inflammatory cells (mainly T-lymphocytes) may be present (18).

The occasional meningioma demonstrating marked nuclear atypia in the absence of other features of malignancy is a potential diagnostic pitfall in smears as well as in histologic sections (181a). As already noted, similar atypical nuclei may be seen in certain categories of glioma, and they occur in schwannomas and other tumors to be discussed. Some very large, bizarre, and hyperchromatic nuclei may raise the question of a malignancy in this setting, and special attention to the presence or absence of nucleoli, mitotic figures, and necrosis, as well as the degree of cellularity (see Malignant Meningiomas, above), is important in the differential diagnosis (Fig. 7.9**E** to **H**). Smears from meningiomas are among the most common illustrations in articles on brain biopsies, owing to the frequency of this tumor type.

Smears of atypical meningiomas may demonstrate smaller polygonal cells with more granular, and often less abundant, cytoplasm. Nuclei are round to oval, more hyperchromatic, and typically smear in fragments with few single cells. Frankly malignant meningiomas may be essentially indistinguishable from poorly differentiated sarcomas of a variety of spindle cell types unless whorls or other more typical features of meningioma are present. While whorls would favor meningioma, they are not exclusive to meningiomas (see above).

Cytologic preparations are infrequently described in hemangiopericytomas of the meninges. Nguyen and Neifer (152) described the typical appearance as that of a spindle cell neoplasm with finely granular chromatin, with or without conspicuous nucleoli. The cells present singly or in loose or dense cellular clusters. Occasionally, gland-like arrangements of tumor cells have been noted. Guarda (68) described an unusual variant of hemangiopericytoma in which epithelioid cells with an alveolar-like architecture produced a very misleading pattern, not only on frozen sections but also on smears. Clearly, this tumor type is readily confused with a variety of other spindle cell and epithelioid lesions, and Nguyen and Neifer (152) discuss the differential diagnosis. Adams et al. (1) have emphasized the papillary appearance of this tumor in smear preparations, due to tumor cell adherence to vessels, and also comment on the frequent presence of mast cells. Russell and Rubinstein (194) note that hemangiopericytoma cells typically contain nuclei similar to those of meningothelial cells, but with a greater percentage of cells containing irregular nuclear outlines and coarser chromatin. Nucleoli are present but not unduly prominent in cells of both tumors (e.g., meningioma and hemangiopericytoma). Cellularity in hemangiopericytoma varies but is usually high, with random nuclear orientation and cells dispersed in sheets more often than in lobules. The cytoplasm in hemangiopericytomas is much less prominent than in either syncytial or fibroblastic forms of meningiomas. Distinction between the two is further aided by the presence of a characteristic "stag-horn" vascular pattern and the absence of whorls or psammoma bodies in the hemangiopericytoma. The absence of whorls or psammoma bodies does not, however, rule out a meningioma. A photograph of an imprint from a hemangiopericytoma is also available in Burger et al. (26, p. 111).

Miscellaneous Meningeal Tumors

Primary Meningeal Melanoma

Mention has already been made of melanin-containing cells in normal leptomeninges (see Chapter 2), and these provide a theoretical source for malignant melanomas that are primary in the neuraxis. They may demonstrate focal or multifocal intra- or extra-axial plaques or nodules or a diffuse leptomeningeal spread. They may metastasize to a variety of extraneural sites. Some, but not all, are associated with one or another of the neuroectodermal dysplasias, and their cytology is consistent with that of extraneural primary melanomas. We call attention to the fact that melanin-containing cells (either neuromelanin or true melanin) may also occur in several other neural neoplasms to greater or lesser degree, as summarized in Table 7.11. Thus, the presence of melanin in tumor cells is a feature common to several benign and malignant neoplasms of presumed neural crest origin.

Table 7.11.
Melanin-Containing Neural Tumors and Cysts

Choroid plexus carcinoma
Ependymal cysts (extraventricular)
Ependymoma
Ganglioglioma (87)
Ganglioneuroblastoma
Malignant peripheral nerve sheath tumor
Medulloblastoma
Medullomyoblastoma
Meningioma
Neurofibroma
Olfactory neuroblastoma
Pineoblastoma
Primary meningeal melanoma
Retinoblastoma
Schwannoma

Other Uncommon Tumors of Meningeal Origin

These include benign fibromas, fibrous histiocytomas, fibro-osseous lesions, and a variety of primary sarcomas. Most of these lesions are far more common in extracranial soft tissues or bone but may also be primary in intracranial or intraspinal locations. The primary sarcoma group includes the malignant fibrous histiocytoma (13), fibrosarcoma, myxochondrosarcoma, chondrosarcoma, osteochondrosarcoma, osteosarcoma, mesenchymal chondrosarcoma, leiomyosarcoma, rhabdomyosarcoma, angiosarcoma (33a), and Ewing's sarcoma. Thus, such tumors are not inevitably the result of blood-borne metastases when encountered within the neuraxis.

Hemangioblastoma and Other Primary Neuraxis Tumors with a Prominent Vascular Component

Hemangioblastoma (Capillary Hemangioblastoma)

This tumor may occur at any age and in a wide variety of CNS locations but is most commonly encountered in the cerebellum or spinal cord, often with an associated cyst in either site (termed syringomyelia in the spinal region). Exceptionally, they may be found extrinsic to neural parenchyma, as masses in the leptomeninges or as extradural masses or attached to spinal or peripheral nerves. Their presence in the retina is well known in the context of von Hippel-Lindau's disease, and a search for stigmata of the latter should always be included in a patient with this neoplasm whatever its site. Another peculiar feature of this lesion is its association with peripheral blood polycythemia, owing to production of an erythropoietin-like substance by tumor cells in an estimated 10 to 20% of cases. This is occasionally reflected histologically by the presence of intratumoral extramedullary erythropoiesis (166, p. 141, Fig. 3.269); the latter may occur even in the absence of erythrocytosis (240).

Histologically, two main variants are described. Both contain a fine capillary network that may resemble the chicken-wire pattern seen in oligodendrogliomas, but usually with smaller cell-filled spaces between the delicate vessels (Fig. 7.10**A** and **B**). The capillaries are variably prominent depending on whether they are filled with erythrocytes or are collapsed. Larger vessels and sinusoidal spaces are common. Hemosiderin-laden macrophages may be variably prominent, and Adams et al. (1) emphasize the presence of mast cells in these tumors as a useful diagnostic feature. It is the character of the stromal cells (i.e., the third major tumor cellular component, in addition to capillary endothelial cells and pericytes) that primarily distinguishes the two histologic varieties of this tumor. In the *reticular type*, vessels are more conspicuous and stain with reticulin stains, and the intervascular stromal cells are round to polygonal and may have a finely to coarsely vacuolated (foamy) cytoplasm that stains variably positive for lipids with oil red O or similar stains. In some tumors, cytoplasmic glycogen may be present to varying degrees. A second type of stromal cell does not stain with neutral lipid stains; is not vacuolated; has variably abundant pale cytoplasm; and has nuclei that are central, spheroidal, and variable in size and appearance. In some cells nuclei are rather small and uniform, with moderately coarse chromatin and indistinct or small nucleoli. In yet others, nuclei may be large, with delicate, finely distributed chromatin, coarse chromatin, or a densely hyperchromatic appearance. Bizarre, irregularly shaped and/or multinucleated forms may be present, and nucleoli may be prominent. As with several tumors previously discussed (i.e., subependymal giant cell astrocytoma, meningioma), the appearance of such bizarre nuclei is not accompanied by a high mitotic index, mitoses being sparse or absent in hemangioblastomas. Further, the nuclear atypia does not correlate with any difference in clinical behavior in this classically indolent, benign neoplasm. Even local spread or tumor deposits at sites other than those accounted for by local recurrence are very rare, and such tumors show no distinguishing histologic features that would allow their separation from the more common benign varieties. While contact with the leptomeninges is nearly always found in careful examination of such tumors, such access is not typically followed by leptomeningeal seeding (194).

In the second histologic variant of hemangioblastoma, termed the *cellular variant*, the stromal cells are rectangular or polygonal, with eosinophilic cytoplasm, and are situated in nests surrounded by compressed, less conspicuous vessels with minimal or no reticulin component, the architectural appearance on routine sections being reminiscent of a paraganglioma. Cytologically, these tumors can also resemble astrocytomas. A reactive astrocyte component is not unusual and is often more prominent in smears than in routine sections (see Cytology, below).

The cell type giving rise to the stromal component is undetermined, and its variable staining with GFAP, lipid stains, glycogen stains, and other markers has not yet settled this question. The tumor commonly presents as a mural nodule within a cyst in the cerebellum. The wall of the cyst beyond the mural nodule is composed of non-neoplastic reactive astrocytes that often display a striking degree of gliosis and Rosenthal fiber formation, with or without evidence of prior hemorrhage. Reactive glia may also penetrate the nonencapsulated tumor mass proper, to lend further variation to the histologic picture. A biopsy of the capsule wall, given this vigorous reactive glial response, may be readily misinterpreted as a cystic astrocytoma. The prominent Rosenthal fiber formation resembles that seen in many pilocytic astrocytomas.

Additional diagnostic pitfalls are associated with this seemingly distinctive tumor (as it is usually illustrated in routine paraffin-embedded sections). For example, cases with a prominent clear cell population may mimic metastatic renal cell carcinoma, with this differential diagnosis further confounded by (*a*) the presence in some examples of both tumor types of stainable glycogen; (*b*) the increased incidence of both tumor types in association with von Hippel-Lindau disease; (*c*) the ability of some examples of both tumor types to produce erythropoiesis (23); and (*d*) the propensity of both tumors to yield frozen sections demonstrating cells with rather homogeneous cytoplasm, since the cytoplasmic vacuoles (or clearing) are largely an artifact of formalin fixation.

The cellular variant may mimic gliomas, as noted above. Certain variants of both astrocytomas and ependymomas may closely mimic hemangioblastomas, even with careful examination of multiple permanent sections (94). In frozen sections, the obscuration of the architecture and of the stromal cell vacuolization, the difficulty in defining the vascular component, and the occasionally striking nuclear pleomorphism may result in appearances that mimic low- or high-grade gliomas or even metastatic carcinoma. This discrepancy in some cases between the appearance of the frozen sections and smears (Fig. 7.10**C**, **D**, **E**, and **F**) and the permanent sections received the following day (Fig. 7.10**A** and **B**) (the latter often revealing classic histologic features of hemangioblastoma, including conspicuous foamy stromal cells) can be disconcerting until experience with several of these tumors is obtained.

Cytology of Hemangioblastoma (1, 14, 57) (Fig. 7.10D, E, and F). Hemangioblastomas may smear easily or with difficulty, depending on the extent of the glial and fibrous tissue components. Capillaries and capillary buds may be more obvious on smears than on frozen sections, but the appearance of stromal cells may vary as noted above. For example, stromal cell cytoplasmic vacuolization may not be obvious in smears. Rather, stromal cells often appear more epithelial, or even glial, in appearance. The fibrillar background may be far more conspicuous in smears than in frozen or permanent sections. Occasionally the stromal cells appear as sheets, without acinar structures. Nucleoli may vary from inconspicuous to prominent. While most nuclei are round to ovoid and regular, with fine dispersed chromatin and a delicate nuclear membrane, this is highly variable, as noted above. Thus, despite the more classic appearance on permanent sections, which may be seen in the same tumor, smear preparations may demonstrate benign-appearing round to oval nuclei, a prominent fibrillary background, with varying admixtures of more obvious reactive astrocytes and without a foam cell population, at times mimicking a diagnosis of astrocytoma rather well. While stains for neutral lipid may be positive in both frozen sections and smear preparations, the time requirement of 35 to 45 minutes usually exceeds that suitable for intraoperative consultation. Thus, we simply urge caution in the interpretation of such cases and suggest careful correlation with the clinical setting. In many instances, it may be appropriate to defer final diagnosis and indicate the most likely possibilities in the differential diagnosis on the intraoperative report.

Other Primary Neuraxis Tumors with a Prominent Vascular Component

Angiosarcomas and hemangioendotheliomas (epithelioid hemangiomas) are among the vascular tumors more commonly encountered in extraneural sites that may also arise from vessels within the nervous system and its coverings (33a).

Craniopharyngioma

Craniopharyngiomas are located in the suprasellar area (and at times also in the intrasellar area) and have varying mixtures of cystic and solid components. The cyst fluid may be straw-colored to dark brown and contains cholesterol crystals and parakeratotic and/or anucleate squamous debris. Cholesterol crystals have a characteristic overlapping, large, birefringent rectangular profile best seen with polarized light (illustrated by Burger et al. and Chandrasoma and Apuzzo) (26, 28). The cyst lining is a keratinizing stratified squamous epithelium that irregularly expands to form wider zones of epithelial tissue in sheets or cords. Its components are a basal cell layer, a prickle cell zone above, and a more loosely structured microcystic zone of stellate cells called the stellate reticulum (Fig. 7.11**A** and **B**). Larger cystic spaces, often multiple, are typically randomly distributed in the midst of the epithelial areas, and may or may not also contain keratinaceous debris. The immediately surrounding brain tissue is often densely gliotic, with a prominent population of Rosenthal fibers (Figs. 7.4 **C** and **D**, 7.11**B**). The latter is reminiscent of the florid gliosis surrounding many capillary hemangioblastomas and may mimic pilocytic astrocytomas. Calcification within the tumor is usually prominent and is often in spatial relation to the keratin debris. Lamellar bone may form. Lymphocyte infiltrates often occur at the tumor-brain interface. Slender extensions of tumor in the surrounding gliotic zone may make total surgical resection difficult and results in a significant local recurrence rate (approximately 22%) (194), even when a total gross removal is believed to have been accomplished (Fig. 7.11**B**).

There is some evidence to suggest that a higher recurrence rate accompanies the adamantinomatous, as opposed to squamous papillary, architecture (2). Rupture of cyst contents into the CSF can be expected to produce a chemical (aseptic) meningitis, a well-documented occurrence in dermoid cysts (124) and an event that may produce multinucleated giant cells as well as inflammatory cells in the CSF (164).

Cytology of Craniopharyngioma (1, 14, 28, 39, 57, 76, 88, 119, 188) (Fig. 7.11C, D, and E). Cyst fluid aspirates from craniopharyngiomas, dermoid cysts, and epidermoid cysts will be indistinguishable unless the dermoid cyst aspirate also contains hair shafts. The common aspirate features of these three lesions (or a teratoma with a squamous-lined cystic component) will consist of keratinaceous debris, cholesterol crystals, and parakeratotic or anucleate squamous material and may include fragments of calcified material. It may also contain multinucleated foreign-body type giant cells and histiocytes. Degenerative atypia may occur, with irregular and enlarged, hyperchromatic nuclei and even keratin pearls, making distinction from a well-differentiated squamous cell carcinoma difficult on morphologic grounds alone. Needle biopsies must include the adamantinomatous zones to be diagnostic, since the squamous epithelium alone will not distinguish among these several types of cysts. Another diagnostic pitfall is the dense fibrillar gliosis with Rosenthal fibers that often surrounds craniopharyngiomas, since a biopsy from this zone only could readily be misinterpreted as a pilocytic astrocytoma. Close attention to the cellularity and degree of pleomorphism of the nuclei will be helpful in distinguishing the latter (see Gliosis versus Glioma in Chapter 8). Finally, squamous metaplasia and calcification may occur in otherwise normal pituitary glands in older individuals (175a), but these are unlikely to pose a diagnostic problem if the cautions outlined above are kept in mind.

Choroid Plexus Tumors

Xanthogranuloma

Xanthogranulomas are non-neoplastic nodular masses that generally vary in size from 0.1 to 1.5 cm, with a greasy, yellow to brown cut surface. The degree of brown pigmentation will vary with the amount of hemorrhage that has previously occurred, which can be nil or extensive. The masses are surfaced by choroid plexus epithelium and usually contain a variable admixture of fresh or old hemorrhage (i.e., hemosiderin-laden macrophages), calcification, cholesterol clefts, chronic inflammatory cells, and foreign-body type giant cells. Xanthomatous cells are often a prominent component. The most common location is in the glomus of the choroid plexus within the trigone of the lateral ventricle. They may be unilateral or bilateral. When large, their main significance is that they may mimick a neoplastic mass lesion on imaging studies. They increase in frequency with age. Hyperlipemic states are associated features in some patients but are not a necessary predisposing factor for the development of a xanthogranuloma (143).

Choroid Plexus Papilloma

This lesion closely resembles normal choroid plexus and in many cases is distinguished more by gross size and clinical characteristics (i.e., associated hydrocephalus) than by histologic features. As with normal choroid plexus, calcifications and xanthogranulomas may occur in the lesion, with foam cells in the papillary stroma. Rarely, melanin pigment is prominent (181).

Histologic features are not a completely reliable guide to clinical behavior, since cytologically benign lesions may rarely demonstrate widespread leptomeningeal seeding as well as focal microscopic invasion of an adjacent ventricular wall. Further, some cellular crowding and pseudostratification, tall columnar cells, acinar profiles, oncocytic change, and cartilaginous or osseous foci may be present. In general, however, the presence of the following features should be brought to the clinician's attention as suspicious (albeit not pathognomonic) for a more aggressive course: frequent mitoses, microscopic invasion of normal brain, and/or cellular pleomorphism and atypia short of criteria for unequivocal carcinoma.

The differential diagnosis includes the papillary ependymoma. Papillary ependymomas may occur in similar locations, and the diagnosis is based primarily on the presence of a neuroglial, rather than fibrovascular, stroma within the papillary fronds in the ependymoma. There is also an increased likelihood of ependymal perivascular rosettes and true rosettes in ependymomas. In addition, cells surfacing the papillae are more often in multiple, rather than single, layers in ependymomas although (as noted above) this may also be a finding in choroid plexus papillomas.

Cytology of Choroid Plexus Papilloma (1, 14, 28, 39, 50, 57, 88, 106, 188). The increased volume of choroid plexus papillae and their fragile nature results in spinal fluid samples from patients with choroid plexus papilloma occasionally containing choroid plexus epithelium or even relatively intact papillae. Depending on the degree of atypia of the choroid plexus papillary fronds the cytology may differ in no significant way from normal choroid plexus, or may show varying degrees of epithelial stratification and atypia. On cytologic grounds alone the differential diagnosis would also include metastatic carcinomas with papillary configuration such as renal cell carcinoma, ovarian papillary serous carcinoma, etc., although this is rarely a practical question due to the difference in age groups in which these various lesions occur, choroid plexus carcinomas being rare beyond the first few years of life.

In the choroid plexus papilloma the nuclear features will generally be bland and uniform and essentially indistinguishable from normal choroid plexus (see Chapter 2). It should also be noted that the presence of choroid and/or ependymal epithelium has been described in spinal fluid samples from children or adults with hydrocephalus or other conditions (i.e., post-traumatic), so that demonstration of choroid plexus epithelium or papillary fronds does not unequivocally indicate that a papilloma is present (see Chapter 3, Table 3.6).

Choroid Plexus Carcinoma

This tumor is almost, if not entirely, limited to children. Similar lesions in adults have nearly always proved to be examples of metastatic carcinoma of lung origin, and the diagnosis of a choroid plexus carcinoma in an adult requires confirmation by a careful autopsy to exclude an occult primary extraneural source for the lesion. The diagnosis is based on usual criteria for carcinoma, including cytologic evidence of pleomorphism, hyperchromicity, coarse chromatin of irregular distribution, high N/C ratio, and frequent mitoses, as well as architectural features including sheets, nests, columns, and individual neoplastic cells extensively infiltrating adjacent normal brain parenchyma (Fig. 7.11**F** and **G**). Loss of the regular papillary architecture is often seen. Differential diagnostic possibilities in this age group also include medulloepithelioma, immature teratoma, and other germ cell tumors that may occasionally demonstrate papillary folds (i.e., yolk sac tumor). Ancillary studies (e.g., immunohistochemistry, ultrastructure) may be helpful in distinguishing between papillomas and carcinomas in questionable cases (30, 132).

Cytology of Choroid Plexus Carcinoma (14, 57). Choroid plexus carcinoma cells spontaneously exfoliated in the spinal fluid resemble adenocarcinoma, and we are not aware of any features that would allow distinction from the latter by morphology alone (Fig. 7.11**F** and **G**). Ancillary studies (e.g., electron microscopy) may be helpful in such cases.

Pineal Body Tumors

Primary pineal body tumors include astrocytomas and glioblastomas, meningiomas, germ cell tumors, malignant melanomas, hemangiopericytomas, chemodectomas, epidermoid cysts, pineal cysts, and craniopharyngiomas (26, 194). The tumors believed to originate from the pinealocyte or its precursor cell, however, are pineoblastoma and pineocytoma.

Pineoblastoma

The predominant cell type and architectural and cytologic features of this tumor are essentially the same as those described above under Cerebellar Medulloblastoma, with a few exceptions. Homer Wright rosettes may occur in both tumor types, as may a suggestion of perivascular pseudorosettes. They may be distinguished from medulloblastomas by several features, although these features are not always readily apparent. The distinguishing features include areas of transition to a more classic pineocytoma (see below), a rare mosaic pattern with the more typical small hyperchromatic tumor cells surrounding zones of cells with similar nuclei but with much lower N/C ratios (194, pp. 384-385), and neural differentiation along retinal lines with Flexner-Wintersteiner rosettes and fleurettes. Differentiation along lines also shared by medulloblastomas, however, include ganglion cell, astrocytic cell, and melanin-producing cell variants.

Pineocytoma

These tumors tend to occur in older age groups than the pineoblastoma and are better differentiated than pineoblastomas, as the name would imply. There is a less striking cellularity, infrequent hemorrhage or necrosis, a lower nuclear to cytoplasmic ratio, inconspicuous nucleoli, and less hyperchromatic—but still moderately coarse—chromatin. Nests of cells surrounded by capillaries, and with capillary end-feet recapitulating the general structure of the normal pineal gland (see Chapter 2), are typical. The rosettes, while usually having a fibrillar center analogous to the Homer Wright type of rosette, are often larger and more elliptical than the classic Homer Wright rosettes encountered in medulloblastomas or pineoblastomas, for example (see Table 7.9). Differentiation along neuronal, astrocytic, or both neuronal and astrocytic (ganglioglioma) lines have been described. A rare papillary variant of pineocytoma has also been described that would result in a wider spectrum of differential diagnostic possibilities (e.g., metastatic carcinoma, papillary ependymoma, atypical choroid plexus papilloma, germ cell tumors, and papillary meningiomas) (226).

Cytology of Pineoblastoma and Pineocytoma (28, 57). Few descriptions of the cytology of the primary pineal tumors exist. The pineoblastoma is virtually indistinguishable from the medulloblastoma unless one of the more specific differentiating features is encountered (see above). Franks (57) indicates that the pleomorphism is usually greater in a pineoblastoma than in a medulloblastoma. The cells are typically smaller and more hyperchromatic than in germinomas (the most common tumor in this location), and one is unlikely to have an admixture of lymphocytes (also characteristic of germinoma) in the pineoblastoma.

Pineocytomas demonstrate a more lobular architecture in thicker areas of the smear, probably corresponding to the larger Homer Wright-type rosettes described above. The cells are small, regular, round, with variable chromatin content but often appearing rather bland. There is a rather uniform nuclear population, and naked nuclei or nuclei with scant associated cytoplasm are common. Chromatin is usually fine and evenly distributed, and nucleoli are small.

Germ Cell Tumors

Germ cell tumors most commonly occur in children, with pineal examples having a striking male preponderance (90%). Sites of predilection are midline, with pineal body and suprasellar areas being the most common. Germinomas are the most common histologic subtype, and previous designations of this tumor as a pinealoma (when located in the pineal body region) and ectopic pinealoma (when located in the suprasellar region) are obsolete. Embryonal carcinoma, endodermal sinus tumor (yolk sac tumor), polyembryoma, choriocarcinoma, mature and immature teratoma, teratoma with malignant transformation, and mixed germ cell tumors may also occur as primary CNS lesions.

The source of such tumors is presumed to be totipotential germ cells in ectopic CNS sites (see Pineal Body in Chapter 2). Their histology does not differ from the same tumors in gonadal or other extragonadal sites and is only briefly described below. For a more detailed review of histologic variations in such tumors the reader is referred to standard texts (26, 194) and well-illustrated monographs on these lesions (140, 205, 235).

Germinoma

This is the most common pineal neoplasm and the most common type of intracranial germ cell tumor. Tumor architecture is usually characterized by lobules of neoplastic cells, divided from one another by fibrovascular trabeculae in the pineal region. In the suprasellar region the architecture is often a more diffuse, rather than lobular, pattern. The neoplastic cell is a large, polygonal to round cell with a high N/C ratio and with a round to irregular nucleus completely surrounded by a thin to moderately sized rim of pale, eosinophilic, vacuolated, or clear cytoplasm (Fig. 7.12**A**).

The nucleus has a distinct nuclear membrane, fine to coarse chromatin with several small chromocenters, and one (or a few) nucleoli that may be spherical or mildly elongated. Mitotic figures are usually readily found. Calcification within the tumor is variable but may be prominent. In most cases there is an infiltrate of non-neoplastic small lymphocytes with or without associated plasma cells. Such infiltrates are irregularly distributed within the tumor, but tend to be in loosely organized groups of inflammatory cells surrounding aggregates rather than single tumor cells. A granulomatous reaction with multinucleated foreign-body giant cells, histiocytes, and epithelioid cells may be prominent. Isolated syncytiotrophoblasts may occur, as in gonadal germinomas, and should not be interpreted as a mixed tumor (i.e., with choriocarcinoma) in the absence of cytotrophoblastic and/or intermediate trophoblastic cellular components. Germinomas in contact with the CNS parenchyma may stimulate a florid gliosis.

Cytology of Germinoma (10, 14, 28, 50, 57, 62, 76, 111, 188) (Fig. 7.12A and B). A small biopsy demonstrating only the granulomatous component of a germinoma is a potential diagnostic pitfall. This finding should prompt a recommendation that additional tissue be obtained, since granulomas in tissue from a pineal mass are likely to be within a germinoma (111, 174a).

The cytology of the neoplastic cell is characterized by cells in the range of 50 μm diameter, singly or in pairs or fragments, with large round nuclei and dispersed, clumped peripheral chromatin or a more irregular chromatin distribution throughout the nucleus. One to three prominent nucleoli, moderately enlarged and usually without angulation, are present. The nuclear to cytoplasmic ratio is high. The cytoplasm is sparse and vacuolated in some examples and more abundant in others. Varying admixtures of lymphocytes and epithelioid histiocytes are described (28, 57).

Immunohistochemical studies may be helpful in the distinction of some of the germ cell tumors. Positivity for ferritin and placental alkaline phosphatase has been described in germinomas, α-fetoprotein in embryonal carcinoma and yolk sac carcinoma, and human chorionic gonadotrophin in choriocarcinoma. Human chorionic gonadotrophin may also be present in the occasional syncytiotrophoblast that may be seen in germinomas or other germ cell tumors in the absence of cytotrophoblasts and may account for the human chorionic gonadotrophin positivity in the germinoma reported by Stark et al. (62, 212). Germinomas in intracranial sites, particularly in atypical locations other than the pineal body or suprasellar region, may also result from metastatic tumor arising in gonadal or extraneural, extragonadal sites and must be included in the differential diagnosis (70).

Embryonal Carcinoma

This tumor is composed of primitive epithelial cells not always readily distinguishable from those in germinomas but usually larger, more hyperchromatic, and less uniform than the germinoma's neoplastic cells. Further distinguishing features are the more common presence (in embryonal carcinoma) of glands and of tubular or papillary formations, all of which are rare or absent in germinomas. There is also an absence of the lymphoplasmacytic infiltrates and granulomas that are more commonly seen in germinomas. Syncytiotrophoblasts, necrosis, and a high mitotic rate occur in both tumors, but all are more frequent in embryonal carcinomas than in germinomas.

Endodermal Sinus Tumor (Yolk Sac Tumor)

The dominant form of endodermal sinus tumor cell shares many cytologic features with germinoma and embryonal carcinoma. They are moderate to large in size, contain clear to amphophilic or mildly basophilic cytoplasm, and have large atypical nuclei. Mitoses are usually abundant. A variety of architectural patterns may occur, including papillary, glandular, solid, and mixed patterns. Stroma is variable in amount, but microcystic change is common. The two most helpful distinguishing features, if present, are (*a*) Schiller-Duval bodies, consisting of a central vessel surrounded by a connective tissue core, both contained within a round or elongate papillary process surfaced by flat, cuboidal, or columnar, primitive-appearing cells. The space into which the papilla projects is lined by similar cells, and these spaces vary in size and are sometimes rather elongate; (*b*) the presence of round, eosinophilic hyalin-like globules that are PAS positive and usually positive for α-fetoprotein. While neither feature is invariably present and the latter is nonspecific, they are nonetheless more typical of the endodermal sinus tumor than any other germ cell tumor.

Choriocarcinoma

These tumors are composed of a mixture of cytotrophoblasts or intermediate trophoblasts, and syncytiotrophoblast cells. They tend to be very vascular and often hemorrhage spontaneously. Most occur in the pineal body, with the second most frequent site being the region of the sella. Syncytiotrophoblast cells vary considerably in appearance, at times having relatively few nuclei and abundant cytoplasm and in other instances having numerous closely packed, uniform nuclei with relatively scant cytoplasm (235). Syncytiotrophoblasts may be more readily identified with human chorionic gonadotrophin staining than by routine histologic methods, both in choriocarcinoma and in other germ cell tumors in which they occasionally occur.

Teratoma

These tumors consist of elements of all three germ cell layers. In mature (and often cystic) teratomas, all contained elements resemble adult tissue. In immature teratomas, one or more components are of embryonic or fetal appearance. Common intracranial sites are the same as for the other germ cell tumors (i.e., pineal body and suprasellar area). Occasionally one component will transform to a cancer of somatic type (e.g., squamous cell carcinoma, adenocarcinoma). CNS *cytologic* findings in an immature teratoma have recently been reported (90a).

Mixed Germ Cell Tumor

Any of the germ cell tumors described above may occur in combination with one another, as is often seen in germ cell tumors primary in gonadal or other extragonadal, non-neural sites.

Lipoma

This tumor is usually situated in the midline over the corpus callosum (where it may be associated with partial or complete agenesis of the corpus callosum) or in the quadrigeminal plate or suprasellar area. It is seen less often at other CNS sites (including intraspinal). Components of the so-called "lipoma" may include not only mature adipose cells but also (less frequently) variable collagen, blood vessels, neurites myelinated by Schwann cells, ganglion cells, fibrillary astrocytic gliosis, smooth or striated muscle, cartilage, fibro-osseous tissue, hematopoietic tissue, and other components (194). Budka's article illustrates many of these features (22).

Pituitary Tumors

Pituitary Adenoma

Until recently, this group of tumors was grouped into three main categories by routine histologic stains (acidophilic, basophilic, and chromophome adenomas) (see Chapter 2). The contemporary classification system, based on more recent ultrastructural and immunohistochemical studies, is now approaching that of non-Hodgkin's lymphomas in complexity. As noted in Chapter 2, this degree of precision in diagnosis is not achieved by the stains employed in the intraoperative consultation setting, but an appreciation of such details and the relevant clinical data enables the pathologist to most appropriately prioritize the ancillary studies that may be necessary to categorize the neoplasm accurately in a given case, depending on the amount of tissue received. The advantages of tissue conservation provided by cytologic smear techniques and the high percentage of pituitary mass lesions in which smears alone are sufficient for intraoperative diagnosis combine to make smear preparations the initial procedure of choice in this tumor category by some workers (26, p. 505). Clinical symptoms will vary with the size, direction of growth, and presence (and type) or absence of endocrinologic activity of the tumor. Recent, well-illustrated reviews of the various pituitary tumor types, including light microscopic, ultrastructural, histochemical, and/or touch preparations are available (26, pp. 503-536; 28; 57; 110; 198). Adenomas are generally recognized histologically by the presence of a uniform cell population causing compression of adjacent, more normal-appearing pituitary tissue. The separation of adenomas from hyperplasias may be aided by a reticulin stain (110). The uniformity of cytoplasmic staining within an adenoma differs from the two- or three-cell population seen in normal portions of the anterior pituitary (Fig. 7.12**C** to **F**; see also Fig. 2.13**A** to **D**). It should be noted, however, that mixed adenomas may uncommonly occur and are an exception to this general rule. Oncocytic change may occur in the presence of several functional types of pituitary adenoma or as a separate histologic type (i.e., pituitary oncocytoma, or oncocytic variant of null cell adenoma) (110). It should also be noted that oncocytic cells have been described in several other types of neuraxis tumors (including choroid plexus papillomas, occasionally in normal choroid plexus epithelium and in cauda equina paragangliomas).

The nuclei of adenoma cells are, in many cases, quite similar to those in the normal adenohypophysial cells (i.e., finely distributed speckled chromatin in a "dusty" nuclear sap;

a central or eccentric location of nuclei within the cells; and small nucleoli). From the review of normal histology in Chapter 2 it may be anticipated that several diagnostic pitfalls may occur, including (*a*) the tendency of normal pituitary gland to demonstrate increased concentrations of certain cell types in certain locations, giving a false impression of a monomorphic cell population in very small specimens; (*b*) overinterpretation of the presence of trophic cell aggregates, multinucleation, nuclear pleomorphism, salivary gland rests, basophil invasion of pars nervosa, and squamous metaplasia that may be present in normal glands (175a); (*c*) patchy oncocytic change in an adenoma giving a two-cell population; (*d*) misinterpretation of granular cell tumors for adenomas; and (*e*) confusion with other tumors that may occasionally appear in the sella or suprasellar area (e.g., metastatic carcinoma, lymphoproliferative lesions, meningiomas, germinoma, olfactory neuroblastoma, and [rarely] glioma). Ectopic suprasellar adenohypophysial tissue has also been reported (26). Multinucleated cells and nuclear pleomorphism can be seen to a degree in normal pituitary tissue, but if these features are prominent—and especially if accompanied by increased mitotic activity and a monomorphic staining population of cells—they tend to favor a diagnosis of adenoma.

Cytomorphologic features provide few clues as to the local invasive tendency of a given tumor, aside from the acidophilic stem cell adenoma (which requires immunohistochemical and ultrastructural criteria for diagnosis). A possible exception is the presence of a high mitotic rate, which is more likely to be present in the rare cases that demonstrate discontinuous spread within the CNS or extracranial metastases (referred to as pituitary carcinomas).

Cytology of Pituitary Adenomas (1, 14, 26, 28, 39, 50, 57, 88, 110, 155, 164, 188, 198) (Fig. 7.12C, D, E, and F). Features helpful in diagnosis include a monomorphic population of cells (with regard to cytoplasmic staining characteristics) and a tendency for adenoma cells (in comparison to normal anterior pituitary cells) often to have somewhat more coarse chromatin, larger and less regular nucleoli, mitotic figures, and somewhat more pleomorphism and multinucleation than would be expected in the normal pituitary gland. Some reports mention a slightly higher N/C ratio. Touch preparations will typically yield a much more cellular slide from adenomas than from normal anterior pituitary tissue. The cells may be polygonal, cuboidal, or columnar. In smear preparations they are discohesive and the cytoplasm is often fragile, with the result that many bare nuclei are seen in a granular background representing cytoplasmic remnants. Burger et al. (26, p. 505) note that assessment of tumor margins is more difficult than the diagnosis of adenoma versus normal tissue, and is probably best assessed on permanent sections. An additional pitfall in diagnosis may occur when smears of pituitary adenomas are made with excessive pressure. This results in the (often prominent) vasculature being even more conspicuous and the fragile cells becoming smudged, and may superficially resemble a highly vascular small-cell malignancy. For this reason and others, we prefer (*a*) to make smears with graded pressure, so that we have both thicker and thinner areas to examine in all cases, and (*b*) to do frozen sections simultaneously as a more accurate guide to cellularity and architectural features. This has helped us to avoid this potential diagnostic error, especially in adenomas with prominent cytologic atypia. The uniformity of the pituitary adenoma cells in many cases, on the other hand, can closely resemble an oligodendroglioma or neurocytoma on smears, but knowledge of the radiographic features and the exact site of the biopsy will generally lead to the proper intraoperative diagnosis.

Tumors of the Neurohypophysis

Astrocytoma

The neurohypophysis consists of the posterior lobe of the pituitary (infundibular process), the infundibular stem, and the median eminence of the tuber cinereum. It is largely composed of modified astrocytes with fibrillary processes (e.g., pituicytes). Occasional round to oval cells with dusky granular cytoplasm may also be present, some of which may represent displaced adenohypophysial basophils and others possibly representing altered pituicytes. Their relation to the nests and frank tumors composed of granular cells is uncertain. The most common primary tumor is the pilocytic astrocytoma, often of the juvenile type (see prior description of this tumor type, above). Morphologic similarities between normal posterior pituitary and astrocytoma are discussed in Chapter 2.

Granular Cell Tumor

These infrequent tumors are believed to arise from small nests of similar-appearing cells seen incidentally in presumably normal neurohypophysial zones. They have also been referred to as choristomas, myoblastomas, and pituicytomas. The granular cells are virtually identical by light and electron microscopy (i.e., abundant cytoplasmic lysosomes) and by histochemical methods to cells in the subcutaneous tumor of the same name. They are round to polygonal cells with abundant granular eosinophilic cytoplasm and small, often eccentrically situated, round nuclei. The latter contain a small nucleolus, fine chromatin, and a well-defined nuclear membrane. Although these tumors are considered most likely to be of Schwann cell origin in peripheral locations, evidence has also been presented to support an origin from altered pituicytes in this location (154) (including the occasional presence of prominent PAS-positive cytoplasmic granules in non-neoplastic astrocytes, in astrocytomas [144], and in oligodendroglioma cells). Examples of similar tumors have occurred in the cerebral hemispheres and meninges (72a).

Other Sellar Area Mass Lesions

Biopsies of sellar mass lesions clinically felt to be neoplastic may yield necrotic tissue (pituitary apoplexy); inflammatory infiltrates consisting of lymphocytes, plasma cells, and histiocytes (lymphocytic hypophysitis); non-caseating granulomas with variable lymphocytic and giant-cell components (giant-cell granuloma of pituitary; sarcoidosis); or purulent material (in the rare abscesses occurring in the sella). These and other unusual lesions are reviewed by Burger et al. (26).

Peripheral Nervous System Tumors

Tumors of the Nerve Sheath Elements

Schwannoma

Schwannomas are derived from the Schwann cell, which is the myelin-forming cell of the peripheral nervous system. Conversion from oligodendrocyte-derived myelin to Schwann cell-derived myelin occurs close to the exit of cranial and spinal nerves from the central nervous system at the Obersteiner-Redlich zone, grossly evident as a slight constriction of the nerve. Schwannomas occur in a wide variety of sites within the neuraxis (even within cerebral and spinal parenchyma, presumably from Schwann cells accompanying vascular-associated nerves) (203), and in peripheral nerves (including intraosseous and visceral sites). Their frequent association with von Recklinghausen's neurofibromatosis is well known.

The classical histologic form of schwannoma consists of two types of architecture in the same tumor. The Antoni type A zones (Fig. 7.13**A**) are composed of compact, interwoven bundles of spindle cells with ovoid or elongate (cigar-shaped) nuclei. One end of the nucleus may be more pointed than rounded. Slightly curved or wavy profiles of the elongated nuclei are also common, though the latter tend to be better developed in neurofibromas (see below). Chromatin content varies in amount and coarseness, but nucleoli are inconspicuous. In addition to this type of nuclear profile, it is not uncommon to find a smaller population of more elliptical or rounded nuclei, not all of which can be ascribed to cross-sectional profiles of elongate nuclei. Cytoplasm tends to be pale and fibrillar. Collagen is usually sparse or absent, but reticulin is often present in the tumor tissue, and a variable (but frequent) architectural feature is nuclear palisading (in a narrow, rather than broadly distributed zone). The nuclear palisading occurs on either side of a nuclear-free fibrillar zone, and such areas may consist of only two narrow zones of nuclear palisades separated by one clear zone, or may demonstrate alternating nuclear-rich and nuclear-poor zones sequentially repeated two or more times before blending imperceptibly into the surrounding fascicular bundles of spindle cells. These focal collections of palisades, called Verocay bodies, are much more likely to be found in peripheral rather than in central (e.g., acoustic nerve) schwannomas but may occasionally occur in the latter.

The second admixed architectural pattern typically present in schwannomas is Antoni type B tissue (Fig. 7.13**B**), which has a looser fibrous texture, more polymorphic cells, and a vacuolated, lightly eosinophilic to somewhat mucinous-appearing background matrix that is often microcystic. The tumor cells in such areas may be only slightly more variable than in Antoni type A areas. In some schwannomas, nuclei may be enlarged, hyperchromatic, and occasionally bizarre or giant (termed "ancient" schwannomas, due to their prevalence in longstanding lesions). However, in the absence of hypercellularity or more than rare mitotic figures, this is not to be misinterpreted as evidence of a more aggressive lesion (in analogy to similar "atypical" nuclei seen in other benign tumors such as meningiomas, subependymal giant-cell astrocytoma, symplastic leiomyomas, etc.). Indeed, malignant change in schwannomas, in contrast to neurofibromas, is exceptionally rare (126, 237).

Other features may also occur in schwannomas, including very prominent cystic and/or mucinous change, hyalinization and thickening of walls of intratumoral vessels, and—less frequently—mast cells, prominent fibrous connective tissue, calcification, xanthomatous change, vascular thromboses and hemorrhage, and variable size, shape, and aggregation of large and small vascular profiles. Osseous, cartilaginous, or lipomatous metaplasia may occur. Rare variants include melanotic, plexiform, and cellular schwannomas, the latter probably representing an intermediate-grade tumor between classic benign schwannomas and clearly malignant peripheral nerve sheath tumors, discussed below. The most common intracranial location of a schwannoma is the vestibular portion of the acoustic nerve, arising at a point just within the internal acoustic meatus.

Cytology of Schwannoma (1, 10, 14, 28, 39, 57, 88, 155) (Fig. 7.13C and D). We have a definite impression, based on a review of publications describing "schwannomas," that a clear histologic distinction between schwannoma and neurofibroma is not invariably made in all reports. We also recognize that mixed types occur and agree with the often-repeated statement in the literature concerning cytologic preparations of benign peripheral nerve neoplasms that schwannomas and neurofibromas are often indistinguishable on cytologic (e.g., smear) preparations. Both may show cohesive clusters of spindle cells, admixed to varying degrees with collagen fibers (the latter would be more common in neurofibromas), rather uniform nuclei with only occasional large or atypical nuclei, and delicate chromatin. Schwannomas are typically very difficult or impossible to smear and consist of thick, irregular cell fragments with sharp borders (Fig. 7.13**C**). Cytoplasm is ill-defined, as are cell membranes. A varying admixture of foamy histiocytes can be present (although they can be difficult to appreciate on smear preparations), but isolated spindle cells are rare due to marked tumor cell cohesiveness. Nuclei may be ovoid, elongate, curved, or wavy, as described in histologic sections, above.

Distinction from gliomas may be possible by the generally more ovoid to round to angular nuclei of glial cell types, the absence in schwannomas of the delicate fibrillar network upon which the nuclei rest in gliomas, and the greater ease with which most gliomas smear. Distinction from fibrous meningiomas is generally based on the nuclei of meningiomas being more plump, with cytoplasmic nuclear pseudoinclusions and the tendency of meningioma cells to occasionally show nuclear clefts. In addition, the absence of whorls and psammoma bodies, characteristic of meningiomas but rare in schwannomas and/or neurofibromas, are helpful distinguishing features (28, 151, 155). A rare exception to these general statements is the psammomatous melanotic schwannoma recently described as an additional component of Carnoy's complex by Martin-Reay et al. (129). These authors define Carnoy's complex as including (*a*) bilateral primary pigmented, nodular, adrenocortical hyperplasia; (*b*) multiple lentigines, particularly of the head and neck, and blue nevi; (*c*) cutaneous myxomata; (*d*) large-cell calcifying Sertoli cell tumors of the testis; (*e*) cardiac myxomata; (*f*) myxoid fibroadenomas of the breast; and (*g*) pituitary tumors. They emphasize the importance of its recognition due to the possibility of presenting a fatal outcome. Schwannoma and neurofibroma cells have not, to our knowledge, been described as spontaneously exfoliated cells in CSF.

Neurofibroma

Also considered to be of Schwann cell origin, this tumor is distinguished by its more sparse cellularity, looser texture, and presence of more frequent bipolar or tripolar cells, as well as a nuclear shape that is likely to be more elongate and hyperchromatic, and with more pronounced curved, wavy, or twisted profiles than in most schwannomas. The nuclei closely accompany loosely packed, wavy, separate collagen bundles that course through a pale, often lightly basophilic, mucinous-appearing background matrix material. The latter may be metachromatic with appropriate stains. Occasional lymphocytes, foam cells, and mast cells may be seen. This more irregular nuclear appearance, the absence of a biphasic architecture (i.e., Antoni types A *and* B), usual lack of cystic change, less prominence of thickened vessel walls, and the occasional presence of axons coursing through the tumor are features that—in most cases—usually suffice to distinguish the neurofibroma from the schwannoma. Transitional forms do occasionally occur, however, making the distinction between the two common benign peripheral nerve tumors difficult or impossible. A smear preparation of a neurofibroma is illustrated by Adams et al. (1).

The gross appearance of a neurofibroma may be ovoid, lobulated, or plexiform, the latter far more common in neurofibromas than schwannomas. Nuclear palisades are rarely encountered in otherwise typical neurofibromas. Other infrequent or rare features include the presence of lamellar stacks resembling Meissner's corpuscles, and the presence of melanin-forming cells (i.e., melanotic neurofibroma). Malignant forms occur (features are discussed under Malignant Peripheral Nerve Sheath Tumors, below). In this context, it should be noted that sparse mitotic activity in a schwannoma (i.e., 1 to 2 mitotic figures per high-power field) does not correlate nearly as well with malignant behavior (54) as it does in a neurofibroma.

Malignant Peripheral Nerve Sheath Tumors ("Malignant Schwannoma")

The term malignant peripheral nerve sheath tumor (MPNST) is currently the preferred nomenclature, since tumors considered by light microscopy to be "malignant schwannomas" have been found by ultrastructural study to be composed in some cases of malignant perineurial elements, in other cases of Schwann cell elements, and in yet other cases of admixtures of the two or of intermedial cell forms (49). Further, evidence favors an origin de novo or from a neurofibroma to be more common than from a pre-existing schwannoma (237). Histologically, they are characterized by an infiltrative growth pattern. Tumor cellularity is high and spindle cells predominate (Fig. 7.13**E**). Tumor cells are arranged in irregular intersecting bundles, herringbone patterns, or (less frequently) storiform patterns. Tumor cell nuclei are ovoid to elongate, are slightly pleomorphic, and have sharp nuclear outlines. A high mitotic index, necrosis with or without surrounding nuclear pseudopalisading, and a peculiar form of perivascular increased tumor cell density with more polygonal than spindle-shaped cells in the immediate perivascular area (reminiscent of either the biphasic pattern of synovial sarcoma or the vascular endothelial proliferation seen in glioblastoma) may occur (Fig. 7.13**F**). Nuclear palisading unrelated to necrotic foci is more prominent in this tumor than in other peripherally situated spindle cell tumors with which it may be confused (e.g., leiomyosarcoma, fibrous synovial sarcoma). In addition, metaplastic features (particularly cartilage) are more commonly encountered in MPNST than in any other spindle cell sarcoma. Other metaplastic features may include bone, rhabdomyoblastic foci (i.e., Triton tumor), or epithelial (including glandular) differentiation (44, 57, 81). The latter can be readily misinterpreted as a metastatic carcinoma or melanoma. The question of melanoma is also raised when rare clear cell or melanotic variants of MPNSTs occur.

Although malignant peripheral nerve sheath tumors are the neural tumors perhaps most likely to demonstrate a variety of metaplastic elements, such elements can occur in several other neural tumors (194). For example, cartilage has been described in astrocytomas, primary CNS sarcomas, ependymomas, gliosarcomas, lipomas, medulloepitheliomas, meningiomas, and, as noted above, in schwannomas. Muscle cells have also been reported in medulloepitheliomas, primary CNS sarcomas, gliosarcomas, medullomyoblastomas, and lipomas.

Table 7.12.
Multiple Endocrine Neoplasia (MEN) Syndromes

MEN I (Werner's syndrome)
- a. Polyendocrine neoplasms and/or hyperplasias (e.g., pituitary, parathyroid, adrenal cortex, and pancreatic islets [nesidioblastosis]) ± thyroid neoplasms and cerebellar hemangioblastoma
- b. Peptic ulcers

MEN II (or MEN IIA) (Sipple's syndrome)
- a. Polyendocrine neoplasms and/or hyperplasias (e.g., thyroid, pheochromocytoma [bilateral in 60-100% of cases]) ± parathyroids
- b. *No* peptic ulcer

MEN III (or MEN IIB) (Gorlin's syndrome)
- a. As in MEN II (IIA) *plus*
- b. Mucocutaneous lesions, including neuromas of eyelids, tongue, lips, intestinal ganglioneuromatosis, bronchus, and bladder
- c. May have marfanoid habitus

Other Primary Peripheral Nerve Tumors

These include granular cell tumors, neurothekeomas (dermal nerve sheath myxomas), neurotropic melanomas, hamartomas, benign and malignant vascular tumors related to the nerve sheath, multiple mucosal neuromas (related to type IIB or 3 MEN syndrome) (see Table 7.12), neuroepitheliomas, and paragangliomas. These tumors are all relatively rare. The reader is referred to the general references and elsewhere in this chapter for further details of this group (26, 194).

Tumors of Peripheral Neuronal and Neuroendocrine Elements

Peripheral Neuroblastoma

This tumor is essentially identical in histologic and cytologic appearance to the central neuroblastoma described previously, including the tendency to show maturation to ganglion cells in some examples, which is seen to greater or lesser extent. Such maturation may be sufficient to designate the tumor a ganglioneuroblastoma or a ganglioneuroma. Rarely, however, differentiation toward a pheochromocytoma is seen.

Also included in this general group of tumors is the olfactory neuroblastoma (esthesioneuroblastoma), with many architectural similarities to neuroblastomas at other sites but cytologically less anaplastic (or primitive) in appearance. Tumor cells are characterized by round nuclei, fine chromatin, and inconspicuous nucleoli, resting in a variable amount of neuropil-like background.

Tumor rosettes in neuroblastomas are usually of the Homer Wright type, but rarely are of the Flexner-Wintersteiner type. Rare examples of neuroblastomas with prominent melanin pigment can occur (35).

The differential diagnosis of peripheral neuroblastoma, which is more common in children, includes Ewing's sarcoma, soft tissue sarcomas (especially rhabdomyosarcoma), and non-Hodgkin's lymphomas, and—less frequently—might include metastatic medulloblastoma, Wilms' tumor, monophasic synovial sarcoma, and germ cell tumors. Distinction among these various neoplasms may at times be extremely difficult, requiring a wide variety of ancillary studies (4, 172, 223). Among the procedures that can be critical diagnostically at the time fresh tissue is obtained is the preparation and saving of touch preparations, smears, and/or frozen sections for later application of formaldehyde-induced fluorescence or glyoxylic acid fluorescence techniques (223).

Cytology of Neuroblastoma. Smear preparations of neuroblastomas have been described by Akhtar et al. (4), among others. Such tumors are cellular, the cells distributed singly or in small clusters, with variable size and shape. Nuclei are generally round with single nucleoli. Many cases will demonstrate a fine fibrillary background material, and rosette formation may occasionally be encountered in smears.

Peripheral Neuroepithelioma

A type of neurogenic tumor with poorly differentiated small round cells growing in sheets, with a pronounced propensity to form Homer Wright type rosettes, is referred to as the peripheral neuroepithelioma. One variation of this tumor tends to occur in relation to the thoracic cage in younger individuals (Askin tumor). Occasional ganglion cell differentiation is seen. We have not seen cytologic preparations of this tumor but would anticipate findings being essentially indistinguishable from neuroblastomas and related tumors. The histologic appearance and differential diagnosis has recently been discussed by Llombart-Bosch et al. (120).

Ganglioneuroblastoma and Ganglioneuroma

These differ from gangliogliomas in two important respects. In ganglioneuromas the neoplastic ganglion cells may be associated with capsular (satellite) cells and the neurites are associated with abundant Schwann cell and connective tissue elements. They are to be excluded from schwannomas and neurofibromas that have infiltrated spinal or autonomic ganglia. If an immature (neuroblastic) element persists they are termed ganglioneuroblastomas; if there is complete maturation and absence of neuroblastic elements the tumor is termed a ganglioneuroma.

Pheochromocytoma and Paraganglioma

Tumors arising in paraganglia and from adrenal medulla are referred to by a variety of confusing terms. The terminology used herein is based on that recommended by Rosai (186). Thus, neuroendocrine tumors arising in the adrenal medulla are termed pheochromocytomas (170). Morphologically indistinguishable tumors arising in extra-adrenal paraganglia are termed paragangliomas. Both demonstrate an affinity for stains containing silver salts, may produce varying neuropeptide secretory products, and have varying associations with other tumor types (e.g., multiple endocrine neoplasia syndrome [Table 7.12], von Hippel-Lindau disease) depending on the site of origin. The term chemodectoma is traditionally restricted to carotid and aortic body tumors, and the term extra-adrenal pheochromocytoma probably serves no useful purpose other than to remind one to look elsewhere when no adrenal mass is identified in a patient with the classic clinical syndrome one associates with a functioning pheochromocytoma.

Histologically, the spectrum of possible findings can include well-defined cell nests (Zellballen) separated by highly vascularized connective tissue septi (65). The polygonal cells within such nests tend to have round nuclei and abundant granular cytoplasm, but varying degrees (at times considerable) of atypia and bizarre forms may occur (Fig. 7.14**A**, **B**, and **C**). Mitoses are rare. Histologic features (e.g., anaplasia, local vascular invasion) are not a guide to malignant potential, the only proof of malignancy being demonstration of distant metastases. The latter occurs in about 10% of pheochromocytomas and paragangliomas.

Peculiar sites of predilection for paragangliomas include duodenum (199) and cauda equina, despite the lack of evidence for the presence of normal paraganglia in the cauda equina area. Those in the cauda equina, in particular, may mimic other tumors, including ependymoma and metastatic carcinoma (161). At either duodenal or cauda equina sites the histologic appearance may be classic but there is an unexplained increased incidence of ganglion cell and spindle-shaped Schwann cell elements (termed gangliocytic paragangliomas) in these two sites. Illustrations of this uncommon lesion are found in several references (26, 65, 194, 198).

There exists a curious association between peripheral ganglion cell tumors, several other (predominantly endocrine) neoplasms and hyperplasias, and neurofibromatosis (see Neuroectodermal Dysplasias). Several of these are described in the recent literature under the general heading of multiple endocrine neoplasia (MEN) syndromes. Examples of some of the more common associations are summarized in Table 7.12. A recent article on intestinal ganglioneuromatosis (which includes 83 references) provides access to a rapid survey of recent literature relevant to this interesting group of disorders (36).

Cytology of Paragangliomas (57) (Fig. 7.14A, B, and C). Franks (57) demonstrates a smear of a paraganglioma that shows sparse cells that tend to be uniform in appearance (cuboidal or columnar) and tend to remain in small groups, correlating with the nesting characteristics of this cell type seen histologically in most cases. Our illustrated case was much more pleomorphic and discohesive (Fig. 7.14**A**, **B**, and **C**).

Carcinoid Tumor

Although not traditionally included in neuropathology textbooks under the heading of neural neoplasia, these tumors arise from enterochromaffin cells of neural crest origin, demonstrate varying degrees of affinity for silver salts, may produce a variety of neuropeptides, and ultrastructurally contain neurosecretory granules. They are histologically similar to islet cell tumors (which are not of proven neural crest origin) and are most commonly encountered in gastrointestinal tract and lung. As with paragangliomas, malignancy is determined by documentation of metastatic deposits and not by histologic criteria, despite the marked atypia that may sometimes be seen. Metastatic sites from extraneural carcinoid tumors may also include the brain (168).

Architectural patterns in carcinoid tumors may include prominent cell nests surrounded by capillaries (Fig. 7.14**D**), but trabeculae and/or sheets of cells may also occur. Thus, they must be included in the differential diagnosis of paragangliomas. Distinguishing features that may be helpful include the presence, in at least many carcinoids, of greater tumor cell uniformity, elliptical cell shape, the polarization of nuclei toward the vascular margin of cell nests, the presence of pseudoacini, and the occasional tendency for some of the cells most peripheral in the nests to demonstrate greater nuclear hyperchromatism (65, 156). Illustrations of many of the histologic features of such tumors are present in the recently published atlas by Colby et al. (31). Rare variants exist that further broaden the differential diagnostic possibilities, in that they may mimic a number of other tumor types (e.g., goblet cell carcinoids) (65). *Cytologically,* typical carcinoids have round nuclei with punctate chromatin, eccentrically placed in the soma (Fig. 7.14**E** and **F**). Nuclei are not readily separated from cytoplasm even in smear preparations (Fig. 7.14**E**).

Neuroectodermal Dysplasias (Phakomatoses; Neurocutaneous Syndromes)

This group of disorders is included in the present review because of the propensity of several members of this group to be associated with an increased incidence of neoplasia and hamartomas of the nervous system. This is a large and complex topic, and the reader is referred to standard textbooks for a more detailed introduction to the various syndromes included in this category (26, 36a, 194). For our purposes, it will suffice to call attention to the disorders that are associated with an increased incidence of one or more neurological tumors. These are summarized in Table 7.13, which excludes vascular malformations but includes nonneural tumors (including hamartomas) that may also occur in association with these syndromes (also see Cowden disease, p. 95).

Cytologic Components of Benign Cystic Lesions of the Neuraxis

Several types of benign cystic lesions occur within the neuraxis, aspiration of which will yield a variety of cell types depending on the cyst origin (194). The types of cyst lining most frequently occurring in the various types of neuraxis cysts are outlined below, for comparison with specimens that may be obtained from cysts of unknown origin. It is also to be noted that cysts frequently accompany true neoplasms in the nervous system, summarized in Table 7.4.

a. *Arachnoidal cysts.* Arachnoid cysts are lined by normal-appearing pia-arachnoid cells (1).
b. *Cerebellar (simple glial) cysts.* These are typically lined by astrocytic gliosis, with or without Rosenthal fibers.
c. *Choroid plexus cysts.* These may be lined by ependymal cells, choroid plexus epithelium, both, or—alternatively—may be a cystic component of a xanthogranuloma. In the latter case, aspirates may contain fibroblastic elements, hemosiderin-containing macrophages, cholesterol crystals, etc. (see Choroid Plexus Lesions) (61, 69, 131).
d. *Colloid cysts of the third ventricle.* The lining epithelium is of variable type. Simple low columnar or cuboidal epithelium with round nuclei and vacuolated cytoplasm is most common. Cilia may be present. More complex, multilayered epithelium with tubular profiles containing a colloid-like eosinophilic material may occur. Mucin-producing cells or xanthomatous cells are also occasionally present (124a, 201a). Infrequently, the epithelium may be pseudostratified or

Table 7.13.
Selected Features of Neuroectodermal Dysplasias Related to Neural and Extraneural Neoplasia

Tuberous sclerosis (Bourneville's disease)
1. Small benign aggregates of gliosis containing altered cellular architecture and abnormal neuronal and glial forms in cortex (tubers) and subependymal areas (candle gutterings)
2. Subependymal giant cell astrocytoma
3. Malignant giant cell tumors (resembling giant cell glioblastoma)
4. Fibrillary astrocytoma
5. Gliomatosis cerebri
6. Retinal glioma and glial hamartoma
7. Benign angiomyolipoma of kidney
8. Cardiac rhabdomyoma
9. Pulmonary cystic hamartoma
10. Adenoma sebaceum (skin)

Von Recklinghausen's neurofibromatosis
1. Neoplasms:
   a. Neurofibroma
   b. Schwannoma
   c. Malignant peripheral nerve sheath tumor
   d. Meningioma
   e. Optic nerve glioma
   f. Cerebellar astrocytoma
   g. Cerebral glioma (several types)
   h. Spinal astrocytoma
   i. Ependymoma
   j. Retinal astrocytoma
   k. Pheochromocytoma
   l. Peripheral neuroblastoma
   m. Peripheral ganglioneuroma
   n. Diffuse intestinal ganglioneuromatosis
   o. Paraganglioma
   p. Carcinoid tumor (especially duodenal)
   q. Hemangioblastoma
   r. *Possibly* Wilms' tumor, rhabdomyosarcoma, and some childhood leukemias
2. Hamartomas ("dysplastic" lesions):
   a. Lisch nodule of iris
   b. Intramedullary schwannosis
   c. Perivascular schwannosis
   d. Meningiomatosis
   e. Angiomatosis
   f. Atypical glial cell nests
   g. Cellular ependymal ectopias

Von Hippel-Lindau disease
1. Hemangioblastoma
2. Pheochromocytoma
3. Renal cell carcinoma
4. *Possibly* ependymoma, astrocytoma, and pancreatic islet cell tumor

Ataxia-telangectasia (187)
Tumors in this group are presumably related to the associated immunologic deficiency with an increased incidence of:
1. Leukemia
2. Non-Hodgkin's lymphoma
3. Carcinoma

Neurocutaneous melanosis
1. Malignant meningeal melanoma
2. Congenital nevi

Encephalocraniocutaneous lipomatosis (8)
1. Hamartomatous aggregates of adipocytes, fibroblasts, blood vessels and mesenchymal cells in meninges
2. Heterotopic gray matter, calcifications, micropolygyria and porencephalic cysts may be associated neural tissues findings

stratified. Cyst contents may include eosinophilic colloid-like material, amorphous debris, lipid droplets, degenerating leukocytes, and occasionally degenerate eosinophilic proteinaceous material mimicking fungal hyphae (especially *Actinomyces* species). Evidence of prior hemorrhage in the form of golden-brown (hemosiderin) pigment, often within macrophages, may be present.

e. *Epidermoid cysts*. Anucleate squamous cells, parakeratotic squamous cells, and cholesterol crystals as well as amorphous keratin debris are the most common cyst contents.

f. *Dermoid cysts*. Contents are identical to the epidermoid cysts; hair shafts are also typically present.

g. *Enterogenous cysts*. Usually located in the spinal canal, exceptionally these cysts may occur in the posterior fossa or elsewhere in the neuraxis. They are lined by low to high columnar epithelium of intestinal type, occasionally pseudostratified. PAS-positive goblet cells and focal squamous metaplasia may occur, as may ciliated cells (124a, 162, 225a).

h. *Ependymal cysts*. These may occur in various sites, including extraventricular locations. They may be lined by simple, ciliated columnar epithelium with rare, mild stratification. One case is described in which the lining cells were heavily laden with melanin pigment (194).

i. *Intrasellar cysts*. These may be of several types, including cystic change following previous pituitary apoplexy, following previous pituitary hemorrhage, and Rathke cleft cysts. The Rathke cleft cyst is lined by cuboidal or columnar epithelium, often ciliated, with or without mucus-producing goblet cells and/or squamous metaplasia.

j. *Neuroepithelial cysts of the fourth ventricle*. The cyst lining may resemble ependyma, choroid plexus epithelium, or a combination of both.

k. *Paraphyseal cysts*. This term is used to designate a cyst of presumed derivation from the paraphysis cerebri, seen in fetal life as a pouch from the telencephalon just rostral to the ditelencephalic boundary (194, p. 722). It subsequently disappears in later fetal life. This term has sometimes been applied to colloid cysts of the third ventricle in which the epithelium forms more complex, stratified epithelial formations and tubular formations.

l. *Pineal cysts*. The lining of the cyst is composed of dense astroglial fibrils, although pinealocytes may also be present (221a). Rosenthal fibers may occur.

m. *Respiratory epithelial cysts*. These cysts are generally located adjacent to the brainstem, and are lined by respiratory-type mucosa with or without squamous metaplasia.

n. *Miscellaneous cysts*. Cysts may occur following trauma or vascular accidents and are lined by astroglial processes. Foamy macrophages may persist, with or without hemosiderin-laden macrophages, depending on the amount of preceding hemorrhage.

Cytology of Benign Neuraxis Cysts. The literature contains meager reference to cytologic preparations of cyst walls or contents. The appearance in smears of colloid cysts and dermoid cysts is commented on by Chandrasoma and Apuzzo (28) and of colloid cysts and Rathke's cleft cysts by Franks (57). Adams et al. (1) illustrate smear preparations from an arachnoidal cyst.

Patterns of Spread of Primary CNS and PNS Tumors

Primary CNS tumors may demonstrate local extraparenchymatous invasion of the leptomeninges, and upon gaining access to the latter may also diffusely seed the neuraxis via the subarachnoid space (Table 7.14). Leptomeningeal spread, at times, may lead to a significant desmoplastic response that may grossly and microscopically mimic meningiomas or sarcomas (Table 7.15). Less frequently, direct invasion of adjacent bone or even extraneural metastases may occur (Tables 7.16 and 7.17). The latter is more common following surgical therapy of the primary CNS tumor but is also well documented in the absence of surgery. Additional information concerning these modes of spread can be obtained from several

Table 7.14.
Tumors in Which Diffuse Leptomeningeal and/or Ependymal Spread May Occur

Astrocytoma
Cerebral neuroblastoma
Primary CNS lymphoma
Ganglioglioma
Glioblastoma
Optic nerve glioma
Pituitary carcinoma
Meningioma
Leukemia
Medulloblastoma
Ependymoblastoma
Malignant (anaplastic) ependymoma
Multiple myeloma
Choroid plexus carcinoma
Oligodendroglioma
Germ cell tumors
Primary intracranial sarcoma
Primary meningeal melanoma
Retinoblastoma

Table 7.15.
Primary Neuraxis Tumors That May Elicit a Prominent Desmoplastic Leptomeningeal Reaction

Pleomorphic xanthoastrocytoma
Desmoplastic infantile ganglioglioma
Ganglioglioma
Gliosarcoma
Oligodendroglioma
Gliofibroma
Medulloblastoma
Primary CNS sarcoma
Glioblastoma
Astrocytoma (83)

Table 7.16.
Primary Neuraxis Tumors That May Directly Invade Bone

Primary CNS lymphoma
Glioblastoma
Invasive pituitary adenoma/carcinoma
Medulloblastoma
Meningioma
Myxopapillary ependymoma
Germ cell tumors
Oligodendroglioma
Retinoblastoma

Table 7.17.
Primary Neuraxis Tumors That May Metastasize to Extraneural Sites

Cerebral medulloepithelioma
Cerebral neuroblastoma
Choroid plexus carcinoma
Germ cell tumors
Malignant ependymoma
Glioblastoma
Gliosarcoma
Medulloblastoma
Anaplastic astrocytoma
Primary meningeal melanoma
Primary CNS sarcomas
Retinoblastoma
Oligodendroglioma

sources (12, 26, 123, 139, 142, 167, 176, 194, 214, 229).

In tumors that do demonstrate extraneural spread, lymph node metastases have been described in cerebral medulloepithelioma, cerebral neuroblastoma, ependymoma, glioblastoma, medulloblastoma, primary CNS melanoma, oligodendroglioma, retinoblastoma, and primary sarcomas of the neuraxis. Bone metastases have occurred from primary neuroblastomas, glioblastomas, medulloblastomas, primary CNS melanoma, mesenchymal chondrosarcoma, oligodendroglioma, peripheral neuroblastoma, pituitary adenoma, polymorphic chondrosarcoma, and retinoblastoma. Lung metastases have occurred in ependymoma, glioblastoma, intracranial primary choriocarcinoma, choroid plexus carcinoma, malignant peripheral nerve sheath tumor, medulloblastoma, primary CNS melanoma, meningioma (220a), oligodendroglioma, pineal germinoma, and primary cerebral sarcomas. Ventriculoperitoneal shunts may provide a route by which neoplastic cells seeding the CSF can directly enter the peritoneal cavity (12a, 170a) or soft tissues (215a); they may also provide a route for benign and reactive cells (e.g., ependymal and choroid plexus epithelial cells, multinucleated foreign body-type giant cells, histiocytes), which may be mistaken for malignant cells (13c).

Secondary Tumors of the Nervous System

This category of tumors involves the CNS by means of direct extension or by bloodborne metastases. Lymphatic spread is precluded by the absence of lymphatic drainage channels in the CNS, a characteristic shared by only a few other body sites (i.e., cornea and lens of the eye, epithelial tissue, cartilage, and the inner region of the arterial wall) (34).

Direct tumor extension may occur from skull or vertebral column osseous and soft tissue structures, with nearly unlimited possibilities as to histologic types of primary tumors, and is the main mechanism of tumor spread to peripheral nerves. Chordomas, in particular, may demonstrate this tendency (Fig. 7.15**D** to **H**). Chordomas may mimic several other tumor types (26, 85) and can be diagnosed or at least strongly suspected on the basis of cytologic findings (1, 50, 128, 157). In addition to the cytologic features, the metachromatic staining of the matrix material with appropriate dyes can be a helpful clue to the diagnosis on smear preparations.

Blood-borne metastases also provide an access route to the CNS for a long list of tumor types originating in extraneural sites (Fig. 7.15**A** to **C**). While a complete list of all tumors reported to metastasize to the nervous system would be of little practical use, an appreciation of certain patterns of spread as well as the tumors most prone to spread to CNS sites is useful. Certain tumors demonstrate a predilection for the CNS or its coverings (Table 7.18). Included in this list are tumors that—although infrequent—demonstrate spread to the CNS in a significant proportion of cases. Some demonstrate a marked proclivity to spontaneous hemorrhage. Among the most common in this latter group are choriocarcinoma, melanoma, and small-cell undifferentiated carcinoma of the lung. Of primary CNS tumors, the highest rate of massive spontaneous hemorrhage is seen in mixed oligoastrocytomas (107).

At times an occult primary tumor presents clinically with CNS metastatic disease (15, 75). A systematic approach to the diagnosis of the unknown primary tumor, including a review of tumor markers commonly employed in this setting, has been recently summarized by Ultmann and Phillips (225). Even in surgical pathology specimens in which tumor would not usually be expected, vigilance for tumor cells is occasionally rewarded. For example, tumor cell emboli may occasionally be seen within vessels in patients with strokes, and tumor cells in subdural hematoma specimens have been described (29).

Also included in Table 7.18 is a brief summary of uncommon features of metastatic tumors to the CNS, including the rare finding of metastatic deposits of systemic cancers within primary CNS tumors (26, 45, 63, 118, 147, 194, 196, 216, 219, 225, 241).

An altered frequency of secondary tumors in the CNS may be expected as newer therapeutic regimens prolong survival in

Table 7.18.
Secondary Tumors of the Neuraxis—Selected Features

Tumors prone to metastasize to CNS parenchyma
1. Bronchogenic carcinoma
2. Breast carcinoma
3. Renal carcinoma
4. Prostatic carcinoma
5. Pancreatic carcinoma
6. Melanoma
7. Gastric carcinoma and other GI tract sites
8. Thyroid carcinoma
9. Lymphoma and leukemia
10. Sarcoma (including Kaposi's sarcoma in AIDS patients)
11. Other—rare examples of Merkel cell carcinoma, etc.

Tumors most likely to metastasize to spinal cord
1. Rostral spinal cord—lung and breast carcinoma
2. Caudal spinal cord—retroperitoneal lymphoma and prostatic carcinoma

Tumors most likely to demonstrate leptomeningeal spread
1. Gastric adenocarcinoma (less often gallbladder carcinoma or other GI sites)
2. Bronchogenic carcinoma
3. Breast carcinoma
4. Ovarian carcinoma

Tumors most likely to demonstrate dura mater spread (± prominent desmoplasia)
1. Breast carcinoma
2. Prostatic carcinoma
3. Lymphoma
4. Peripheral neuroblastoma

Unusual sites of metastasis (26, 194)
1. Choroid plexus
2. Pineal body (most often from bronchogenic or breast carcinoma)
3. Optic nerve (breast carcinoma, melanoma)
4. Metastases into an existing primary cerebral tumor:
    a. Most common tumor hosts are meningioma, glioma, schwannoma, and pituitary adenoma.
    b. Most common primary sites of metastasis to a primary CNS tumor are breast carcinoma, lung carcinoma, prostate carcinoma, renal carcinoma, and malignant melanoma.

various tumor types, as has been observed in the past (3). Finally, if faced with a small biopsy from a ring-enhancing intracerebral mass, we believe the diagnosis of cerebral endometriosis could prove quite challenging (221). Endometriosis may also involve the leptomeninges and exfoliate typical endometrial cells into the CSF (109, pp. 972-973).

Cytology of Secondary Tumors of the Neuraxis (1, 10, 14, 26, 28, 39, 50, 57, 76, 88, 104, 106, 109, 119, 155, 164, 188, 218) (Fig. 7.15B to H). Given the variety of secondary tumors that may involve the nervous system, only a few general points are in order. The majority of secondary tumors are carcinomas. In comparison with primary CNS tumors, metastatic carcinoma is less likely to have the fibrillar background typical of glial tumors and is usually sharply demarcated from adjacent neural tissue (Fig. 7.15**A**) rather than diffusely infiltrating the neuropil as single cells (the latter is more characteristic of primary glial tumors). Further, the propensity of cells to adhere to blood vessels in smear preparations of many of the glial tumors, giving a pseudopapillary appearance, is not characteristic of secondary neural tumors. Imprints of secondary tumors will generally reveal an epithelial appearance with round or polygonal cells, moderate cytoplasm, and distinct cellular borders without conspicuous processes extending well beyond the parakaryon. Prominent single or multiple nucleoli, irregular shape of nucleoli, frequent mitoses, and the presence of both cohesive cell clusters and individual cells may occur, depending on the primary tumor. In our experience, breast carcinomas, melanomas, sarcomas, and lymphomas are the tumor types most likely to produce primarily or exclusively single cells within the spinal fluid, without cohesive groups, making diagnosis more difficult. Glands, papillae, intercellular bridges, and intracytoplasmic mucin may occur, depending on tumor type.

Chordomas tend to smear poorly but, if present, physaliferous cells are easily recognized in smears (Fig. 7.15**D** to **H**). A large population of chordoma cells may have a more uniformly eosinophilic cytoplasm, however, rather than the typical vacuolated cytoplasm. Diagnosis of chordoma, particularly in isolated cerebrospinal fluid cells, would be tentative owing to the number of other tumors in which bizarre vacuolated cells may appear (e.g., liposarcoma) (128, 157).

Rosenthal (188) emphasizes some important points with regard to metastatic carcinoma in the spinal fluid. Carcinoma cells in spinal fluid may appear more pale-stained than is generally evident in carcinoma cells within other body fluids. In addition, carcinoma cell nuclei are usually round. If bean-shaped nuclei are seen, the possibility of monocytes or other reactive elements must be considered with more than usual care.

Lymphoma, Leukemia, and Related Disorders

Primary Cerebral Lymphomas

This term replaces the now obsolete terms microglioma and reticulum cell sarcoma of the nervous system, and refers to non-Hodgkin's lymphomas arising in the CNS with no, or late, systemic involvement. Most are of B-cell origin, and most arise in immunocompromised hosts (i.e., organ transplant recipients, AIDS patients, etc.). Grossly, appearances may vary considerably. Some present as focal mass lesions, others as areas of softening without significant mass effect, and yet others simply as hemorrhagic foci. Often there is a discrepancy between the gross appearance and the degree of microscopic distribution of tumor cells, the latter far more than might be expected from the gross appearance. Neoplastic infiltrates are typically angiocentric, the perivascular atypical lymphocytes arranged concentrically and irregularly separated by an "onion skin" arrangement of reticulin fibers (Fig. 7.16**A**). More prominent fibrosis, gliosis, and perivascular cuffing by morphologically benign-appearing lymphoplasmacytic infiltrates are common accompaniments. These tumors are also a rare exception to the rule that Scherer's secondary structures (200) are exclusive to primary neuroectodermal tumors, since the neoplastic lymphocytes may also demonstrate a tendency to aggregate preferentially in perivascular, subpial, and subependymal sites (see also Chapter 8). To our knowledge, however, the perineuronal satellitosis seen in neuroectodermal tumors has not been a feature of lymphomas. Concentrations of tumor cells in these areas may be far out of proportion to their presence in the intervening neuropil. Although large-cell types of lymphoma predominate, a wide variety of lymphomas (including signet-ring forms) (171) may occur as primary CNS tumors, and their discohesive character and tendency to involve (or even be essentially limited to) the subarachnoid space (113a) provides a useful means of accessibility to tumor cells for diagnostic and therapeutic purposes (see Chapters 4 and 5) (Fig. 7.16**B**, **C**, **D**, and **E**). A single report describes the occurrence of Homer Wright rosettes in lymph nodes in non-Hodgkin's malignant lymphoma (59a), but to our knowledge such rosettes have not been described in primary (or secondary) CNS lymphomas.

A recent reference that provides a very useful summary of the classification, histology, and imprint cytology of the non-Hodgkin's lymphomas is that of Koo et al. (108). Air-dried Diff-Quik-stained sections are extremely valuable in the diagnosis of lymphoproliferative disorders, since this stain provides a ready means of identifying lymphoid versus carcinoma cells (i.e., the presence of lymphoglandular bodies in the former but not the latter) and also can facilitate the classification of lymphomas within the spectrum of non-Hodgkin's lymphomas in combination with immunohistochemical typing and other ancillary techniques.

CNS symptoms in such patients, while often the result of direct infiltration of the neuraxis by neoplastic cells, may also result from paraneoplastic syndromes (see below), opportunistic infections (see Chapter 7), and various hematologic complications of such tumors (5), accounting in part for those cases in which clinical suspicion of neuraxis neoplastic disease is high but remains unconfirmed despite repeated CSF cytologic studies. Rare cases may demonstrate tumor cell localization to leptomeningeal and perivascular spaces, devoid of a parenchymatous mass lesion component.

Secondary Non-Hodgkin's Lymphomas of the Nervous System

Involvement patterns of secondary lymphomas often differ topographically from those of primary lymphomas of the CNS, in that spread is from without inward more often than focal or multifocal and intraparenchymatous. Thus, extradural (especially spinal), dural, leptomeningeal, or parenchymatous perivascular extensions may occur alone or in combination with a variety of lymphoma subtypes. One unusual variant receiving considerable attention in the recent literature is described under a variety of names, our preference being intravascular malignant lymphomatosis. This morphologically striking lesion consists of a preferential accumulation of malignant lymphocytes, most often of B-cell origin, within capillaries and postcapillary venules. Involvement may be systemic, but the most common symptoms relate to skin and central nervous system. The latter are due to ischemic lesions resulting from vascular occlusion by tumor cells (43, 179, 206, 215, 232, 236).

Cytology of Non-Hodgkin's Lymphomas (1, 14, 28, 39, 50, 57, 104, 106, 164, 188, 198) (Fig. 7.16A to E). Cytologic features of non-Hodgkin's lymphomas are varied, depending on the neoplastic cell type.

The diagnosis of malignant lymphoma is based on data obtained from a variety of sources, which may include clinical features, paraffin-embedded lymph node sections stained with H&E, imprint or smear preparations stained with Diff-Quik or similar stains, immunocytochemical studies, peripheral blood and bone marrow findings, biopsy of extranodal sites of involvement, and cytogenetic and gene rearrangement studies. This complex subject defies brief summary, but work in recent years provides convincing evidence for the contributory role cytologic methods may play in improving the accuracy of diagnostic classification in these disorders. Immunocytochemical studies performed on cells retrieved from CSF are now routine in many laboratory protocols (see Chapters 3 to 5). Imprints made from tissue biopsy samples and stained with Diff-Quik or other Romanowski-type procedures can provide diagnostic information not apparent on H&E-stained imprints or smears or in routine paraffin sections (e.g., lymphoglandular bodies). They are especially useful in cases where routine sections are suboptimal technically and in certain categories of lymphoma that are difficult to distinguish by routine histologic methods (e.g., plasmacytoma versus plasmacytoid immunoblastic lymphoma versus plasmacytoid T-cell lymphoma). The recently published color atlas of imprint cytology of non-Hodgkin's lymphomas by Koo et al. is, in our opinion, an excellent resource for current and detailed information in this difficult diagnostic area (108).

Imprint cytology preparations of lymphomas, with regard to general features, typically demonstrate noncohesive cells with a high nuclear to cytoplasmic ratio, prominent nucleoli, and often (in those that most frequently involve the nervous system) irregularities in nuclear membrane outline. The differential diagnosis includes virtually all types of highly anaplastic CNS neoplasms, but the presence of lymphoglandular bodies on air-dried imprints or smears stained with Diff-Quik can be useful as a preliminary distinguishing feature from poorly differentiated carcinomas. A large body of literature has accumulated on this subject, selected examples of which are included in the references cited (47, 67, 77, 101, 145, 146, 158, 159, 160, 230).

Hodgkin's Disease

CNS involvement by Hodgkin's disease is, with rare exceptions, a result of systemic disease with secondary spread to the CNS. The most common sites of involvement are epidural, dural or subdural, and less frequently leptomeningeal (see Case Report, Chapter 5), with CNS parenchymatous involvement rare.

A detailed description of the cytopathology of Hodgkin's disease is beyond the scope of this review. A useful observation by Frable (56) is that differential staining of the nucleolus with the Diff-Quik stain may sometimes be helpful in making the distinction between morphologically similar T-cell lymphomas (blue nucleolus with Diff-Quik) and Hodgkin's cell nucleoli (more likely to be red with Diff-Quik). Confirmatory studies by appropriate ancillary techniques are always indicated for the initial diagnostic workup in lymphomas, due to the many categories that are morphologically similar. In addition, patients with Hodgkin's disease may develop a non-Hodgkin's lymphoma of the central nervous system following therapy of the Hodgkin's disease (136). Thus, the cytologist must be alert to a change in morphologic features that may be the first indication of the emergence of a new tumor category, since the latter may require an altered therapeutic approach. CSF cytology may be useful not only in the diagnosis of CNS involvement by Hodgkin's disease, but also in the monitoring of such patients (207) (also see Chapter 5).

Multiple Myeloma and Related Disorders

Plasmacytoma

These solitary lesions may involve cranial bones, rarely penetrating the dura to involve underlying brain, and may also occur in the spinal canal. Histologic and cytologic features may vary depending on the varied appearance of the neoplastic plasma cells that form such masses. Several examples are given in the reference by Koo et al. (108).

Multiple Myeloma

Involvement of bones of the skull and spine are commonplace in this form of plasmacytoid malignancy, and leptomeningeal involvement has been reported. Thus, neurologic involvement is more often the result of cranial nerve palsies and spinal cord compression from bony mass lesions and/or vertebral pathologic fractures, respectively, than from direct invasion of neoplastic cells. Once again, the spectrum of cytologic appearance of malignant plasma cells in multiple myeloma is quite varied, and reference should be made to the appropriate hematologic literature (92). Cytologic appearance may vary from relatively well-differentiated plasma cells to anaplastic cells unrecognizable as plasmacytoid in origin, and may also include flame cells and Mott cells. Illustrations of myeloma cells in smears or imprints from CNS tissues (1, 50, 88) or from CSF (14, 164) are relatively infrequent in the literature (Fig. 7.17**E** and **F**).

Heavy Chain Disease

These are rare lymphoplasmacytic malignancies in which the abnormal cells secrete a defective heavy chain isotype. The most common of this group is α-heavy chain disease (Seligmann's disease). Central nervous system involvement has been reported in this disorder, and Kumar et al. (113) have described the presence of atypical, immature plasmacytoid cells in the cerebrospinal fluid of one such case. Well-preserved plasma cells were also described in that report but were sparse.

Histiocytosis X

This complex disorder is a spectrum of conditions ranging from focal lesions resembling inflammatory scars or masses (eosinophilic granuloma) with a sparse Langerhans cell component to an aggressive systemic form with clinical features of a malignancy, more common in children (Letterer-Siwe disease), as well as variants with prominent cranial bone and orbital involvement (Hand-Schüller-Christian disease) (51). Whether histiocytosis X represents a true malignancy or is a non-neoplastic disorder is still controversial. CNS involvement may occur by a variety of mechanisms. Bone involvement and adjacent pressure effects, leptomeningeal involvement, and direct parenchymatous involvement (e.g., hypothalamic region) may occur. A smear preparation of an eosinophilic granuloma of the skull, for example, is illustrated by Adams et al. (1). The leptomeningeal infiltrate, as well as mass lesions occurring in this disorder, consist predominantly of Langerhans cells, eosinophils, and plasma cells in varying proportions. The Langerhans cell origin of the histiocytic component may not always be obvious (e.g., classically consisting of large cells with round to elongate nuclei containing a prominent longitudinal fold or cleft), and a differential diagnosis would include other granulomatous processes in the CSF spaces such as those due to acid-fast bacteria, fungi, sarcoidosis, rheumatoid arthritis, foreign-body reactions, etc. The reader is referred to reviews by Kepes on CNS involvement in this group of disorders (97, 98).

Leukemia and the Nervous System

Leptomeningeal involvement by leukemia, both lymphocytic and myelocytic, has increased as treatment protocols have improved the duration of survival (Fig. 7.17**A** to **D**). Direct neoplastic cell infiltration (microscopic, or as grossly apparent masses such as chloromas), vascular insults as a consequence of vessel lumen obstruction by neoplastic cells, hemorrhage secondary to attendant coagulopathies that are often present in such patients, and complications resulting from therapeutic efforts and/or the immunocompromised state resulting from the disease itself provide more than sufficient differential diagnostic possibilities to challenge the clinician and pathologist when leukemic patients develop CNS symptomatology. Cytologic methods play a key role in such cases, not only by determining the presence or absence of neoplastic cells in CSF or tissue biopsy samples but also by providing the first concrete evidence of an inflammatory or infectious disorder, often to the point of morphologically identifying a specific pathogen (see Chapter 8). Peripheral nerves may also be involved, but occasions for applying cytologic methods to this situation are likely to be infrequent and are more often in the context of previously diagnosed, widespread systemic disease. Occasionally, neuropathic involvement may be the presenting symptom. Direct neoplastic cell infiltrates in the peripheral nerve must be distinguished from neuropathies due to associated nutritional, toxic, or paraneoplastic mechanisms that may develop in such patients.

Familiarity with the cytologic appearance of various leukemias will minimize the possibility of confusing leukemic infiltrates with reactive conditions, whether in CSF or tissue biopsy samples (Fig. 7.17**C** and **D**). Representative examples of hematologic atlases are included in the references (11, 92).

CNS involvement with leukemia is relatively common in acute lymphocytic leukemia and undifferentiated stem cell leukemia, particularly in childhood. However, a variety of other leukemic types may involve the CNS (13b). The incidence of symptomatic meningeal involvement with certain leukemias is unusual, for example in chronic lymphocytic leukemia, but it is also true that the resemblance of such cells to normal lymphocytes would make that diagnosis difficult without immunotyping in the presence of low cell counts (19). Although an elevated CSF mononuclear cell count in patients of this type should result in a suspicion of opportunistic infection, rather than direct CNS involvement by chronic lymphatic leukemia, we also recommend screening studies for infection in those types of leukemia that more frequently involve the neuraxis, since CNS involvement by leukemia and infectious agents may co-exist.

Cytology of CNS Leukemia. Examples of leukemic cells in cerebrospinal fluid (Fig. 7.17**A** to **D**) are illustrated in many of the standard reference works previously cited (13b, 14, 39, 106, 164, 188). Several additional citations dealing with selected aspects of leukemic involvement of the nervous system are also included (17, 19, 32, 42, 64, 105, 114, 180, 191).

The Problem of Blast-Like Cells in the CSF

Cytologic studies of CSF are frequently performed in patients with leukemia to determine the presence or absence of blast forms as an indicator of CNS leukemic involvement, since the latter is often asymptomatic in early stages.

Terminal deoxynucleotidyl transferase (TdT) and common acute lymphocytic leukemia antigen (CALLA, also designated CS 10) are two of the markers most frequently utilized to increase the sensitivity of such screening studies, since they may demonstrate the presence of leukemic cells with greater sensitivity than morphologic methods alone. Curiously, TdT- and CALLA-positive cells also occur in patients with acute lymphatic leukemia who do not subsequently develop CNS leukemia, even in the absence of follow-up treatment (80, 82, 117, 133, 163). Cytologic studies using cytocentrifuge preparations have also demonstrated the presence of blasts in patients with acute lymphoblastic leukemia (ALL) who did not subsequently develop CNS leukemia.

It has also been found that similar blast-type cells may be present in the bone marrow in a variety of disorders. These disorders include not only ALL (pre- or post-treatment) but also non-Hodgkin's malignant lymphoma after treatment comparable to that utilized in ALL, in post-therapeutic bone marrow of children with non-lymphoid malignancies, and in the marrow of children under 2 years of age with non-malignant diseases (213).

Since cells with identical immunotyping characteristics to those described above (i.e., CALLA and TdT positive) have been described in the bone marrow, not only in ALL patients but also in the absence of hematologic malignancy, it has been suggested that such cells represent hematogones (122, 141). Hematogones—morphologically distinct lymphoid cells with homogeneous, condensed chromatin and scant cytoplasm—may occur in the bone marrow of children with a variety of hematologic and non-hematologic disorders, occasionally accounting for more than 50% of the bone marrow cells. This can pose differential diagnostic problems, since the histologic appearance can mimic ALL or metastatic tumor.

Hematogones are virtually absent from peripheral blood, and typically lack nucleoli but are often confused with blasts because of their general nuclear appearance and high N/C ratio. They increase in the bone marrow of children under many of the same circumstances in which the TdT- and CALLA-positive cells appear in the CSF, as described above (122). We suggest that this may be more than coincidence, and consider it theoretically possible that hematogones may also, at times, enter the CSF. This would provide an explanation for the presence of TdT- and CALLA-positive cells in the CSF in normal children and in a variety of disease states, including lymphoid malignancies, in which there is an apparent discrepancy between the presence of such cells and the appearance of subsequent CNS lymphoid malignancy. This hypothesis may be testable, given recent evidence that CALLA-positive reactive bone marrow cells may be differentiated from leukemic blasts by peanut agglutinin (78, 79, 182) and that other sensitive means for identifying leukemic versus non-leukemic cells (e.g., polymerase chain reaction) may soon become practical (208). We also note the possibility that, under certain special circumstances, blast-like cells in the cerebrospinal fluid of neonates may be of germinal matrix origin, as suggested in four infants with hydrocephalus examined by Fischer et al. (53).

Tumors of the Eye and Orbit

The topic of eye and orbital tumors is included in this chapter in a restricted, rather than broad, sense. That is, our review is largely confined to those tumors of the eye and orbit that are believed to be of neural (including neural crest) origin, and only briefly comments on a few of the other possible lesions in this anatomic area that are discussed elsewhere in this chapter or that are important as differential diagnostic considerations. The aspects of ophthalmic pathology that are most likely to be encountered by the general surgical pathologist are reviewed in several recent texts and articles, to which the reader is referred for a broader perspective of this complex subject (46; 73; 95; 186, pp. 1791-1848). Table 7.19 summarizes the primary neural tumors that may involve the eye and orbit (38, 46, 73, 186). Non-neural tumors discussed elsewhere in this text that may also be primary in the eye and orbit include germ cell tumors, hemangiopericytomas, and lymphomas (38, 102, 210).

Table 7.19.
Primary Neural Tumors of the Eye and Orbital Area

Eyelid
Nevi
Melanoma
Schwannoma
Neurofibroma
Merkel cell tumor
Conjunctiva
Nevi
Melanoma
Neurofibroma
Globe
Nevi
Melanoma
Ocular medulloepithelioma (dictyoma)
Retinoblastoma
Neurofibroma
Gliomas and glial (± neuronal) hamartomas
Hemangioblastoma
Orbit (including optic nerve and its sheath)
Optic nerve glioma (astrocytoma, anaplastic astrocytoma, glioblastoma)
Neurofibroma
Schwannoma
Granular cell tumor
Paraganglioma

The accuracy, indications, contraindications, and safety of needle aspiration of the orbit and eye are not yet as precisely defined for this anatomic area as they are, for example, for intracranial lesions. However, some of the recent attempts to examine these questions suggest that an important role for the application of cytohistologic methods to selected lesions in these sites will likely emerge in the near future (7, 93, 96, 112, 134, 189, 202, 204, 233, 238).

Nevi and Melanomas

Melanocytic nevi of a variety of types may involve the eyelids. Among these, the nevus of Ota (congenital oculodermal melanosis) is not only of interest because of its association with an increased incidence of ocular and orbital melanoma (186), but also because of its occasional association with leptomeningeal melanomatosis and with primary meningeal melanomas (20, 48, 84, 194). It should also be emphasized that specialized experience in the interpretation of ocular pigmented lesions is critical to avoid possibly unnecessary enucleations due to a mistaken diagnosis of melanoma. Eagle and Yanoff (46) indicate that about 5% of eyes enucleated for presumed melanoma contain a variety of lesions, both benign (e.g., choroidal or subretinal pigment epithelial hemorrhages, retinal detachments, disciform macular degeneration, benign choroidal hemangiomas, and nevi) and occasionally other malignancies (e.g., metastatic carcinoma, other rare intra-ocular tumors). Sanderson et al. (195) also comment upon benign ocular lesions that may cause confusion with melanoma.

The prognosis of melanomas varies not only with their site within the eye or orbit but also with their cytohistologic features, size, and stage. Familiarity by the pathologist with these unique characteristics of ocular melanomas is essential for proper clinical decision making. For example, melanomas of the eyelid tend to metastasize early and have a less favorable prognosis than those arising in the bulbar conjunctiva (possibly excluding the fornix and caruncle region) or uveal tract.

Cytology of Melanomas (189, 204, 233). The cytologic appearance of melanomas of the eyelids and conjunctivae does not differ significantly from that of the common cutaneous melanomas. Uveal tract melanomas, on the other hand, are commonly divided into three main cytologic varieties (186). The *spindle A cell type* is composed of bland, slender spindle cells with relatively small fusiform nuclei without nucleoli evident. The chromatin is frequently arranged in linear fashion along the central axis of the elongate nucleus, somewhat reminiscent of the Aschoff (or Anitschkow) cell in cardiac Aschoff bodies of rheumatic heart disease. The *spindle B cell type* is composed of larger, more plump and pleomorphic spindle cells with large ovoid nuclei that contain prominent nucleoli. Mitoses are generally more prominent in this variety than in the spindle A cell type. The *epithelioid cell type* consists of large (even giant and bizarre), more pleomorphic cells with abundant cytoplasm, large nuclei (often multinucleated), and very prominent nucleoli. This variety is typically more discohesive than the spindle cell varieties and tends to have more prominent necrosis. Mixtures of two or more cell types are not unusual. The prominence of melanin pigment is quite variable from case to case, and even from cell to cell within the same tumor. Melanin pigment may also be free in the background of the smear and within macrophages. The tumor architecture is variable and may include sheets of cells and fascicular and trabecular (or ribbon-like) arrangements of cells. The latter tend to be oriented along blood vessels.

Retinoblastoma

Retinoblastoma tumor cells closely resemble those of the medulloblastoma. The retinoblastoma is a cellular tumor containing cells with a high N/C ratio, narrow rims of cytoplasm, dense chromatin, a high mitotic rate, and frequent necrosis. The nuclei in retinoblastomas may have a tendency to be more round to oval than angular or carrot-shaped, and true rosettes (Flexner-Wintersteiner type) are more likely to be present than Homer Wright rosettes. Indeed, true rosettes are present in about 70% of cases and are often lined by cells with basally situated nuclei and a lower N/C ratio. The cells forming the rosette may also demonstrate mitotic figures. Such rosettes are less often a conspicuous feature in extra-ocular extensions or metastatic deposits of tumor than in the primary tumor (194). Hematoxyphilic deposits in and around blood vessels (i.e., Azzopardi effect) may be seen in areas of necrosis in retinoblastomas (38, 186). A variant of rosette formation is seen in retinoblastomas in which the rosette is larger and is associated with broad, distinct cytoplasmic processes that traverse a fenestrated membrane side by side in linear or arc-like configurations; these are termed fleurettes. They have been interpreted as evidence of photoreceptor differentiation and may occur not only in retinoblastomas but also in pineocytomas and pineoblastomas (see Table 7.9) (166, 194). Perivascular pseudorosettes may also occur but are typically in the form of residual viable tumor cells clustered around vessels in zones of extensive necrosis, rather than attached to vessel walls by fibrillary processes in viable portions of the tumor. Reactive astrocytic fibrillary gliosis is a common tumor accompaniment, but melanin production by tumor cells is exceptional. Retinoblastomas may invade the optic nerve and thus gain access to the cerebrospinal fluid and neuraxis (Fig. 7.7**E**) and may also metastasize to distant extraneural sites (see Tables 7.14, 7.16, and 7.17).

The differential diagnosis of retinoblastoma, in addition to other small, blue-cell tumors, includes retinal dysplasia (Fig. 7.7**F**). Retinal dysplasia may be a sporadic and uniocular phenomenon or may occur as a component of Norrie's disease (X-linked bilateral ocular anomalies, deafness, and mental retardation) or of trisomy 13-15 (Patau's syndrome, which may include microphthalmos and a variety of other ocular, optic nerve, and CNS developmental defects) (73, 115, 186). Histologically, retinal dysplasia consists of a disordered retinal architecture, which may be focally hypercellular, with many branching tubular profiles that, on cross-section, have the appearance of Flexner-Wintersteiner rosettes.

Also included in the differential diagnosis are retinocytomas, which are benign retinal plaque-like lesions that are non-invasive, contain numerous fleurettes, and are without necrosis or mitotic activity (127).

Retinoblastomas may be bilateral (30% of all cases and over 90% of familial cases). The inherited (familial) form not only demonstrates a greater degree of bilaterality (which may be synchronous or metachronous) but is also associated with a higher incidence of second primary tumors. The latter most often are osteosarcomas, but may also include rhabdomyosarcoma, fibrosarcoma, sebaceous carcinoma, epidermoid carcinoma, melanoma, and Hodgkin's disease (6). These second primary tumors may occur in the field of radiation treatment of the original retinoblastoma, but there is also an increased incidence of such tumors in nonradiated patients (38).

The association of bilateral retinoblastomas with a morphologically similar-appearing neoplasm in the pineal or suprasellar region has also been described and is referred to as a "trilateral retinoblastoma" (26, 186).

Cytology of Retinoblastoma (39, 188, 189, 204, 233) (Fig. 7.7E). Many of the cytologic features discussed under the heading of Medulloblastoma also apply to retinoblastoma, the cytology alone of these tumors being essentially indistinguishable. Smears are highly cellular, with small tumor cells demonstrating hyperchromatic nuclei that are round to angular and generally with inconspicuous or small nucleoli. Cytoplasm is very sparse and poorly defined in these cells, giving a high N/C ratio. Necrosis and calcification may be present in the smear background. The diagnostically more useful architectural features (e.g., Flexner-Wintersteiner rosettes, Homer Wright rosettes, and fleurettes) are better appreciated on tissue sections than on smears or other cytopreparatory techniques.

Ocular Medulloepithelioma (Dictyoma)

This rare tumor develops in the ciliary body and is composed of sheets and convoluted ribbons of mitotically active columnar to small ovoid cells enclosing spaces of variable size and shape. Rosettes resembling the Flexner-Wintersteiner rosettes may occur, as may papillary configurations. This lesion has cytologic features in common with the cerebral medulloepithelioma, including a tendency to differentiate along neural, astrocytic, ependymal, choroid plexus, or mesenchymal lines (e.g., cartilage, skeletal muscle, etc.). The term "teratoid medulloepithelioma" is sometimes used for tumors with mesenchymal differentiation. Thus, confusion with choroid plexus carcinoma and certain germ cell tumors (e.g., immature teratoma, endodermal sinus tumor, combined forms) may occur.

We have not had occasion to examine this tumor using cytopreparatory methods and are not aware of a published report demonstrating the application of these techniques to the ocular medulloepithelioma.

Glial and Other Miscellaneous Primary and Secondary Ocular and Orbital Tumors

Astrocytomas, capillary hemangioblastomas, and possibly oligodendrogliomas may occur as primary ocular tumors (194).

Astrocytomas most commonly arise from the optic nerve and chiasm and typically are of the pilocytic variety. The latter are composed of predominantly spindle-shaped cells with or without associated vacuolated cells with mucinous change (myxomatous appearance), cystic changes, Rosenthal fiber formation, perivascular pseudorosettes, and cells resembling oligodendroglial cells. Anaplastic astrocytomas and glioblastomas may infrequently involve these structures, but high-grade gliomas of the optic nerve and chiasm are more commonly seen in adults than children.

Several of these ocular and optic nerve tumors are more likely to occur in the context of certain neuroectodermal dysplasias (i.e., phakomatoses). These include optic nerve gliomas, meningiomas, and benign peripheral nerve sheath tumors in neurofibromatosis; retinal astrocytic tumors in tuberous sclerosis; and capillary hemangioblastomas and hemangiomas in von Hippel-Lindau disease. Indeed, the presence of any of the glial tumors or hamartomas, vascular tumors, nerve sheath tumors, or meningiomas in the eye or orbit should prompt studies to rule out an occult neuroectodermal dysplasia syndrome, due to the frequency with which such associations occur (see Table 7.13). The optic nerve sheath meningiomas may be of several histologic types but are most often of the meningothelial (syncytial) variety.

The differential diagnosis of retinal astrocytomas or hamartomas also includes massive retinal gliosis, which is a reactive, elevated scar developing near the optic disc following prior hemorrhage or inflammation (186).

It should also be kept in mind that, in children, rhabdomyosarcomas (usually embryonal type) are the most common orbital tumors (209) and retinoblastomas the most common intraocular tumors. The retinoblastoma is the third most common ocular malignancy overall, after choroidal melanoma and metastatic carcinoma (194). The most common metastatic orbital lesion in children is the neuroblastoma, with Ewing's sarcoma somewhat less frequent.

In white adults, the most common orbital tumor is a metastasis from a primary systemic tumor (e.g., carcinoma, lymphoma, leukemia, melanoma, or sarcoma) (186, 197, 217). The most common primary site for a metastatic lesion to the eye or orbit in females is a breast carcinoma, and in males a bronchogenic carcinoma. Less commonly renal, testicular, and gastrointestinal tract primary tumors metastasize to the eye or orbit, and rarely even carcinoid tumors are seen as metastatic or primary orbital tumors (186). Direct spread into the orbit from adjacent structures occasionally serves as a route for meningiomas, chordomas, pituitary adenomas, and other primary tumors within the cranial vault. The most common primary intraocular tumor in white adults is a melanoma of uveal tract origin.

Exceptionally, developmental anomalies presenting in the orbital region (e.g., encephalocele) may mimic a primary neural tumor (38).

Cytology of Miscellaneous Orbital Tumors. The cytology of most of these tumors is discussed elsewhere in this chapter (i.e., pilocytic astrocytoma, hemangioblastoma, schwannoma, neurofibroma, and meningioma).

A few illustrations of ocular region meningiomas (189, 233), histiocytosis X (189), metastatic tumors (204, 233), and lymphoma (204, 233) have been published in the cytologic literature.

Radiation and Chemotherapeutic Effects on CNS Tumors and Adjacent Tissue

Effects on Neural Tumors

Tumor cell necrosis and cyst formation is a common sequel to radiation therapy of radiosensitive CNS tumors. Recurrences, not unexpectedly, will typically occur at the periphery of such cysts. Intralesional vascular and connective tissue changes include vascular wall hyalinization, vascular occlusion, and increased collagen deposition. In nonneural tissue, changes in fibroblasts characteristic—although not pathognomonic—of prior radiation include enlarged, atypical, and often irregularly shaped and vacuolated nuclei. This may or may not be associated with cytoplasmic vacuolization. Although it is not emphasized in the reports on CNS radiation effects, we have observed similar changes in fibroblasts associated with connective tissue proliferation in CNS sites.

Effects on Adjacent Neural Tissues

Early delayed radiation effects include foci of demyelination resembling multiple sclerosis plaques and perivascular lymphoplasmacytic infiltrates (194). Late delayed radiation effects, generally more pronounced in white matter, may include cystic change, coagulative necrosis, demyelination, lymphoplasmacytic perivascular infiltrates, presence of lipid macrophages, occasional presence of eosinophils, perivascular and vascular wall hyalinization and fibrinoid necrosis, endothelial swelling and proliferation, thromboses, presence of amyloid-like material, calcifications, capillary telangiectasias, collagenous fibrosis, fibrillary gliosis, and bizarre or binucleated ganglion cells. Of these, fibrinoid necrosis is the most specific for radionecrosis effect. Intracerebral hemorrhage rarely occurs (175).

There is also some evidence to suggest that the prolonged survival resulting from more effective radiation and/or chemotherapeutic treatment measures may, in some patients, result in the emergence of an increased incidence of neoplasms different than the original tumor type. These may either occur within the irradiated field and/or be secondary to systemic immunosuppressive effects. Within the former group are infrequent examples of meningiomas, sarcomas, and occasional gliomas (86, 103, 130, 194, 211, 220, 239). Within the latter group the situation is more complex, since combination therapy (local radiation plus local or—more commonly—systemic chemotherapy) and a variety of agents with different neoplastic associations may be utilized in various chemotherapeutic protocols. Although effects of systemic radiation in producing secondary neoplasia are theoretically relevant here, systemic chemotherapy is the most common manner of delivery of chemotherapy, and examples of secondary cancers reported with the latter are summarized in Table 7.20.

A mechanism of chemotherapeutic agent delivery unique to the nervous system is the intrathecal route, either via lumbar puncture or implantation of an Ommaya reservoir, with or without combined radiotherapy. In some patients receiving this form of treatment periventricular demyelination, or a more disseminated necrotizing leukoencephalopathy, has been reported (52). A more detailed discussion of these and similar events is reported in Russell and Rubinstein (194). The immunocompromised status of such patients associated with the basic underlying disease state and/or secondary to therapy may also result in a variety of opportunistic infections, which are reviewed in Chapter 8.

Table 7.20A.
Secondary Neoplasms Following Local or Systemic Chemotherapy (30a, 33, 91, 125, 157a, 159, 228)

Acute non-lymphocytic leukemia
Non-Hodgkin's lymphoma
Bone sarcoma
Soft tissue sarcoma (including Kaposi's sarcoma)
Gliomas and other primary neuroepithelial tumors
Skin cancer (including melanoma)
Thyroid carcinoma
Breast carcinoma
GI tract carcinoma
Uterine cervix in situ carcinoma (rarely invasive carcinoma)
Hepatocellular carcinoma
Other miscellaneous tumors

Table 7.20B.
Other Secondary Effects of Anti-neoplastic Therapy on the Nervous System (Radiation and/or Chemotherapy) (30a, 194)

Calcification
White matter gliosis
Diffuse cortical atrophy
Subacute leukoencephalopathy
Cerebellar sclerosis
Wernicke's encephalopathy
Central pontine myelinolysis
Neuroaxonal dystrophy
Neurofibrillary tangles
Necrotic myelopathy and encephalopathy
Spinal subpial demyelination and spinal nerve demyelination
Transverse myelopathy
Vasculopathies

Cytology of Tumor Therapy. In addition to the effects of chemotherapy in neural tissue, which can result in a number of cytologic changes mimicking malignancy, effects of chemotherapy in non-neural tissues must be kept in mind. As noted previously (Table 7.17), primary CNS tumors occasionally, even in the absence of prior surgery, metastasize to extraneural sites such as lung, lymph nodes, etc. Chemotherapy-induced cytologic changes mimicking malignancy may occur in pulmonary cytologic specimens (e.g., due to bleomycin, busulfan), as well as in pituitary tissue (228). Since hypophysectomy is sometimes used as a palliative treatment for certain tumors (i.e., breast carcinoma), the possibility of atypical cells in either pulmonary or pituitary cytologic specimens being related to therapy, rather than metastatic disease, should be kept in mind.

The differential diagnosis of radiation cerebritis versus recurrent neoplasm may also confront the surgical pathologist, since it may be virtually impossible to clinically distinguish these two conditions. Both may be associated with a mass effect, edema, and contrast-enhancing lesions on neuroimaging (CT or MRI) techniques, and both may occur months after therapy is completed (16). Further, both problems may co-exist (24). Although recent advances in positron emission tomography give promise for an eventual noninvasive means of solving this dilemma (16), biopsy is currently utilized in selected cases to plan the most appropriate therapy. Chandrasoma and Apuzzo (28) report that radiated brain tissue usually does not smear well, but smears may display many of the features noted in histologic sections (see above), including gliosis, necrosis, astrocyte atypia, irregular and smudged nuclear chromatin, and vascular hyalinization. They regard cellularity and the degree of cytologic atypia as the most helpful distinguishing features.

The cellularity is described as being mild to moderate in radiation cerebritis and moderate to high in recurrent neoplasia. The degree of cytologic atypia is typically more marked in recurrent neoplasia than in radiation cerebritis. Clearly, caution in interpreting occasional bizarre cells in a moderately cellular specimen, due to the degree of atypia that may occur in benign CNS cells after irradiation, is appropriate. Ancillary studies (i.e., immunohistochemical markers) may be decisive in cases where only occasional neoplastic cells are present, depending on the tumor type (i.e., lymphoma, metastatic carcinoma). However, final distinction between radiation necrosis and recurrent glioma may be impossible without a large number of obviously malignant cells on the smear, and sectioning of the entire sample in permanent sections may be required (155).

Paraneoplastic Syndromes (Remote Effects of Cancer on the Nervous System)

This term encompasses a group of conditions etiologically related to tumors but not resulting from contiguous invasion, metastases, or pressure effects from local mass lesions. While such syndromes are by no means limited to the nervous system, neurological manifestations have thus far dominated the literature on this subject. They may be the presenting sign of an occult tumor, and can cause difficulties in the clinical determination of symptom etiology in known cancer patients (thus complicating treatment decisions). Also, such mechanisms may provide chemical markers identifiable as clues to the underlying tumor type or to the presence of tumor recurrence. An excellent recent review of this topic, which includes 524 references, is that of Bunn and Ridgway (23). These authors indicate that mechanisms of production of such syndromes, where defined, have included:

1. Effects of tumor cell-produced biologically active proteins or polypeptides, their precursors, growth factors, interleukins, cytokines, prostaglandins, fetal proteins (e.g., CEA, AFP), other

Table 7.21.
CSF Abnormalities in Paraneoplastic Syndromes[a]

Paraneoplastic Syndrome	CSF Abnormality
Subacute cerebellar degeneration	Lymphocytosis and increased protein
Dementia	Pleocytosis
Subacute necrotic myelopathy	Pleocytosis may occur; increased protein
Neuropathy (sensory, sensorimotor, or acute ascending forms)	Increased protein
Stroke (related to emboli, hypercoagulable states, etc.)	Variable, depending on whether ischemic or hemorrhagic, proximity to CSF, etc.

[a] Modified from Bunn, P.A. Jr., and Ridgway, E.C.: Paraneoplastic syndromes. Chapter 55 in: De Vita, V.T. Jr., Hellman, S., and Rosenberg, S.A. (Eds.): Cancer. Principles and Practice of Oncology. Ed. 3. J.B. Lippincott Co., Philadelphia, 1989, pp. 1896–1940.

proteins (e.g., immunoglobulins), and enzymes.

2. Autoimmunity or immune complex production and immunosuppression.
3. "Ectopic receptor" production or a competitive blockade of normal hormone action by tumor-produced biologically inactive hormones.
4. "Forbidden contact" in which release of enzymes or other products normally inaccessible to the circulation gain access to the intravascular space via abnormally permeable vasculature (e.g., abnormal tumor vessels or antigenically injured vessels), allowing antigenic reactions, inappropriate initiation of normal physiologic functions, or toxic manifestations to occur.

The importance of these syndromes to the cytopathologist lies in the frequent inclusion of CSF cytologic examinations in the clinical evaluation of such patients and the presence of CSF abnormalities in several of the known syndromes. Examples of such associations are listed in Table 7.21.

References

1. Adams, J.H., Graham, D.I., and Doyle, D.: Brain Biopsy. The Smear Technique for Neurosurgical Biopsies. J.B. Lippincott Co., Philadelphia, 1981.
2. Adamson, T.E., Wiestler, O.D., Kleihues, P., and Yasargil, M.G.: Correlation of clinical and pathological features in surgically-treated craniopharyngiomas. J. Neurosurg. 73:12–17, 1990.
3. Aisner, J., Aisner, S.C., Ostraw, S., Govindan, S., Mummert, K., and Wiernik, P.: Meningeal carcinomatosis from small cell carcinoma of the lung. Consequence of improved survival. Acta Cytol. 23:292–296, 1979.
4. Akhtar, M., Ali, M.A., Sabboh, R., Bakry, M., and Nash, J.E.: Fine-needle aspiration biopsy diagnosis of round cell malignant tumors of childhood. A combined light and electron microscopic approach. Cancer 55:1805–1817, 1985.
5. Arber, D., Bilbao, J., and Bassion, S.: Large-cell anaplastic (Ki-1-positive) lymphoma complicated by disseminated intravascular coagulation. Arch. Pathol. Lab. Med. 115:188–192, 1991.
6. Arya, S., Gilbert, E.F., and Wiedrich, T.A.: Complications of treatment of neoplasia in childhood, including second malignancies. Chapter 17 in: Finegold, M. (Ed.): Pathology of Neoplasia in Children and Adolescents. W.B. Saunders Co., Philadelphia, 1986, pp. 433–464.
7. Augsburger, J.J., Shields, J.A., Folberg, R., Lang, W., O'Hara, B.J., and Claricci, J.D.: Fine needle aspiration biopsy in the diagnosis of intraocular cancer. Cyto-histologic correlations. Ophthalmology 92:39–49, 1985.
8. Bamforth, J.S.G., Riccardi, V.M., Thisen, P., Chitayat, D., Friedman, J.M., Caruthers, J., and Hall, J.G.: Encephalocraniocutaneous lipomatosis. Report of two cases and a review of the literature. Neurofibromatosis. 2:166–173, 1989.
9. Barbosa, M.D., Balsitis, M., Jaspan, T., and Lowe, J.: Intraventricular neurocytoma: a clinical and pathological study of three cases and review of the literature. Neurosurgery 26:1045–1054, 1990.
10. Barnard, R.O.: Smear preparations in the diagnosis of malignant lesions of the central nervous system. In: Koss, L.G., and Coleman, D.V. (Eds.): Advances in Clinical Cytology. Butterworths, London, 1981, pp. 254–269.
11. Begmann, H., and Rastetter, J.: Atlas of Clinical Hematology. Ed. 4. Springer-Verlag, New York, 1989.
12. Bell, W.O., Packer, R.J., Seigel, K.R., Rorke, L.B., Sutton, L.N., Bruce, D.A., and Schut, L.: Leptomeningeal spread of intramedullary spinal cord tumors. Report of three cases. J. Neurosurg. 69:295–300, 1988.

12a. Berger, M.S., Baumeister, B., Geyer, J.R.,

Milstein, J., Kanev, P.M., and LeRoux, P.D.: The risks of metastases from shunting in children with primary central nervous system tumors. J. Neurosurg. 74:872–877, 1991.
13. Berry, A.D. III, Reintjes, S.L., and Kepes, J.J.: Intracranial malignant fibrous histiocytoma with abscess-like tumor necrosis. Case report. J. Neurosurg. 69:780–784, 1988.
13a. Bertoni, F., Unni, K.K., Dahlin, D.C., Beabout, J.W., and Onofrio, B.M.: Calcifying pseudoneoplasms of the neural axis. J. Neurosurg. 72:42–48, 1990.
13b. Bigner, S. Central nervous system. Chapter 18 in: Bibbo, M. (Ed.): Comprehensive Cytopathology. W.B. Saunders, Philadelphia, 1990, pp. 473–478.
13c. Bigner, S.H., Elmore, P.D., Dee, A.L., and Johnston, W.W.: The cytopathology of reactions to ventricular shunts. Acta Cytol. 29:391–396, 1985.
14. Bigner, S.H., and Johnston, W.W.: Cytopathology of the Central Nervous System. In: W.W. Johnston (Ed.): Monographs in Diagnostic Cytopathology, Vol. 3. Masson Publishing USA, Inc., New York, 1983.
15. Bigner, S.H., and Johnston, W.W.: The diagnostic challenge of tumors manifested initially by the shedding of cells into cerebrospinal fluid. Acta Cytol. 28:29–36, 1984.
16. Black, K.L., Mazziotta, J.C., and Becker, D.P.: Brain tumors. West. J. Med. 154:186–197, 1991.
17. Bleyer, W.A.: Biology and pathogenesis of CNS leukemia. Am. J. Pediatr. Hematol. Oncol. 11:57–63, 1989.
18. Bo, L., Mork, S.J., and Nyland, H.: Mononuclear cells in meningiomas. J. Neuropathol. Exp. Neurol. 50:372, 1991.
19. Boogerd, W., and Vroom, T.M.: Meningeal involvement as the initial symptom of B cell chronic lymphatic leukemia. Eur. Neurol. 25:461–464, 1986.
20. Botticelli, A.R., Villani, M., Angiori, P., and Peserico, L.: Meningeal melanocytoma of Meckel's cave associated with ipsilateral Ota's nevus. Case report. Cancer 51:2304–2310, 1983.
21. Bruner, J.M.: Oligodendroglioma: diagnosis and prognosis. Semin. Diagn. Pathol. 4:251–261, 1987.
22. Budka, H.: Intracranial lipomatous hamartomas (intracranial "lipomas"). A study of 13 cases including combinations with medulloblastoma, colloid and epidermoid cysts, angiomatosis and other malformations. Acta Neuropathol. (Berl.) 28:205–222, 1974.
23. Bunn, P.A. Jr., and Ridgway, E.C.: Paraneoplastic syndromes. Chapter 55 in: De Vita, V.T. Jr., Hellman, S., and Rosenberg, S.A. (Eds.): Cancer. Principles and Practice of Oncology. Ed. 3. J.B. Lippincott Co., Philadelphia, 1989, pp. 1896–1940.
24. Burger, P.C.: Malignant astrocyte neoplasms: classification, pathologic anatomy, and response to treatment. Semin. Oncol. 13:16–26, 1986.
25. Burger, P.C., and Kleihues, P.: Cytologic composition of the untreated glioblastoma with implications for evaluation of needle biopsies. Cancer 63:2014–2023, 1989.
26. Burger, P.C., Scheithauer, B.W., and Vogel, F.S.: Surgical Pathology of the Nervous System and Its Coverings. Ed. 3. Churchill Livingstone, New York, 1991.
27. Burger, P.C., Vogel, F.S., Green, S.B., and Strike, T.A.: Glioblastoma multiforme and anaplastic astrocytoma. Pathologic criteria and prognostic implications. Cancer 56:1106–1111, 1985.
28. Chandrasoma, P.T., and Apuzzo, M.L.J.: Stereotactic Brain Biopsy. Igaku-Shoin, New York, 1989.
29. Cheng, C.L.Y., Greenberg, J., and Hoover, L.A.: Prostatic adenocarcinoma metastatic to chronic subdural hematoma membranes. J. Neurosurg. 68:642–644, 1988.
30. Coffin, C.M., Wick, M.R., Brawn, J.T., and Dehner, L.P.: Choroid plexus neoplasms. Clinicopathologic and immunohistochemical studies. Am. J. Surg. Pathol. 10:394–404, 1986.
30a. Cohen, M.E., and Duffner, P.K.: Long-term consequences of CNS treatment for childhood cancer. Part I: Pathologic consequences and potential for oncogenesis. Pediatr. Neurol. 7:157–163, 1991.
31. Colby, T.V., Lombard, C., Yousem, S.A., and Kitaichi, M.: Atlas of Pulmonary Surgical Pathology. W.B. Saunders Co., Philadelphia, 1991, pp. 84–88.
32. Coleman, A., and Schumann, G.B.: Cytodiagnosis and monitoring of acute lymphocytic leukemia and eosinophilia in cerebrospinal fluid. Diagn. Cytopathol. 3:330–334, 1987.
33. Coleman, C.N., and Tucker, M.A.: Secondary cancers. Section 7, Chapter 60, in: De Vita, V.T. Jr., Hellman, S., and Rosenberg, S.A. (Eds.): Cancer. Principles and Practice of Oncology. Ed. 3. J.B. Lippincott Co., Philadelphia, 1989, pp. 2181–2190.
33a. Cookston, M., Cotter, G.W., Schlitt, M., and Bastian, F.O.: Primary angiosarcoma of the brain. South. Med. J. 84:517–520, 1991.
34. Cormack, D.H.: Ham's Histology. Ed. 9. J.B. Lippincott Co., Philadelphia, 1987, p. 447.
35. Curtis, J.L., and Rubinstein, L.J.: Pigmented olfactory neuroblastoma. A new example of melanotic neuroepithelial neoplasm. Cancer 49:2136–2143, 1982.
36. d'Amore, E.S.G., Manivel, J.C., Pettinato, G., Niehans, G.A., and Snover, D.C.: Intestinal ganglioneuromatosis: mucosal and transmural types. A clinicopathologic and immunohistochemical study of six cases. Hum. Pathol. 22:276–286, 1991.
36a. Davis, R.L., and Robertson, D.M. (Eds.): Textbook of Neuropathology. Ed. 2. Williams & Wilkins, Baltimore, 1991.
37. Dehner, L.P.: Peripheral and central primitive neuroectodermal tumors. A nosologic concept

seeking a consensus. Arch. Pathol. Lab. Med. 110:997–1005, 1986.
38. Dehner, L.P.: Pediatric Surgical Pathology. Ed. 2. Williams & Wilkins, Baltimore, 1987, pp. 199–228.
39. den Hartog Jager, W.A.: Color Atlas of C.S.F. Cytopathology. J.B. Lippincott Co., Philadelphia, 1980.
40. Deutsch, M.: Medulloblastoma: staging and treatment outcome. Int. J. Radiat. Oncol. Biol. Phys. 14:1103–1107, 1988.
41. DiLorenzo, N., Lunardi, P., and Fortuna, A.: Granulomolecular hypertrophy of the cerebellum (Lhermitte-Duclos disease). Case report. J. Neurosurg. 60:644–646, 1984.
42. Doshi, H.M., Schochet, S.S. Jr., Gold, M., and Nugent, G.R.: Granulocytic sarcoma presenting as an epidural mass with acute paraparesis in an aleukemic patient. Am. J. Clin. Pathol. 95:228–232, 1991.
43. Dozic, S., Suvakovic, V., Cvetkovic, D., Jevtovic, Dj., and Skender, M.: Neoplastic angioendotheliomatosis (NAE) of the CNS in a patient with AIDS subacute encephalitis, diffuse leucoencephalopathy and meningocerebral cryptococcosis. Clin. Neuropathol. 9:284–289, 1990.
44. Ducatman, B.S., and Scheithauer, B.W.: Malignant peripheral nerve sheath tumors with divergent differentiation. Cancer 54:1049–1057, 1984.
45. Dudley, T.H. Jr., and Moinuddin, S.: Cytologic and immunohistochemical diagnosis of neuroendocrine (Merkel cell) carcinoma in cerebrospinal fluid. Am. J. Clin. Pathol. 91:714–717, 1989.
46. Eagle, R.C. Jr., and Yanoff, M.: The eye. Chapter 51 in: Silverberg, S.G. (Ed.): Principles and Practice of Surgical Pathology. John Wiley and Sons, New York, 1983, 2:1547–1578.
47. Efremidis, A.P., Sabato, U., Taff, I., Krieger, H., and Bekesi, J.G.: Diagnosis of CNS lymphoma using immunofluorescent phenotyping of CSF mononuclear cells. Clin. Neurol. Neurosurg. 88:101–107, 1986.
48. Enriquez, R., Egbert, B., and Bullock, J.: Primary malignant melanoma of central nervous system. Pineal involvement in a patient with nevus of Ota and multiple pigmented skin nevi. Arch. Pathol. 95:392–395, 1973.
49. Erlandson, R.A., and Woodruff, J.M.: Peripheral nerve sheath tumors: an electron microscopic study of 43 cases. Cancer 49:273–287, 1982.
50. Esiri, M.M., and Oppenheimer, D.R.: Diagnostic Neuropathology. A Practical Manual. Blackwell Scientific Publications, Oxford, 1989.
51. Favara, B.E., McCarthy, R.C., and Mierau, G.W.: Histiocytosis X. Chapter 6 in: Finegold, M. (Ed.): Pathology of Neoplasia in Children and Adolescents. Vol. 18 in: Bennington, J.L. (Ed.): Major Problems in Pathology. W.B. Saunders Co., Philadelphia, 1986, pp. 126–144.
52. Filloux, F.M., and Townsend, J.J.: Subacute leukoencephalopathy complicating acute lymphoblastic leukemia. West. J. Med. 146:207–212, 1987.
53. Fischer, J.R., Davey, D.D., Gulley, M.L., and Goeken, J.A.: Blast-like cells in cerebrospinal fluid of neonates. Possible germinal matrix origin. Am. J. Clin. Pathol. 91:255–258, 1989.
54. Flinner, R.L., and Hammond, E.H.: Pathology of the Mediastinum. American Society of Clinical Pathologists Press, Chicago, 1989, pp. 61–83.
55. Flynn, S.D., and Yousem, S.A. Pulmonary meningiomas: a report of two cases. Hum. Pathol. 22:469–474, 1991.
56. Frable, W.J.: Lecture on "Lymph node aspirates." In: 35th Tutorial on Clinical Cytology. Universal City, Calif., Jan. 26, 1991.
57. Franks, A.J.: Diagnostic Manual of Tumours of the Central Nervous System. Churchill Livingstone, New York, 1988.
58. Friede, R.L.: Developmental Neuropathology. Ed. 2. Springer-Verlag, New York, 1989.
59. Friede, R.L., and Pollak, A.: The cytogenetic basis for classifying ependymomas. J. Neuropathol. Exp. Neurol. 37:103–118, 1978.
59a. Frizzera, G., Gajl-Peczalska, K., Sibley, R.K., Rosai, J., Cherwitz, D., and Hurd, D.D.: Rosette formation in malignant lymphoma. Am. J. Pathol. 119:351–356, 1985.
60. Frost, J.K.: The Cell in Health and Disease. Karger, New York, 1986.
61. Gherardi, R., Nguyen, J.P., Gaston, A., and Poirier, J.: Symptomatic xanthogranuloma of the third ventricle: a clinicopathological report. Eur. Neurol. 23:156–162, 1984.
62. Gindhart, T.D., and Tsukahara, Y.C.: Cytologic diagnosis of pineal germinoma in cerebrospinal fluid and sputum. Acta Cytol. 23:341–346, 1979.
63. Glass, J.P., Melamed, M., Chernik, N.L., and Posner, J.B.: Malignant cells in cerebrospinal fluid (CSF): the meaning of a positive CSF cytology. Neurology 29:1369–1375, 1979.
64. Glass, J.P., Van Tassel, P., Keating, M.J., Cork, A., Trujillo, J., and Holmes, R.: Central nervous system complications of a newly recognized subtype of leukemia: AMML with a pericentric inversion of chromosome 16. Neurology 37:639–644, 1987.
65. Glenner, G.G., and Grimley, P.M.: Tumors of the Extra-Adrenal Paraganglion System (Including Chemoreceptors). Atlas of Tumor Pathology. Second Series. Fascicle 9. Armed Forces Institute of Pathology, Washington D.C., 1974.
66. Goldwein, J.W., Glauser, T.A., Packer, R.J., Finlay, J.L., Sutton, L.N., Curran, W.J., Laehy, J.M., Rorke, L.B., Schut, L., and D'Angio, G.J.: Recurrent intracranial ependymomas in children. Survival, patterns of failure, and prognostic factors. Cancer 66:557–563, 1990.

67. Grote, T.H., Grosh, W.W., List, A.F., Wiley, R., Cousar, J.B., and Johnson, D.H.: Primary lymphoma of the central nervous system. A report of 20 cases and a review of the literature. Am. J. Clin. Oncol. (CCT), 12:93–100, 1989.
68. Guarda, L.A.: Intraoperative cytologic diagnosis. Evaluation of 370 consecutive intraoperative cytologies. Diagn. Cytopathol. 6:235–242, 1990.
69. Hadfield, M.G., Ghatak, N.R., and Wanger, G.P.: Xanthogranulomatous colloid cyst of the third ventricle. Acta Neuropathol. (Berl.), 66:343–346, 1985.
70. Hafiz, M.A., and Ekanem, I.-O. A.: Cytologic diagnosis of seminoma metastatic to the central nervous system. A case report. Acta Cytol. 27:663–665, 1983.
71. Hardman, J.M., Schochet, S.S. Jr., and Libcke, J.H.: Rosenthal fibers in ovarian teratomas. Arch. Pathol. Lab. Med. 93:448–452, 1972.
72. Harms, D., Janig, U., and Gobel, U.: Gliomatosis peritonei in childhood and adolescence. Clinicopathological study of 13 cases including immunohistochemical findings. Pathol. Res. Pract. 184:422–430, 1989.
72a. Harris, C.P., Townsend, J.J., Brockmeyer, D.L., and Heilbrun, M.P.: Cerebral granular cell tumor occurring with glioblastoma multiforme: case report. Surg. Neurol. 36:202–206, 1991.
73. Harry, J.: The eye and associated structures. Chapter 24 in: Weller, R.O. (Ed.): Nervous System, Muscle and Eyes. Vol. 4 of: Symmers, W. St. C. (Ed.): Systemic Pathology. Ed. 3. Churchill Livingstone, New York, 1990, pp. 668–753.
74. Hassoun, J., Gambarelli, D., Grisoli, F., Pellet, W., Salamon, G., Pellissier, J.F., and Toga, M.: Central neurocytoma. An electron microscopic study of two cases. Acta Neuropathol. (Berl.), 56:151–156, 1982.
75. Heimann, A., and Merino, M.J.: Carcinomatous meningitis as the initial manifestation of breast cancer. Acta Cytol. 30:25–28, 1986.
76. Herndon, R.M., and Brumback, R.A. (Eds.): The Cerebrospinal Fluid. Kluwer Academic Publishers, Boston, 1989.
77. Hoefnagels, W.A.J., Speelman, J.D., and Hische, E.A.H.: Diagnosis of a primary non-Hodgkin's lymphoma of the central nervous system by examination of the cerebrospinal fluid. Clin. Vol. Neurol. Neurosurg. 88:45–48, 1986.
78. Hogeman, P.H.G., Veerman, A.J.P., Huismans, D.R., and Van Zantwijk, I.H.: Common acute lymphoblastic leukemia antigen-positive cells in normal bone marrow. Blood 66:246, 1985.
79. Hogeman, P.H.G., Veerman, A.J.P., Van Zantwijk, C.H., and Huismans, D.R.: Peanut agglutinin distinguishes CALLA positive reactive bone marrow cells from leukaemic blasts. Br. J. Hematol. 59:392–394, 1985.
80. Homans, A.C., Barker, B.E., Forman, E.N., Cornell, C.J., Dickerman, J.D., and Truman, J.T.: Immunophenotypic characteristics of cerebrospinal fluid cells in children with acute lymphoblastic leukemia at diagnosis. Blood 76:1807–1811, 1990.
81. Honma, K., Watanabe, H., Ohnishi, Y., Tachikawa, S., and Tachikawa, K.: Epithelioid malignant schwannoma. A case report. Acta Pathol. Jpn. 39:195–202, 1989.
82. Hooijkaas, H., Hählen, K., Adriaansen, H.J., Dekker, I., van Zanen, G.E., and van Dongen, J.J.M.: Terminal deoxynucleotidyl transferase (TdT)-positive cells in cerebrospinal fluid and development of overt CNS leukemia: a 5-year follow-up study in 113 children with a TdT-positive leukemia or non-Hodgkin's lymphoma. Blood 74:416–422, 1989.
83. Horoupian, D.S., Lax, F., and Suzuki, K.: Extracerebral leptomeningeal astrocytoma mimicking a meningioma. Arch. Pathol. Lab. Med. 103:676–679, 1979.
84. Horsey, W.J., Bilbao, J.M., Nethercott, J., Myers, R., and Hoffman, H.J.: Oculodermal melanosis (naevus of Ota) complicated by multiple intracranial tumors. Le Journal Canadien des Sciences Neurologique 7:101–107, 1980.
85. Hruban, R.H., Traganos, F., Reuter, V.E., and Huvos, A.G.: Chordomas with malignant spindle cell components. A DNA flow cytometric and immunohistochemical study with histogenetic implications. Am. J. Pathol. 137:435–447, 1990.
86. Huang, C-I., Chiou, W-H., and Ho, D.M.: Oligodendroglioma occurring after radiation therapy for pituitary adenoma. J. Neurol. Neurosurg. Psychiatry 50:1619–1624, 1987.
87. Hunt, S.J., and Johnson, P.C.: Melanotic ganglioglioma of the pineal region. Acta Neuropathol. (Berl.), 79:222–225, 1989.
88. Jane, J.A., and Yashon, D.: Cytology of Tumors Affecting the Nervous System. Charles C. Thomas, Springfield, Ill, 1969.
89. Johannsson, J.H., Rekate, H.L., and Roessmann, U.: Gangliogliomas: pathological and clinical correlation. J. Neurosurg. 54:58–63, 1981.
90. Kalyan-Raman, U.P., and Olivero, W.C.: Ganglioglioma: a correlative clinicopathological and radiological study of ten surgically treated cases with follow-up. Neurosurgery 20:428–433, 1987.
90a. Kamiya, M., Tateyama, H., Fujiyoshi, Y., Tada, T., Eimoto, T., Shibata, H., and Hashizume, Y.: Cerebrospinal fluid cytology in immature teratoma of the central nervous system. A case report. Acta Cytol. 35:757–760, 1991.
91. Kanakura, Y., Yonezawa, T., Hamaguchi, Y., Otsuka, A., Matayoshi, Y., Kondoh, H., Tamaki, T., Katagiri, S., Kanayama, Y., Nishiura, T., Aozasa, K., and Tarui, S.: Acute promyelocytic

leukemia with an intracranial mass and meningeal involvement after treatment of non-Hodgkin's lymphoma. Cancer 59:94–98, 1987.
92. Kapff, C.T., and Jandl, J.H.: Blood. Atlas and Sourcebook of Hematology. Little, Brown and Co., Boston, 1981.
93. Karcioglu, Z.A., Gordon, R.A., and Karcioglu, G.L.: Tumor seeding in ocular fine needle aspiration biopsy. Ophthalmology 92:1763–1767, 1985.
94. Kawano, N., Ito, H., Yada, K., and Yagishita, S.: Presence of gliomas mimicking cerebellar hemangioblastoma. J. Neuropathol. Exp. Neurol. 49:274, 1990.
95. Kennedy, R.E.: An evaluation of 820 orbital cases. Trans. Am. Ophthalmol. Soc. 82:134–154, 1984.
96. Kennerdell, J.S., Dubois, P.J., Dekker, A., and Johnson, B.L.: CT-guided fine needle aspiration biopsy of orbital optic nerve tumors. Ophthalmology 87:491–496, 1980.
97. Kepes, J.J.: "Xanthomatous" lesions of the central nervous system: definition, classification and some recent observations. In: Zimmerman, H.M. (Ed.): Progress in Neuropathology. Vol. 4. Grune & Stratton, New York, 1979, pp. 179–213.
98. Kepes, J.J.: Histiocytosis X. In: Vinken, P.J., and Bruyn, G.W. (Eds.): Handbook of Clinical Neurology, Vol. 38. North-Holland Publishing, Amsterdam, 1979, pp. 93–117.
99. Kepes, J.J.: Meningiomas. Biology, Pathology and Differential Diagnosis. Masson Publishing USA, New York, 1982.
100. Kepes, J.J., and Rubinstein, L.J.: Malignant gliomas with heavily lipidized (foamy) tumor cells: a report of three cases with immunoperoxidase study. Cancer 47:2451–2459, 1981.
101. Kerr, R.S.C., Hughes, J.T., Blamires, T., and Teddy, P.J.: Lymphomatoid granulomatosis apparently confined to one temporal lobe. Case report. J. Neurosurg. 67:612–615, 1987.
102. Kirmani, M.H., Thomas, E.L., Rao, N.A., and Laborde, R.P.: Intraocular reticulum cell sarcoma: diagnosis by choroidal biopsy. Br. J. Ophthalmol. 71:748–752, 1987.
103. Kitanaka, C., Shitara, N., Nakagomi, T., Nakamura, H., Genka, S., Nakagawa, K., Akanuma, A., Aoyama, H., and Takakura, K.: Postradiation astrocytoma. Report of two cases. J. Neurosurg. 70:469–474, 1989.
104. Kjeldsberg, C.R., and Knight, J.A.: Body Fluids. Laboratory Examination of Amniotic, Cerebrospinal, Seminal, Serous and Synovial Fluids: A Textbook Atlas. Ed. 2. American Society of Clinical Pathologists Press, Chicago, 1986.
105. Knecht, H., Budmiger, H., Groscurth, P., and Streuli, R.A.: Central nervous system involvement in hairy cell leukemia. Klin. Wochenschr. 63:423–427, 1985.
106. Kölmel, H.W.: Atlas of Cerebrospinal Fluid Cells. Ed. 2. Springer-Verlag, New York, 1977.
107. Kondziolka, D., Bernstein, M., Resch, L., Tator, C.H., Fleming, J.F.R., Vanderlinden, R.G., and Schutz, H.: Significance of hemorrhage into brain tumors: clinicopathological study. J. Neurosurg. 67:852–857, 1987.
108. Koo, C.H., Rappaport, H., Sheibani, K., Pangalis, G.A., Nathwani, B.N., and Winberg, C.D.: Imprint cytology of non-Hodgkin's lymphomas. Based on a study of 212 immunologically characterized cases. Hum. Pathol. 20:1–138 (Suppl. 1), 1989.
109. Koss, L.G.: Diagnostic Cytology and its Histopathological Bases. Ed. 3. J.B. Lippincott Co., Philadelphia, 1979.
110. Kovacs, K., and Howath, E.: Tumors of the Pituitary Gland. Atlas of Tumor Pathology. Second Series. Fascicle 21. Armed Forces Institute of Pathology, Washington D.C., 1986.
111. Kraichoke, S., Cosgrove, M., and Chandrasoma, P.T.: Granulomatous inflammation in pineal germinoma: a cause of diagnostic failure at steretaxic brain biopsy. Am. J. Surg. Pathol. 12:655–660, 1988.
112. Krohel, G.B., Tobin, D.R., and Chavis, R.M.: Inaccuracy of fine needle aspiration biopsy. Ophthalmology 92:666–670, 1985.
113. Kumar, P.V., Esfahani, F.N., Tabei, S.Z., and Malekzadeh, R.: Cytopathology of alpha chain disease involving the central nervous system and pleura. Acta Cytol. 32:902–907, 1988.
113a. Lachance, D.H., O'Neill, B.P., Macdonald, D.R., Jaeckle, K.A., Witzig, T.E., Li, C.-Y., and Posner, J.B.: Primary leptomeningeal lymphoma: report of 9 cases, diagnosis with immunocytochemical analysis, and review of the literature. Neurology 41:95–100, 1991.
114. Lane, P.K., Townsend, R.M., Beckstead, J.H., and Corash, L.: Central nervous system involvement in a patient with chronic lymphocytic leukemia and non-Hodgkin's lymphoma (Richter's syndrome), with concordant cell surface immunoglobulin isotypic and immunophenotypic markers. Am. J. Clin. Pathol. 89:254–259, 1988.
115. Larroche, J.-C.: Malformations of the nervous system. Chapter 10 in: Adams, J.H., Corsellis, J.A.N., and Duchen, L.W. (Eds.): Greenfield's Neuropathology. Ed. 4. John Wiley and Sons, New York, 1984, p. 411.
116. Lattes, R., and Bigotti, G.: Lipoblastic meningioma: "vacuolated meningioma." Hum. Pathol. 22:164–171, 1991.
117. Lauer, S.J., Kirchner, P.A., and Camitta, B.M.: Identification of leukemic cells in the cerebrospinal fluid from children with acute lymphoblastic leukemia: advances and dilemmas. Am. J. Pediatr. Hematol. Oncol. 11:64–73, 1989.

118. Lewis, A.J.: Sarcoma metastatic to the brain. Cancer 61:593–601, 1988.
119. Liwnicz, B.B., and Rodriquez, C.A.: The central nervous system. Chapter 16 in: Koss, L.G., Woyke, S., and Olszewski, W.: Aspiration Biopsy. Cytologic Interpretation and Histologic Bases. Igaku-Shoin, New York, 1985, pp. 457–490.
120. Llombart-Bosch, A., Terrier-Lacombe, J., Peydro-Olaya, A., and Contesso, G.: Peripheral neuroectodermal sarcoma of soft tissue (peripheral neuroepithelioma): a pathologic study of ten cases with differential diagnosis regarding other small, round-cell sarcomas. Hum. Pathol. 20:273–280, 1989.
121. Loesel, L.S.: Fine needle aspiration cytology of a cerebral ganglioglioma. Report of a case. Acta Cytol. 32:391–394, 1988.
122. Longacre, T.A., Foucar, K., Crago, S., Chen, I.-M., Griffith, B., Dressler, L., McConnell, T.S., Duncan, M., and Gribble, J.: Hematogones: a multiparameter analysis of bone marrow precursor cells. Blood 73:543–552, 1989.
123. LoRusso, P.M., Tapazoglou, E., Zarbo, R.J., Cullis, P.A., Austin, D., and Al-Sarraf, M.: Intracranial astrocytoma with diffuse bone marrow metastases: a case report and review of the literature. J. Neurooncol. 6:53–59, 1988.
124. Lunardi, P., Missori, P., Rizzo, A., and Gaglairdi, F.M.: Chemical meningitis in ruptured intracranial dermoid. Case report and review of the literature. Surg. Neurol. 32:449–452, 1989.
124a. Mackenzie, I.R.A., and Gilbert, J.J.: Cysts of the neuraxis of endodermal origin. J. Neurol. Neurosurg. Psychiatry 54:572–575, 1991.
125. Malone, M., Lumley, H., and Erdohazi, M.: Astrocytoma as a second malignancy in patients with acute lymphoblastic leukemia. Cancer 57:1979–1985, 1986.
126. Marcus, P.B., Couch, W.D., and Martin, J.H.: Crystals in a gastric schwannoma. Ultrastruct. Pathol. 2:139–145, 1981.
127. Margo, C., Hidayat, A., Kopelman, J., and Zimmerman, L.E.: Retinocytoma. A benign variant of retinoblastoma. Arch. Ophthalmol. 101:1519–1531, 1983.
128. Marigil, M.A., Pardo-Mindan, F.J., and Joly, M.: Diagnosis of chordoma by cytologic examination of cerebrospinal fluid. Am. J. Clin. Pathol. 80:402–404, 1983.
129. Martin-Reay, D.G., Shattuck, M.C., and Guthrie, F.W. Jr.: Psammomatous melanotic schwannoma: an additional component of Carnoy's complex. Report of a case. Am. J. Clin. Pathol. 95:484–489, 1991.
130. Marus, G., Levin, C.V., and Rutherfoord, G.S.: Malignant glioma following radiotherapy for unrelated primary tumors. Cancer 58:886–894, 1986.
131. Matsushima, T., Fukui, M., Kitamura, K., Soejima, T., Ohta, M., and Okano, H.: Mixed colloid cyst - xanthogranuloma of the third ventricle. A light and electron microscopic study. Surg. Neurol. 24:457–462, 1985.
132. McComb, R.D., and Burger, P.C.: Choroid plexus carcinoma. Report of a case with immunochemical and ultrastructural observations. Cancer 51:470–475, 1983.
133. McIntosh, S., and Ritchey, A.K.: Diagnostic problems in cerebrospinal fluid of children with lymphoid malignancies. Am. J. Pediatr. Hematol. Oncol. 8:28–31, 1986.
134. Midena, E., Segato, T., Piermarocchi, S., and Boccato, P.: Fine needle aspiration biopsy in ophthalmology. Surv. Ophthalmol. 29:410–422, 1985.
135. Milbouw, G., Born, J.D., Martin, D., Collignon, J., Hans, P., Reznik, M., and Bounal, J.: Clinical and radiological aspects of dysplastic gangliocytoma (Lhermitte-Duclos disease); a report of two cases with review of the literature. Neurosurgery 22:124–128, 1988.
136. Miller, D.C., Knee, R., Schoenfeld, S., Wasserstrom, W.R., and Karp, G.: Non-Hodgkin's lymphoma of the central nervous system after treatment of Hodgkin's disease. Am. J. Clin. Pathol. 91:481–485, 1989.
137. Miller, R.R., Lin, F., and Mallonee, M.M.: Cytologic diagnosis of gliomatosis cerebri. Acta Cytol. 25:37–39, 1981.
138. Mork, S.J., and Rubinstein, L.J.: Ependymoblastoma. A reappraisal of a rare embryonal tumor. Cancer 55:1536–1542, 1985.
139. Moseley, R.P., Davies, A.G., Bourne, S.P., Popham, C., Carrel, S., Monro, P., and Coakham, H.B.: Neoplastic meningitis in malignant melanoma: diagnosis with monoclonal antibodies. J. Neurol. Neurosurg. Psychiatry 52:881–886, 1989.
140. Mostofi, F.K., and Price, E.B. Jr.: Tumors of the Male Genital System. Atlas of Tumor Pathology. Second Series. Fascicle 8. Armed Forces Institute of Pathology, Washington D.C., 1973.
141. Muehleck, S.D., McKenna, R.W., Gale, P.F., and Brunning, R.D.: Terminal deoxynucleotidyl transferase (TdT)-positive cells in bone marrow in the absence of hematologic malignancy. Am. J. Clin. Pathol. 79:277–284, 1983.
142. Myers, T., Egelhoff, J., and Myers, M.: Glioblastoma multiforme presenting as osteoblastic metastatic disease: case report and review of the literature. Am. J. Neuroradiol. 11:802–803, 1990.
143. Nag, S.: The ependyma and choroid plexus. Chapter 2 in: Davis, R.L., and Robertson, D.M. (Eds.): Textbook of Neuropathology. Ed. 2. Williams & Wilkins, Baltimore, 1991, pp. 95–114.
144. Nakamura, T., Hirato, J., Hotchi, M., Kyoshima, K., and Nakamura, Y.: Astrocytoma with granular cell tumor-like changes. Report of a case with histochemical and ultrastructural characterization of granular cells. Acta Pathol. Jpn. 40:206–211, 1990.

145. Nakhleh, R.E., Manivel, J.C., Hurd, D., and Sung, J.H.: Central nervous system lymphomas. Immunohistochemical and clinicopathologic study of 26 autopsy cases. Arch. Pathol. Lab. Med. 113:1050–1056, 1989.
146. Namiki, T.S., Nichols, P., Young, T., Martin, S.E., and Chandrasoma, P.: Stereotaxic biopsy diagnosis of central nervous system lymphoma. Am. J. Clin. Pathol. 90:40–45, 1988.
147. Naylor, A.R., MacGregor, J.E., Hutcheon, A.W., and Best, P.V.: Meningeal carcinomatosis from a clinically undiagnosed signet-ring cell primary in the gallbladder. Surg. Neurol. 29:315–318, 1988.
147a. Neglia, J.P., Meadows, A.T., Robison, L.L., Kim, T.H., Newton, W.A., Ruymann, F.B., Sather, H.N., and Hammond, G.D.: Second neoplasms after acute lymphoblastic leukemia in childhood. N. Engl. J. Med. 325:1330–1336, 1991.
148. Nelson, J.S., Tsukada, Y., Schoenfeld, D., Fulling, K., Lamarche, J., and Peress, N.: Necrosis as a prognostic criterion in malignant supratentorial, astrocytic gliomas. Cancer 52:550–554, 1983.
149. Ng, T.H.K., and Poon, W.S.: Gliosarcoma of the posterior fossa with features of a malignant fibrous histiocytoma. Cancer 65:1161–1166, 1990.
150. Ng, T.H.K., Fung, C.F., and Ma, L.T.: The pathological spectrum of desmoplastic infantile gangliogliomas. Histopathology 16:235–241, 1990.
151. Nguyen, G.-K., Johnson, E.S., and Mielke, B.W.: Cytology of meningiomas and neurilemmomas in crush preparations. A useful adjunct to frozen section diagnosis. Acta Cytol. 32:362–366, 1988.
152. Nguyen, G.-K., and Neifer, R.: The cells of benign and malignant hemangiopericytomas in aspiration biopsy. Diagn. Cytopathol. 1:327–331, 1985.
153. Nishio, S., Mizuno, J., Barrow, D.L., Takei, Y., and O'Brien, M.S.: Intracranial extracerebral glioneural heterotopia. Child's Nerv. Syst. 4:244–248, 1988.
154. Nishioka, H., Ii, K., Llena, J.F., and Hirano, A.: Immunohistochemical study of granular cell tumors of the neurohypophysis. J. Neuropathol. Exp. Neurol. 50:363, 1991.
155. Nochomovitz, L., Sidawy, M., Silverberg, S., Jannotta, F., and Schwartz, A.: Intraoperative Consultation. A Guide to Smears, Imprints and Frozen Sections. American Society of Clinical Pathologists Press, Chicago, 1989.
156. Norton, J.A., Doppman, J.L., and Jensen, R.T.: Cancer of the endocrine system. Chapter 39 in: De Vita, V.T. Jr., Hellman, S., and Rosenberg, S.A.: Cancer. Principles and Practice of Oncology. Ed. 3. J.B. Lippincott Co., Philadelphia, 1989, pp. 1303–1314.
157. O'Dowd, G.J., and Schumann, G.B.: Aspiration cytology and cytochemistry of coccygeal chordoma. A case report and review of the literature. Acta Cytol. 27:178–183, 1983.
158. O'Hara, M.F., Cousar, J.B., Glick, A.D., and Collins, R.D.: Multiparameter approach to the diagnosis of hematopoietic-lymphoid neoplasms in body fluids. Diagn. Cytopathol. 1:33–38, 1985.
159. O'Neill, B.P., Habermann, T.M., Banks, P.M., O'Fallon, J.R., and Earle, J.D.: Primary central nervous system lymphoma as a variant of Richter's syndrome in two patients with chronic lymphocytic leukemia. Cancer 64:1296–1300, 1989.
160. O'Neill, B.P., Kelly, P.J., Earle, J.D., Scheithauer, B., and Banks, P.M.: Computer-assisted stereotaxic biopsy for the diagnosis of primary central nervous system lymphoma. Neurology 37:1160–1164, 1987.
161. O'Sullivan, M.G., Keohane, C., and Buckley, T.F.: Paraganglioma of the cauda equina: a case report and review of the literature. Br. J. Neurosurg. 4:63–68, 1990.
162. Odaki, G., Yamaki, T., and Naruse, S.: Neurenteric cyst with meningomyelocele. Case report. J. Neurosurg. 45:352–356, 1976.
163. Odom, L.F., Wilson, H., Cullen, J., Bank, J., Blake, M., and Jamieson, B.: Significance of blasts in low-cell-count cerebrospinal fluid specimens from children with acute lymphoblastic leukemia. Cancer 66:1748–1754, 1990.
164. Oehmichen, M.: Cerebrospinal Fluid Cytology. An Introduction and Atlas. W.B. Saunders Co., Philadelphia, 1976.
165. Ojeda, V.J., Spangnolo, D.V., and Vaughan, R.J.: Palisades in primary cerebral neuroblastoma simulating so-called polar spongioblastoma. A light and electron microscopical study of an adult case. Am. J. Surg. Pathol. 11:316–322, 1987.
166. Okazaki, H., and Scheithauer, B.W.: Slide Atlas of Neuropathology. Gower Medical Publishing, New York, 1988.
167. Onda, K., Tanaka, R., Takahashi, H., Takeda, N., and Ikuta, F.: Cerebral glioblastoma with cerebrospinal fluid dissemination: a clinicopathological study of 14 cases examined by complete autopsy. Neurosurgery 25:533–540, 1989.
168. Ozawa, T., Terabayashi, T., Takahashi, H., Tekeda, N., Ito, Y., Saito, A., Sigiyama, Y., and Ikuta, F.: Metastatic intracranial carcinoid with immunohistochemical observation. J. Neurosurg. 73:130–134, 1990.
169. Padberg, G.W., Schot, J.D.L., Vielvoye, G.J., Bots, G.T.A.M., and de Beer, F.C.: Lhermitte-Duclos disease and Cowden disease: a single phakomatosis. Ann. Neurol. 29:517–523, 1991.
170. Page, D.L., DeLellis, R.A., and Hough, A.J. Jr.: Tumors of the Adrenal. Atlas of Tumor Pathology. Second Series, Fascicle 23. Armed Forces Institute of Pathology, Washington D.C., 1986.
170a. Pallini, R., Bozzini, V., Scerrati, M., Zuppi, C., Zappacosta, B., and Rossi, G.F.: Bone metastasis

associated with shunt-related peritoneal deposits from a pineal germinoma. Case report and review of the literature. Acta Neurochir. (Wien) 109:78–83, 1991.
171. Pappas, C.T.E., Johnson, P.C., and Sonntag, V.K.H.: Signet-ring cell lymphoma of the central nervous system. J. Neurosurg. 69:789–792, 1988.
172. Parham, D.M., Thompson, E., Fletcher, B.,and Meyer, W.H.: Metastatic small cell tumor of bone with "true" rosettes and glial fibrillary acidic protein positivity. Am. J. Clin. Pathol. 95:166–171, 1991.
173. Paulis, W., and Peiffer, J.: Intratumoral histologic heterogeneity of gliomas. A quantitative study. Cancer 64:442–447, 1989.
174. Pearl, G.S., Takei, Y., Bakay, R.A.E., and Davis, P.: Intraventricular primary cerebral neuroblastoma in adults: report of three cases. Neurosurgery 16:847–849, 1985.
174a. Peeples, D.M., Stern, B.J., Jiji, V., and Sahni, K.S.: Germ cell tumors masquerading as central nervous system sarcoidosis. Arch. Neurol. 48:554–556, 1991.
175. Pendlebury, W.W., Anderson, M.L., Goldsby, R.E., and Sullivan, J.K.: Intracerebral hemorrhage as a complication of delayed radionecrosis. J. Neuropathol. Exp. Neurol. 50:370, 1991.
175a. Pernicone, P.J., Scheithauer, B.W., Howath, E., and Kovacs, K. Pituitary and sellar region. Chapter 13 in: Sternberg, S.S. (Ed.): Histology for Pathologists. Raven Press, New York, 1992, pp. 279–300.
176. Pezeshkpour, G.H., Henry, J.M., and Armbrustmacher, V.W.: Spinal metastases. A rare mode of presentation of brain tumors. Cancer 54:353–356, 1984.
177. Popoff, N., and Feigin, I.: Heterotopic central nervous tissue in subarachnoid space. Arch. Pathol. 78:533–539, 1964.
178. Raimondi, A.J., Mullan, S., Evans, P.E.: Human brain tumors: an electron-microscopic study. J. Neurosurg. 19:731–753, 1962.
179. Raroque, H.G. Jr., Mandler, R.N., Griffey, M.S., Orrison, W.W., and Kornfeld, M.: Neoplastic angioendotheliomatosis. Arch Neurol. 47:929–930, 1990.
180. Rautonen, J.: Elevated cerebrospinal fluid leukocyte count and protein concentration at diagnosis: independent risk factors in children with acute lymphoblastic leukemia. Blut 56:265–268, 1988.
181. Reimund, E.L., Sitton, J.E., and Harkin, J.C.: Pigmented choroid plexus papilloma. Arch. Pathol. Lab. Med. 114:902–905, 1990.
181a. Riazmontazer, N., and Bedayat, G.: Cytodiagnosis of meningioma with atypical cytologic features. Acta Cytol. 35:501–504, 1991.
181b. Riazmontazer, N., and Beddayat, G.R.: A case of calcified cerebral neuroblastoma diagnosed cytologically in intraoperative imprint smears. Acta Cytol. 35:253–254, 1991.
182. Ritz, J.: (Letter to the editor). Blood 66:246–247, 1985.
182a. Rorat, E., Yang, W., and De La Torre, R.: Fine needle aspiration cytology of parapharyngeal meningioma. Acta Cytol. 35:497–500, 1991.
183. Rorke, L.B.: Presidential Address: The cerebellar medulloblastoma and its relationship to primitive neuroectodermal tumors. J. Neuropathol. Exp. Neurol. 42:1–15, 1983.
184. Rorke, L.B.: Relationship of morphology of ependymoma in children to prognosis. Prog. Exp. Tumor Res. 30:170–174, 1987.
185. Rorke, L.B., Gilles, F.H., Davis, R.L., and Becker, L.E.: Revision of the World Health Organization classification of brain tumors for childhood brain tumors. Cancer 56:1869–1886, 1985.
186. Rosai, J.: Ackerman's Surgical Pathology. The C.V. Mosby Co., St. Louis, 1989, pp. 809–813.
187. Rosenblatt, H.M., and Schearer, W.T.: Immunodeficiency and cancer. Chapter 3 in: Finegold, M. (Ed.): Pathology of Neoplasia in Children and Adolescents. W.B. Saunders Co., Philadelphia, 1986, pp. 31–45.
188. Rosenthal, D.L.: Cytology of the central nervous system. In: Wied, G.L. (Ed.): Monographs in Clinical Cytology, Vol. 8, S. Karger, New York, 1984.
189. Rosenthal, D.L., Mandell, D.B., and Glasgow, B.J.: Eye. Chapter 19 in: Bibbo, M. (Ed.): Comprehensive Cytopathology. W.B. Saunders Co., Philadelphia, 1991, pp. 484–501.
190. Ross, G.W., and Rubinstein, L.J.: Lack of histopathological correlation of malignant ependymomas with postoperative survival. J. Neurosurg. 70:31–36, 1989.
191. Roy, E.P. III, Rogers, J.S. II, and Riggs, J.E.: Intracranial granulocytic sarcoma in postpolycythemia myeloid metaplasia. South. Med. J. 82:1564–1567, 1989.
192. Rubinstein, L.J.: Embryonal central neuroepithelial tumors and their differentiating potential: review article. J. Neurosurg. 62:795–805, 1985.
193. Rubinstein, L.J.: Primitive neuroectodermal tumors (Letter). Arch. Pathol. Lab. Med. 111:310–311, 1987 (and reply by Dehner, L.P.: ibid, p. 311; reply by Triche, T.J.: ibid, p. 311–312).
194. Russell, D.S., and Rubinstein, L.J.: Pathology of Tumours of the Nervous System. Ed. 5. Williams & Wilkins, Baltimore, 1989.
195. Sanderson, T.L., Pustai, W., Shelley, L., Gelender, H., and Ng, A.: Cytologic evaluation of ocular lesions. Acta Cytol. 24:391–400, 1980.
196. Schabet, M., Kloeter, I., Adam, T., Heidemann, E., and Wietholter, H.: Diagnosis and treatment of meningeal carcinomatosis in ten patients with breast cancer. Eur. Neurol. 25:403–411, 1986.
197. Schachat, A.P., Markowitz, J.A., Guyer, D.R., Burke, P.J., Karp, J.E., and Graham, M.L.: Ophthalmic manifestations of leukemia. Arch. Ophthalmol. 107:697–700, 1989.

198. Scheithauer, B.W.: Central nervous system and pituitary. Chapter 8 in: Silva, E.G., and Kraemer, B.B. (Eds.): Intraoperative Pathologic Diagnosis. Frozen Section and Other Techniques. Williams & Wilkins, Baltimore, 1987, pp. 167–219.
199. Scheithauer, B.W., Nora, F.E., LeChago, J., Wick, M.R., Crawford, B.G., Weiland, L.H., and Carney, J.A.: Duodenal gangliocytic paraganglioma. Clinicopathologic and immunocytochemical study of 11 cases. Am. J. Clin. Pathol. 86:559–565, 1986.
200. Scherer, H.J.: Structural development in gliomas. Am. J. Cancer 34:333–351, 1938.
201. Schmidbauer, M., Müller, C., Podreka, I., Mamoli, B., Sluga, E., and Deecke, L.: Diffuse cerebrospinal gliomatosis presenting as motor neuron disease for two years. J. Neurol. Neurosurg. Psychiatry 52:275–278, 1989.
201a. Schröder, R., Sanker, P., Thun, F., and Richard, K.-E.: Cysts of the third ventricle. Zentralbl. Neurochir. 51:42–48, 1990.
202. Schumann, G.B., O'Dowd, G.J., and Spinnler, P.A.: Eye cytology. Lab. Med. 11:533–540, 1980.
203. Schwartz, A.M., and Sotrel, A.: Intracerebral and intracerebellar neurilemmoma. South. Med. J. 81:385–388, 1988.
204. Scroggs, M.W., Johnston, W.W., and Klintworth, G.K.: Intraocular tumors. A cytopathologic study. Acta Cytol. 34:401–408, 1990.
205. Scully, R.E.: Tumors of the Ovary and Maldeveloped Gonads. Atlas of Tumor Pathology. Second Series, Fascicle 16. Armed Forces Institute of Pathology. Washington, D.C., 1979.
206. Sepp, N., Schuler, G., Romani, N., Geissler, D., Gattringer, C., Burg, G., Bartram, C.R., and Fritsch, P.: "Intravascular lymphomatosis" (angioendotheliomatosis); evidence for a T-cell origin in two cases. Hum. Pathol. 21:1051–1058, 1990.
207. Shenoy, U.A., Kushner, J.P., and Schumann, G.B.: Cytologic diagnosis and monitoring of Hodgkin's disease in cerebrospinal fluid: a case report. Diagn. Cytopathol. 3:323–325, 1987.
208. Shibata, D., Nichols, P., Sherrod, A. Rabinowitz, A., Bernstein-Singer, L., and Hu, E.: Detection of occult CNS involvement of follicular small cleaved lymphoma by the polymerase chain reaction. Mod. Pathol. 3:71–75, 1990.
209. Shields, J.A., Bakewell, B., Augsburger, J.J., Donoso, L.A., and Bernardino, V.: Space-occupying orbital masses in children. A review of 250 consecutive biopsies. Ophthalmology 93:379–384, 1986.
210. Siegel, M.J., Dalton, J., Friedman, A.H., Strauchen, J., and Watson, C.: Ten-year experience with primary ocular "reticulum cell sarcoma" (large cell non-Hodgkin's lymphoma). Br. J. Ophthalmol. 73:342–346, 1989.
211. Soffer, D., Gomori, J.M., Siegal, T., and Shalit, M.N.: Intracranial meningiomas after high-dose irradiation. Cancer 63:1514–1519, 1989.
212. Stark, E., Knehaus, A., Wurster, U., and Patzold, U.: Primary germinoma of the brain. Immunocytochemical demonstration of tumor cells in the cerebrospinal fluid. Clin. Neurol. Neurosurg. 88:263–265, 1986.
213. Stekhoven, J.H.S., Langenhuysen, C.A.M., Bakkeren, J.A.J.M., Holland, R., Höller, I., DeVaan, G.A.M., and Schretlen, E.D.A.M.: Morphology and incidence of the "posttherapeutic lymphoid cell" in the bone marrow of children with acute lymphoblastic leukemia. Am. J. Pathol. 124:46–52, 1986.
214. Stoller, J.K., Kavuru, M., Mehta, A.C., Weinstein, C.E., Estes, M.L., and Gephardt, G.N.: Intracranial meningioma metastatic to the lung. Cleve. Clin. J. Med. 54:521–527, 1987.
215. Stroup, R.M., Scheibani, K., Moncada, A., Purdy, L.J., and Battifora, H.: Angiotropic (intravascular) large cell lymphoma. A clinicopathologic study of seven cases with unique clinical presentations. Cancer 66:1781–1788, 1990.
215a. Sunita, Kapila, K., Singhal, R.M., and Verma, K.: Extracranial metastasis of an astrocytoma detected by fine-needle aspiration: a case report. Diagn. Cytopathol. 7:290–292, 1991.
216. Tajika, Y., Reifenberger, G., Kiwit, J.C.W., and Wechsler, W.: Metastatic adenocarcinoma in cerebral astrocytoma: clinicopathological and immunohistochemical study with review of the literature. Acta Neurochir. (Wien), 105:50–55, 1990.
217. Takagi, T., Yamaguchi, T., Mizoguchi, T., and Amemiya, T.: A case of metastatic optic nerve head and retinal carcinoma with vitreous seeds. Ophthalmologica 199:123–126, 1989.
218. Takahashi, M.: Color Atlas of Cancer Cytology. Ed. 2, Igaku-Shoin, New York, 1981.
219. Tally, P.W., Laws, E.R. Jr., and Scheithauer, B.W.: Metastases of central nervous system neoplasms. Case report. J. Neurosurg. 68:811–816, 1988.
220. Tamura, T., Nakamura, S., Shirata, K., Sato, K., Tsubokawa, T., and Sawada, T.: Cerebellar malignant glioma after radiation therapy for suprasellar germinoma. Case report. Neurol. Med. Chir. (Tokyo), 29:223–229, 1989.
220a. Tao, L.-C.: Pulmonary metastases from intracranial meningioma diagnosed by aspiration biopsy cytology. Acta Cytol. 35:524–528, 1991.
220b. Tashiro, Y., Kondo, A., Aoyama, I., Nin, K., Shimotake, K., Tashiro, H., and Nishioka, T.: Calcified metastatic brain tumor. Neurosurgery 26:1065–1070, 1990.
221. Thibodeau, L.L., Prioleau, G.R., Manuelidis, E.E., Merino, M.J., and Heafner, M.D.: Cerebral endometriosis. Case report. J. Neurosurg. 66:609–610, 1987.

221a. Todo, T., Kondo, T., Shinoura, N., and Yamada, R. Large cysts of the pineal gland: report of two cases. Neurosurgery 29:101–106, 1991.
222. Townsend, J.J., and Seaman, J.P.: Central neurocytoma—a rare benign intraventricular tumor. Acta Neuropathol. (Berl.), 71:167–170, 1986.
223. Triche, T.J., Askin, F.B., and Kissane, J.M.: Neuroblastoma, Ewing's sarcoma, and the differential diagnosis of small-, round-, blue-cell tumors. Chapter 7 in: Finegold, M. (Ed.): Pathology of Neoplasia in Children and Adolescents. Vol. 18 in: Bennington, J.L. (Ed.): Major Problems in Pathology. W.B. Saunders Co., Philadelphia, 1986, pp. 145–195.
224. Truong, L.D., Jurco, S. III, and McGavran, M.H.: Gliomatosis peritonei. Report of two cases and review of literature. Am. J. Surg. Pathol. 6:443–449, 1982.
225. Ultmann, J.E., and Phillips, T.L.: Cancer of unknown primary site. Chapter 56 in: De Vita, V.T. Jr., Hellman, S., and Rosenberg, S.A.: Cancer. Principles and Practice of Oncology. Ed. 3. J.B. Lippincott Co., Philadelphia, 1989, pp. 1941–1952.
225a. Umezu, H., Aiba, T., and Unakami, M.: Enterogenous cyst of the cerebellopontine angle cistern: case report. Neurosurgery 28:462–466, 1991.
226. Vaquero, J., Coca, S., Martinez, R., and Escandón, J.: Papillary pineocytoma. Case report. J. Neurosurg. 73:135–137, 1990.
227. Wald, U., Levy, P.J., Rappaport, Z.H., Michowitz, S.D., Schuger, L., and Shalet, M.N.: Conus ganglioglioma in a two and a half year old boy. Case report. J. Neurosurg. 62:142–144, 1985.
228. Walloch, J.L., Hong, H.Y., and Bibb, L.M.: Effects of therapy on cytologic specimens. Chapter 31 in: Bibbo, M. (Ed.): Comprehensive Cytopathology. W.B. Saunders Co., Philadelphia, 1991, pp. 860–877.
229. Wasserstrom, W.R., Glass, J.P., and Posner, J.B.: Diagnosis and treatment of leptomeningeal metastases from solid tumors: experience with 90 patients. Cancer 49:759–772, 1982.
230. Whelan, H.T., and Moore, P.: Central nervous system lymphomatoid granulomatosis. Pediatr. Neurosci. 13:113–117, 1987.
231. Whittle, I.R., Gordon, A., Misra, B.K., Shaw, J.F., and Steers, J.W.: Pleomorphic xanthoastrocytoma. Report of four cases. J. Neurosurg. 70:463–468, 1989.
232. Wick, M.R., and Rocamora, A.: Reactive and malignant "angioendotheliomatosis": a discriminant clinicopathological study. J. Cutan. Pathol. 15:260–271, 1988.
233. Woyke, S.: The orbit and the eye globe. Chapter 15 in: Koss, L.G., Woyke, S., and Olzewski, W.: Aspiration Biopsy. Cytologic Interpretation and Histologic Bases. Igaku-Shoin, New York, 1984, pp. 442–456.
234. Young, R.H., Kleinman, G.M., and Scully, R.E.: Glioma of the uterus. Report of a case with comments on histogenesis. Am. J. Surg. Pathol. 5:695–699, 1981.
235. Young, R.H., and Scully, R.E. Testicular Tumors. American Society of Clinical Pathologists Press, Chicago, 1990.
236. Yousem, S.A., and Colby, T.V.: Intravascular lymphomatosis presenting in the lung. Cancer 65:349–353, 1990.
237. Yousem, S.A., Colby, T.V., and Urich, H.: Malignant epithelioid schwannoma arising in a benign schwannoma. A case report. Cancer 55: 2799–2803, 1985.
238. Zajdela, A., Vielh, P., Schlienger, P., and Haye, C.: Fine-needle cytology of 292 palpable orbital and eyelid tumors. Am. J. Clin. Pathol. 93:100–104, 1991.
239. Zampieri, P., Zorat, P.L., Mingrino, S., and Soattin, G.B.: Radiation-associated cerebral gliomas. A report of two cases and review of the literature. J. Neurol. Sci. 33:271–279, 1989.
240. Zec, N., Cera, P., and Towfighi, J.: Extramedullary hematopoiesis in cerebellar hemangioblastoma. J. Neuropathol. Exp. Neurol. 50:364, 1991.
241. Zon, L.I., Johns, W.D., Stomper, P.C., Kaplan, W.D., Connolly, J.L., Morris, J.H., Harris, J.R., Henderson, C., and Skarin, A.T.: Breast carcinoma metastatic to a meningioma. Case report and review of the literature. Arch. Intern. Med. 149:959–962, 1989.

8 / Non-Neoplastic Disorders

In this chapter, we review selected aspects of non-neoplastic nervous system disorders that we consider particularly relevant to the cytopathologist and cytotechnologist in a general surgical pathology laboratory setting. Thus, discussion of the following topics is largely excluded in this review: trauma, effects of toxins, metabolic disorders, developmental disorders, epilepsy, peripheral neuropathies, hydrocephalus, and herniation syndromes.

There remain several general categories of non-neoplastic neurological disorders in which CSF samples or CNS tissue biopsies may be sent to a pathologist, either as a routine part of the clinical evaluation of such disorders or as a consequence of an inability to narrow the clinical differential diagnostic possibilities sufficiently without a CSF examination or a tissue diagnosis. The conditions that are discussed in this chapter are summarized in Table 8.1. For a more detailed review of non-neoplastic disorders of the nervous system, including those not reviewed in this chapter, the reader is referred to several standard neuropathology textbooks (2, 22, 30, 129).

General Aspects

Gliosis versus Glioma

This diagnostic dilemma is frequently encountered by the pathologist in small biopsies of CNS tissue. It is analogous to similar problems encountered in other tissues (e.g., reactive versus neoplastic mesothelial cells in body fluid cytology; benign versus malignant ductal epithelial lesions of the breast; atypical small acinar hyperplasia versus well-differentiated adenocarcinoma of the prostate). The distinction between (reactive) gliosis and a well-differentiated glioma (astrocytoma) not only may be difficult but may be impossible in certain cases depending on the spectrum of findings and the size of the tissue sample. Since gliosis, by definition, does not occur de novo but rather is always an astrocyte reaction to some form of neural tissue insult (evidence of which primary process may or may not be histologically apparent), and since some of these processes lead to cytologic atypia that may exceed that of some well-differentiated astrocytomas, it follows that there is currently no single criterion (morphologic or other) that will reliably distinguish gliosis from glioma in every case. Nonetheless, several general principles are reviewed below, application of which will lead to the proper diagnosis in most cases.

Dumas-Duport et al. (29) divide reactive gliosis into three types: acute, subacute, and chronic. In acute stages the astrocyte nuclei are enlarged and regular and have delicate chromatin and often a solitary prominent nucleolus. Cytoplasmic processes are delicate and appear stellate and symmetrical. In subacute gliosis the cell processes are thicker and nuclei are larger and more irregular. Multinucleation may occur. In chronic gliosis the nuclei tend to be small and are superimposed on a rather dense fibrillary background of glial processes. The density of nuclei and glial processes, it should be noted, will vary with the intensity and nature of the instigating process, but regularity of the nuclear arrangement itself is often stressed as being characteristic of reactive gliosis (see below). Several aspects of the

Table 8.1.
Selected Non-Neoplastic Disorders

I. General
a. Gliosis vs. glioma
b. Neuronal and glial cellular inclusions
II. Degenerative disorders
III. Demyelinating disease and leukodystrophies
a. Multiple sclerosis
b. Leukodystrophies
IV. Vascular disorders
a. Cerebral infarction
b. Cerebral amyloid angiopathy
c. Vascular malformations
V. Infectious diseases
a. General considerations
b. Cerebral abscess
c. Progressive multifocal leukoencephalopathy
VI. Inflammatory disorders
VII. Non-neoplastic disorders of the eye and orbit
VIII. Miscellaneous conditions
a. Fetal neural tube defects
b. Extramedullary hematopoiesis
c. Benign lymphoproliferative disorders
d. Cytologic manifestations of ballistic injury

diagnosis of gliosis versus glioma that should be considered are summarized in Table 8.2 and discussed below.

Table 8.2.
Gliosis (i.e., Reactive Astrocytes) versus Glioma (i.e., Low-Grade Astrocytoma): A Checklist of Differential Features

Clinical history (including prior radiation therapy, etc.)
Radiologic findings
Anatomic site of biopsy
Scherer's secondary structures
Cellularity (amount and distribution)
Cytologic features
Rosenthal fibers
Vascularity
Mitoses
Microcystic change
Ease of making smear preparations
Inflammatory cells
Foamy (lipid) macrophages
Hemosiderin-laden macrophages
Necrosis

History and Radiologic Findings

In most neoplastic disorders the course is progressive once symptoms appear, whereas in most vascular and demyelinating disorders the course is either stepwise, or exacerbating and remitting. In degenerative disorders the course is typically progressive once symptoms appear, and neuroimaging techniques will not disclose mass lesions. Unfortunately, frequent exceptions to these generalizations occur. Neoplasms may announce their presence by a sudden hemorrhage or infarction (with subsequent and temporary clinical improvement). Further, infections (e.g., abscess), vascular accidents, acute demyelinating lesions (see below), and neoplasms may occasionally be indistinguishable by all available clinical and neuroimaging techniques, necessitating a tissue diagnosis. Thus, while often helpful, clinical and radiologic data do not always aid the pathologist in distinguishing gliosis from glioma.

Anatomic Site of Biopsy

As already noted in Chapter 2, certain areas of the brain and its direct extensions may normally appear very gliotic, even to the point of resembling a low-grade astrocytoma. This effect often becomes more pronounced with aging. Areas in the normal brain in which particular caution should apply when considering the question of gliosis versus glioma include the subpial, subependymal, and perivascular areas; the hippocampal/Ammon's horn area; the inferior olivary nuclei; and the posterior pituitary. Further, as discussed in Chapter 7, a florid gliosis that may mimic low-grade astrocytomas (and may even include Rosenthal fibers) may occur in the vicinity of benign cysts, neoplasms, and other pathologic processes (see Table 7.6). Gliosis is often quite striking around certain histologic types of tumors such as (but not limited to) craniopharyngiomas and capillary hemangioblastomas. Small biopsies from the more peripheral zone of such neoplasms can cause diagnostic problems because they reflect only the reactive gliosis and not the primary underlying pathologic process to which the astrocytes are reacting.

Scherer's Secondary Structures

The presence of these histologic features provide, in our opinion, one of the most reliable distinguishing features of gliosis versus glioma (114). If one or more of these features is present the diagnosis of glioma is strongly favored. Their absence does not, however, imply that the process under consideration is non-neoplastic. Briefly stated, the secondary structures of particular interest in this context consist of increased concentrations of neoplastic cells (in comparison to their concentration in the intervening neuropil) in perivascular, subpial, subependymal, and/or perineuronal sites (see Figs. 7.3**C**, **D**, **E**, and **F**). The increased concentration of neoplastic cells in perineuronal areas is not to be mistaken for the neuronal satellitosis seen in non-neoplastic conditions (e.g., in certain infectious processes).

Such cellular concentrations may be found within zones of obvious tumor or in more peripheral sites where hypercellularity and pleomorphism is much more subtle and where the distinction of neoplasm versus gliosis is much more difficult. It is in the latter zones that identification of such focal increased cellularity can be most helpful, even when pleomorphism is minimal and true reactive gliosis coexists. The importance of recognizing such structures cannot be overemphasized, and the reader is referred to the original report by Scherer (114) and to the discussions and illustrations by Rubinstein and by Russell and Rubinstein for further study (108, 109). The importance of these structures is not only in their value in distinguishing gliosis from glioma but also in the fact that they tend to occur in a relatively restricted group of CNS neoplasms. These include astrocytomas, oligodendrogliomas, medulloblastomas (especially the desmoplastic variety), and CNS lymphomas. In the latter tumor type perivascular, subpial, and subependymal tumor cell aggregates may occur, but preferential perineuronal aggregation of neoplastic lymphocytes has not, to our knowledge, been described. Of the secondary structures described above, the most common overall are the subpial aggregates. The perivascular aggregates are outside of the Virchow-Robin spaces and are usually confined to gray matter (109).

Cellularity

In the absence of sufficient increased cellularity to allow ready distinction of gliosis from glioma, the *distribution* of the cells can be helpful. Even in the absence of concentration differences of the type described as Scherer's secondary structures, the distribution of nuclei in a given microscopic field tends to be more regular and uniform in gliosis than in gliomas. The greater the variation in cell density the more likely the diagnosis of glioma, other factors being equal.

Although this point is frequently emphasized in standard texts and is often the case, we have occasionally observed areas of reactive gliosis with rather prominent nuclear density variations and have noted selected areas of gliomas with a rather uniform nuclear distribution. Hence, this characteristic is not a completely reliable distinguishing feature. It can also be stated that the cellularity in most cases of reactive gliosis is not as pronounced as in most cases of low-grade astrocytomas. A conscious effort to assess the number of nuclei in relation to the density of astrocytic processes in normal brain tissue and in proven cases of gliosis and low-grade glioma, in sections of varying thickness, can be helpful in improving one's judgment in this important histologic parameter. We have also found reactive gliosis in zones of chronic edema to be among the more difficult conditions to differentiate from low-grade gliomas, and sampling of brain tissue at sites that vary in distance from the center of primary tumors in large surgical resections or in postmortem tissue can be a useful teaching exercise.

Cytologic Features

Most reactive astrocytes contain nuclei with few or no atypical features, but the nuclear atypia of some reactive astrocytes overlaps that of some low-grade astrocytomas. There is, however, a continuum of atypia as one encounters progressively less well differentiated astrocytomas, and the point is reached where the combination of atypia, increased cellularity, and other features are no longer confused with reactive glial changes. Perhaps the most pronounced degree of atypia (and even atypical mitotic figures) seen in non-neoplastic astrocytes occurs in lesions of some cases of progressive multifocal leukoencephalopathy (PML) (see Infectious Diseases in this chapter). However, the accompanying oligodendrocyte nuclear inclusions and other associated changes will usually allow distinction of PML from gliosis or glioma, assuming a representative sample is obtained.

Cytoplasmic characteristics of reactive astrocytes are of some assistance at times. It is generally stated that the processes of reactive astrocytes are (as seen in routine hematoxylin and eosin [H&E]-stained sections) more readily visible, present in larger numbers, longer, distributed in a more symmetrical (i.e., stellate) fashion, and associated with more obvious paranuclear (i.e., soma) cytoplasm than in most gliomas (29) (Fig. 8.1**A**, **B**, and **C**). In gliomas, one more often sees apparently bare nuclei or nuclei with scant cytoplasm and/or asymmetric cytoplasmic processes against a neuropil with variable fibrillar content and less prominent reactive-type astrocytes (22). However, such generalizations do not necessarily apply in many fibrillar astrocytomas or in astrocytomas with a prominent gemistocytic component. Therefore, far more careful scrutiny of cellularity, nuclear atypia, pleomorphism and other features is always appropriate. Once again, the larger the volume of tissue available, the more likely the correct diagnosis can be obtained. Smears facilitate examination of cytologic detail under such circumstances.

Rosenthal Fibers

These may occur in both gliosis and in gliomas (see Table 7.6) and are not a helpful distinguishing feature in this regard (see Fig. 7.4**C** and **D**).

Vascularity

In both reactive processes and low-grade astrocytomas it is unusual for significant vascular and/or endothelial proliferation to occur. Occasionally, vascular changes of this type occur in low-grade gliomas to variable but usually mild degree and may also occur in the zone surrounding abscesses and infarctions (see Table 7.5). Well-developed vascular changes of this type, with glomeruloid formations, typically occur in higher-grade tumors (see Fig. 7.2**B**) in which other features (e.g., cellularity, anaplasia) exist that allow ready distinction from reactive gliosis.

Mitoses

Mitoses are rare in reactive gliosis, and when present are morphologically normal (113). However, the same statement applies to low-grade astrocytomas, and while the presence of one or two mitoses in a small biopsy would tend to favor a glioma, we recommend caution in making a diagnosis of glioma unless other supportive findings are present.

Microcystic Change

This may occur in gliosis (particularly in zones of chronic edema) as well as in gliomas, and is not a helpful distinguishing feature.

Ease of Making Smear Preparations

Many astrocytomas smear more readily than most well-established areas of gliosis. Very gliotic areas tend to be cohesive and resist smearing and thus appear as large clumps of tissue with few or no small fragments or single intact cells. However, the overlap in ease of smearing is sufficiently great in gliosis and gliomas, depending on the stage of gliosis and the amount of reactive gliosis accompanying the glioma, for us to conclude that this is not a reliable guide to distinguishing between gliosis and glioma. The combination of smear preparations and histologic sections, however, has been found to be more accurate than histologic sections alone in making this distinction (29, 113), as discussed in Chapter 7.

Inflammatory Cells, Hemosiderin-laden Macrophages, Foamy (Lipid) Macrophages, and/or Necrosis

Any or all of these features may occur in association with either gliosis or glioma. However, they are still very important observations for the following reasons. First, in association with astrocytosis of the "reactive versus low-grade glioma" type, the presence of any of these features should make the pathologist very reluctant to diagnose a low-grade glioma in a smear preparation or frozen section. Significant numbers of inflammatory cells are, with infrequent exceptions (e.g., ganglioglioma), rare in low-grade gliomas. Second, significant numbers of hemosiderin-laden macrophages and foamy macrophages are rare in low-grade gliomas and are uncommon even in malignant CNS tumors. However, they are not uncommon in other more rapidly progressive tissue-destructive lesions such as cerebral hemorrhage, cerebral infarction, abscesses, and some types of demyelinating plaques (Fig. 8.1**D** and **E**). Thus, the presence of a polymorphous cell population that includes not only glial forms but also inflammatory cells, foamy macrophages, hemosiderin-laden macrophages, and/or evidence of necrosis will nearly always be an indicator that: (*a*) the lesion is not a low-grade glioma; (*b*) there is a definite possibility that the lesion is non-neoplastic (e.g., infarction, multiple sclerosis plaque, abscess), and microbiologic studies as well as consideration of additional biopsies from the peripheral zone of the lesion may be appropriate; and (*c*) if a high-grade tumor is considered likely on the basis of clinical and radiologic features, the initial sample is probably non-representative of the lesion either because it is too deep (e.g., necrosis) or too superficial (e.g., in the gliotic, compressed zone just outside the tumor).

Radiation Cerebritis

Prior radiation may produce a number of additional confounding tissue alterations, which can make the distinction between reactive gliosis and tumor recurrence difficult. This is discussed in Chapter 7.

In summary, we believe the more helpful guides to the distinction between gliosis and glioma to be the presence in gliomas of Scherer's secondary structures, clearly increased cellularity (particularly when irregularly distributed) and nuclear pleomorphism (i.e., anaplasia), particularly when the latter consists of "bare" nuclei without obvious paranuclear cytoplasm and/or numerous elongate cell processes. By the time criteria for anaplastic astrocytoma are met (see Table 7.2), confusion with gliosis is no longer an issue. The presence of inflammatory cells, foamy macrophages, hemosiderin-laden macrophages and/or necrosis, seen either in isolation or in the presence of only reactive or mildly atypical astrocytes (i.e., where the question of gliosis versus glioma arises), should raise doubt that one is dealing with a low-grade glioma. We also urge caution in offering a preliminary diagnosis of glioma whenever there is a discrepancy between clinical and radiologic data and results from smears or frozen sections, unless the latter two are in agreement and are unequivocally diagnostic.

In order that the distinction between gliosis and glioma not be considered inviolate, we also note that certain conditions in which reactive astrocytosis occurs may subsequently become the site of glial neoplastic change. This sequence of events has been described in post-traumatic glial scars, progressive multifocal leukoencephalopathy, multiple sclerosis plaques (1), Alexander's disease, neurofibromatosis, and tuberous sclerosis, among other conditions (109).

Cytology (3, 13, 22, 26, 29, 32, 61, 68, 76, 78, 87, 93, 95, 113). The references cited above demonstrate histologic sections and/or smear preparations of reactive gliosis (Fig. 8.1**B**) (3, 22, 26, 29, 68, 87, 93, 113), inflammatory cells, erythrophagocytosis and/or hemosiderin-laden macrophages (3, 13, 32, 61, 78, 95), foamy (lipid) macrophages (Fig. 8.1**E**) (3, 26, 68, 76, 78, 95, 113), and CNS necrosis (26, 68). The inflammatory cell spectrum will vary with the nature and chronological stage of the underlying disorder and may include neutrophils, lymphocytes and monocytes demonstrating varying degrees of reactive change, plasma cells, and/or eosinophils. The cytologic features of reactive astrocytes have been described above, and those of Rosenthal fibers in Chapter 7. The vacuoles of foamy (lipid) macrophages vary in size but are generally multiple and small, rather than few and large. Macrophages typically have bland-appearing round to bean-shaped nuclei, single nucleoli of variable prominence, and distinct cell membranes. The appearance of hemoglobin-derived pigment in macrophages (Fig. 8.1**F**) will vary with the stain employed and the stage of hemoglobin breakdown. For example, hemosiderin will be seen as golden-brown granules in H&E-stained material, and as medium to dark blue granules with Diff-Quik. The latter should not be erroneously interpreted as basophils. Hematoidin pigment generally appears as bright yellow rhomboidal crystals in the cytoplasm of macrophages with both of these stains. The prominence of lipid-laden macrophages in CNS processes associated with tissue destruction is a consequence of the high lipid content of CNS tissues.

Neuronal and Glial Cellular Inclusions

A number of nuclear and cytoplasmic inclusions occur in neurons and glia, some of which are very characteristic of certain diseases while others are present in several different diseases or are without pathologic significance (except when misinterpreted as a pathologic finding). Many of these inclusions are visible by light microscopy with routine H&E stains. For a detailed review of the staining characteristics and the immunochemical and ultrastructural features of these inclusions the reader should consult standard textbooks of neuropathology (2, 22, 30, 44, 109, 129). Our purpose in briefly tabulating such inclusions in the present chapter is primarily to remind the cytopathologist and cytotechnologist that a remarkable number and variety of inclusion bodies may be found in normal and pathologic neural tissues (Table 8.3). Precise classification of several of these inclusions requires ancillary techniques, since their appearance by light microscopy may overlap. For this reason, Table 8.3 also includes a directory to selected references for each inclusion type, to facilitate the reader's acquisition of further descriptive detail and illustrations.

While such inclusions are generally most commonly encountered in non-neoplastic conditions, they may rarely occur in neoplastic cells. For example, several inclusion

Table 8.3.
Light Microscopically Visible Inclusions in Neurons and Glial Cells

Neuronal Inclusions
- Intranuclear
  - a. Cowdry type A and B inclusions (82) (e.g., herpes simplex encephalitis (82), subacute sclerosis panencephalitis) (20, 82).
  - b. Pseudoinclusions (cytoplasmic spurs, or nuclear infoldings resembling inclusions due to plane of section).
  - c. Eosinophilic, fibrillar, lattice-like inclusions (62).
  - d. Eosinophilic inclusions of uncertain significance in rare degenerative diseases (62).
  - e. Marinesco bodies (62).
- Intracytoplasmic
  - a. Lipofuscin (35, 62).
  - b. Neuromelanin (62).
  - c. Alzheimer's neurofibrillary tangles (35, 62, 80, 102).
  - d. Granulovacuolar bodies (35, 62, 80).
  - e. Abnormal lipid or other metabolic product accumulations (e.g., lipidoses, mucopolysaccharidoses, etc.) (11, 62, 79, 90).
  - f. Pick bodies (35, 62, 80, 102).
  - g. Lewy bodies (35, 47, 62, 71, 80, 102).
  - h. Lafora bodies and polyglycosan bodies (35, 62, 80, 102).
  - i. Bunina bodies (35, 62, 80).
  - j. Nigri bodies and lyssa bodies (82).
  - k. Intracytoplasmic hyaline (colloid) bodies (62).
  - l. Eosinophilic rod-like structures (Hirano bodies) (62).
  - m. Eosinophilic granules in pigmented and non-pigmented neurons (62, 119).
  - n. Eosinophilic inclusions in thalamic neurons (62).
  - o. Eosinophilic rod-like inclusions in the caudate nucleus (62).
  - p. Kuru plaques (82).
- Axonal spheroids ("torpedoes") (62).
- Dendritic stellate bodies ("cacti") of Purkinje cells (62).

Oligodendrocyte Inclusions
- Intranuclear
  - a. Progressive multifocal leukoencephalopathy (82, 100).
  - b. Subacute sclerosing panencephalitis (82).
- Intracytoplasmic
  - a. Polygonal crystalline inclusions in oligodendroglioma (99).
  - b. Accumulation of lipids and other metabolic products in enzyme disorders (e.g., lipidoses) (11, 62, 79, 90).

Astrocyte Inclusions
- Intranuclear inclusions
  - a. Progressive multifocal leukoencephalopathy (100).
  - b. Eosinophilic bodies (62).
- Intracytoplasmic
  - a. Corpora amylacea (see Chapter 2) (62, 80).
  - b. Rosenthal fibers (see Chapter 7) (62, 80).
  - c. Eosinophilic hyaline granules (62).

types have been described in neoplastic cells in gangliogliomas (e.g., Hirano bodies, Lafora bodies, curvilinear bodies, zebra bodies, membranous cytoplasmic bodies, neurofibrillary tangles, and granulovacuolar bodies) (65, 109), in ganglioneuromas (e.g., Pick bodies) (109), and in ganglioneuroblastomas (e.g., Hirano bodies, Pick bodies, membranous cytoplasmic bodies, and zebra bodies) (109). We should note that the inclusion types listed in these neoplasms includes forms that are defined by their ultrastructural features, and these are not specifically listed in Table 8.3 (e.g., zebra bodies). The reader will find information concerning them in the references listed in Table 8.3 for accumulations of metabolic products such as in the lipidoses and the mucopolysaccharidoses. There are a number of other cytomorphologic changes that neurons or glia may demonstrate in a variety of pathologic conditions or as a consequence of fixation artifact. These are listed, with selected references, in Table 8.4.

Degenerative Disorders

Degenerative disorders of the nervous system are represented by a variety of conditions affecting various neuroanatomic regions and demonstrating diverse pathologic changes. In many instances, degeneration

Table 8.4.
Miscellaneous Cytomorphologic Changes in Neurons and Glial Cells

Neurons (35, 62, 80)
Simple atrophy
Ischemic cell change
Homogenizing cell change
Neuronophagia
Satellitosis (80)
Vacuolar change
Ferrugination and calcification
Chromatolysis
Oligodendrocytes (80)
Swelling
Vacuolization
Astrocytes (35, 62, 80)
Reactive gliosis
Swelling and clasmatodendrosis (80)
Vacuolization
Alzheimer type I astrocytes (94)
Alzheimer type II astrocytes (94)
Opalski cells (11, 80)

occurs in functionally linked neuronal systems. The classification of these disorders varies from text to text, depending on the identification of new categories of disease and/or the removal and re-categorization of a disease as infectious or metabolic etiologies, for example, are established by new technologies. Many of the neurodegenerative disorders are characterized cytopathologically by a nonspecific simple neuronal atrophy (Table 8.4), but with such atrophy occurring in a relatively specific topographic distribution. Gliosis is a common nonspecific accompaniment of the pathologic process in these disorders. In other instances cellular changes (such as inclusion bodies of more or less specificity for a given disease) may occur (see Table 8.3). Definitive diagnosis of many of these disorders usually requires correlation of clinical and pathological data. The information required may include knowledge of the detailed topographic distribution and the type and intensity of neuropathologic abnormalities, the presence or absence of abnormalities in other body organs, ethnic background and family history of the subject, and results of routine and specialized clinical laboratory and radiologic studies. That is, assignment of the patient to this category of disease is typically a diagnosis of exclusion, necessitating a very thorough clinical investigation for the purpose of ruling out a more specific etiology and, of more practical importance, ruling out treatable disorders. Assuming that routine clinical and radiographic procedures have not yielded a specific diagnosis there are a number of biochemical studies that may be used to screen for specific toxic and metabolic disorders (11, 49, 117).

It follows that CNS tissue biopsies of small size are infrequently indicated in such settings, since a diagnosis of treatable versus currently nontreatable conditions can usually be established by less invasive procedures. Such biopsies are presently, in the United States, essentially limited to two general categories of patients. The first consists of cases in which clinical and/or basic research efforts to establish the etiology in such diseases are being carried out in an appropriate clinical setting, and CNS tissue is utilized for studies not applicable to postmortem tissues. The second setting is those rare instances in which all other diagnostic approaches (for example, analysis of blood, bone marrow, urine, CSF, tears, hair, and/or biopsy study of skin, conjunctivae, muscle, adrenal gland, gastrointestinal tract, liver, and/or nerve) (69) have not yielded sufficient data to make the necessary clinical decisions. In the recent literature, only Alexander's disease and Canavan's disease (and a single case report of late-onset Krabbe's disease) (37a) in children are included in this latter category, primarily because genetic counseling becomes an issue (11, 46a). These three disorders are more commonly classified with the leukodystrophies than with degenerative diseases, although Garcia and Cervós-Navarro (46a) do group the first two in the latter category. While it is true that a specific antemortem diagnosis is not possible in several of the presenile dementias, procedures short of CNS tissue biopsy are sufficient to rule out a treatable disorder and genetic counseling is less likely to be an issue in the age groups so affected. The imprecision of clinical diagnosis in the presenile dementias does complicate, for example, analysis of drug trials, and greater diagnostic accuracy in these groups of patients by the use of stereotactic biopsy has been reported by some workers (127a). There will undoubtedly remain a significant group of patients with presenile dementia in whom the diagnosis remains elusive even after biopsy, however, due to (*a*) the spectrum of pathologic findings in these several diseases even within a given nosologic category and (*b*) the difficulty encountered in establishing a firm diagnosis at autopsy in certain cases, including Alzheimer's disease (the most common and most thoroughly studied of all presenile dementias) (56, 73, 85, 105, 134-136). After reviewing these several references concerning the difficulties involved in obtaining a consensus on the presence or absence of Alzheimer's disease given a whole brain for study, the reader will perhaps forgive our present lack of enthusiasm for stereotactic biopsy as a primary diagnostic tool in this group of disorders. This situation may rapidly change, however, if markers that are sensitive and specific for these various degenerative disorders, and that are adaptable to small tissue samples, become available (see Chapter 10).

Cytology. Neurocytologic methods as presently utilized have little application in neurodegenerative disorders. Familiarity with the pathologic features of these conditions is important, however, for differential diagnostic purposes and for the occasional case in which CNS tissue is obtained for some unrelated purpose (e.g., mass lesion) and histologic features exist (e.g., cellular inclusions) that may provide a clue to a clinically unsuspected disorder. Further information on the pathologic features of the broad group of neurodegenerative diseases can be found in the standard neuropathology textbooks (2, 14, 30, 129).

Reports of CSF cytologic abnormalities in neurodegenerative conditions are very sparse. Rosenthal (107) describes reactive cells (macrophages) in an "acute" episode of Parkinson's disease but does not detail the patient sample size, and we are not aware that this finding has been confirmed elsewhere. Foamy macrophages have been occasionally reported in the CSF in several of the metabolic enzymatic deficiencies that lead to one or another of the storage disorders (e.g., lipidoses, mucopolysaccharidoses) (95, 107).

Demyelinating Disease and Leukodystrophies

Multiple Sclerosis

Receipt of CNS tissue biopsies of multiple sclerosis (MS) plaques are, in current surgical pathology practice, almost invariably a result of the occasional case in which such lesions are clinically and radiographically indistinguishable from neoplastic or inflammatory lesions. Further, the clinical features in these cases are generally such that an urgent diagnosis is believed to be necessary to institute proper therapy as soon as possible (as opposed to, for example, serial clinical and neuroimaging studies). Paty et al. (96) have recently reviewed the diagnostic techniques applicable to MS and reaffirm the fact that none yet exist that are pathognomonic. Magnetic resonance imaging cannot invariably distinguish between brain lesions such as edema, infarction, inflammation, or demyelination (96). In cases in which an MS plaque is solitary or associated with mass effect, neoplasia enters the differential diagnosis. It is not surprising, therefore, that there exist occasional reports of MS plaques mimicking brain tumors (22, 45, 66, 91a, 103).

Since the detailed pathologic features of the MS plaque may vary from case to case, from one plaque to another, and in different zones of the same plaque (excluding variation with time), familiarity with the spectrum of changes seen in such plaques is a necessary foundation for the interpretation of the small biopsies that one may encounter. The classic (i.e., emphasizing paraffin section appearance) neuropathology of MS has been discussed and well illustrated in several reviews over the years (6, 89, 130). A review with greater emphasis on the appearance of MS plaques in 1.0-μm epoxy sections and ultrastructural features has been recently published by Raine (100). To briefly summarize this complex topic it is necessary to make some generalizations, keeping in mind the fact that exceptions will occur. MS plaques tend to demonstrate myelin loss out of proportion to axonal depopulation. Thus, myelin stains are very useful for their identification, often indicating their presence and their limits far more distinctly than, for example, routine H&E stains or axon stains (e.g., Bodian, Bielschowsky). Gliosis is virtually always present but varies in amount. The reactive astrocytes may be plump and conspicuous (i.e., gemistocytic), small and with rather delicate fibrillar processes, or anywhere within these two extremes. At times there may be bizarre and/or multinucleated astrocytes reminiscent of neoplastic cells (100). Foamy (lipid-laden) macrophages that stain positively for neutral lipids are often present even in lesions that otherwise appear inactive, and oligodendrocytes are sparse or absent in demyelinated zones. The presence of chronic inflammatory cells (primarily lymphocytes, but often with some plasma cells and rarely with mast cells) together with more prominent foamy macrophages is generally regarded as evidence of active demyelination in a plaque. Oligodendrocytes may undergo hyperplasia in active plaque margins. Shadow plaques (with sparse myelinated axons, rather than complete absence of myelin) are believed to represent areas of CNS remyelination that occurs in a zone of prior demyelination. In acute MS, the areas of demyelination are characterized by more destructive and inflammatory lesions than those described above, usually with more intense and active-appearing gliosis.

With this brief background, it can be appreciated that biopsy findings in reported cases have not been uniform. It follows that MS plaques may histologically be mistaken for other conditions, particularly infectious or vascular lesions or gliomas (usually gemistocytic astrocytomas or other low-grade astrocytoma variants).

Cytology. One of the most important keys to avoiding the pitfall of mistaking MS plaques for a glioma in the intraoperative consultation setting is, in our opinion, recognizing the presence of foamy (lipid) macrophages. Their recognition is often easier in smear preparations than in frozen sections, especially when they are sparse. While identification of their presence does not allow a diagnosis of MS, it nearly rules out a low-grade glioma, which is the neoplasm most likely to be confused with reactive gliosis in MS plaques or other settings (see Gliosis versus Glioma, above).

The astrocytes in typical plaques will demonstrate morphologic features characteristic of reactive glia, and the foamy macrophages are not associated with evidence of necrosis. Mononuclear inflammatory cells will often be present, but neutrophils are much less likely to be found in MS plaques than, for example, in cerebral infarction or abscess. Myelin and axon stains of permanent sections are helpful for further confirmation of the diagnosis, or at least may allow the diagnosis to be suggested. The clinician may then proceed with other laboratory studies and serial follow-up examinations as indicated, in an effort to establish a firm diagnosis.

CSF cytology in MS has been the subject of extensive investigation, but no findings specific to MS have yet been identified. Depending on the activity of the disease the CSF may contain an increase (usually mild to moderate) in lymphocytes (some of which may be reactive), in monocytes, and (less commonly) in macrophages. Some of the latter may contain myelin debris, and plasma cells and/or eosinophils may occur (61, 76, 78, 95, 107). Neutrophils are an exceptional finding in the CSF in MS, and in significant numbers should raise question about the diagnosis. Herndon and Brumback (61) also describe rare cells undergoing mitosis in the CSF of MS patients. Current trends in the application of CSF cytologic methodology and related techniques in MS patients can be extrapolated from several recent reports (7, 43, 52, 53, 61, 97, 116, 125).

Leukodystrophies

Alexander's disease and Canavan's disease are grouped with the neurodegenerative diseases by Garcia and Cervós-Navarro (46a); under the category of inherited metabolic disease (subcategory leukodystrophies) by Becker and Yates (11); under the category of leukodystrophy by Weller (130, 131); and with demyelinating diseases (subcategory leukodystrophy) by Allen (6). All of the cited authors acknowledge the currently unknown etiology of both disorders, however. Biopsies in such cases are elective procedures and are carried out in settings where a multidisciplinary team, which includes a neuropathologist, is available. This ensures proper handling and disposition of available tissue for routine and special studies so that the maximum possible information is obtainable from the procedure. Intraoperative consultation, if performed in this setting, is for the purpose of ensuring that the tissue sample is appropriate for the planned studies (e.g., for both Alexander's disease and Canavan's disease the sample must include white matter). As already noted above, these represent rare progressive childhood neurologic disorders in which a definite diagnosis still requires brain biopsy (11, 46a), and they are briefly described in the present chapter for this reason only.

Alexander's Disease (6, 11, 131)

This rare form of leukodystrophy (i.e., primarily a white matter degeneration of the CNS) is a progressive disorder affecting a wide age group from infants to adults. Its most distinctive histopathologic feature is the massive accumulation of Rosenthal fibers in subpial, perivascular, and subependymal locations in both gray and white matter. The cerebellar cortex tends to be spared. Cerebral white matter, particularly in infantile cases, demonstrates myelin loss and gliosis and may also include perivascular lymphocytes and histiocytes.

This type of Rosenthal fiber distribution is quite distinctive, but a degree of caution is still appropriate, particularly if tissue sampling is limited. For example, there may exist rare variants of Alexander's disease with the characteristic histologic changes limited to brainstem areas that would be impossible to diagnose by cerebral cortex biopsy (48). Second, some adults with severe medical illness appear prone to develop florid Rosenthal fiber deposition in a pattern resembling that of Alexander's disease, but in the absence of an associated clinical neurologic syndrome. It has been suggested that this latter condition represents a disorder distinct from Alexander's disease (104). Third, Rosenthal fibers associated with other conditions may focally achieve concentrations that overlap their density in Alexander's disease (see Table 7.6), a point to be remembered when examining very small biopsy specimens.

Canavan's Disease (Spongy Degeneration of the Nervous System; Canavan-van Bogaert-Bertrand Spongy Degeneration) (11)

This rare condition may be seen in an infantile form (which typically occurs in an autosomal-recessive inheritant pattern in children of Jewish extraction) and in a juvenile form (in non-Jewish children). The primary microscopic features consist of prominent spongy change, demyelination, proliferation of Alzheimer type II glia, and mild gliosis. The distribution of the spongy change and associated findings is mainly in the immediate subcortical white matter and adjacent deep cortical gray matter, both in cerebrum and cerebellum. Curiously, the expected association of Alzheimer type II glia with liver pathology is not present in Canavan's disease.

Cytology. We have not encountered well-illustrated reports of smear preparations specific to demyelinating diseases or leukodystrophies. There is a rare mention of foamy macrophages and/or inflammatory cells in the CSF in certain leukodystrophies (51, 61, 95), but to our knowledge these have not been confirmed as clinically useful findings.

Vascular Disorders

Vascular disorders of the CNS include vascular malformations; occlusive vascular disease due to local or nearby extracranial vessel involvement (e.g., compressive lesions, atheroma, vasculitis); embolization of various types (e.g., atheromatous plaque constituents, fat, air, neoplastic cells); various hematologic disorders, including coagulopathies; and vascular changes due to hypertension, radiation, drugs, trauma, and a host of interesting and unusual vascular wall diseases (e.g., inherited disorders of connective tissue such as Marfan's syndrome; fibromuscular dysplasia; cerebral amyloid angiopathy; Moyamoya disease). The end result of such processes may vary from subtle degrees of cerebral ischemia to frank infarction and/or hemorrhage. Clinical manifestations may be nil to catastrophic, depending on factors such as lesion type, location, size, and pace of development (i.e., abrupt versus a pace permitting development of collateral circulation). These topics are discussed in many general pathology and neuropathology texts (2, 14, 30, 129). Our emphasis in this section is to review selected vascular disorders the surgical pathologist may encounter in routine practice via either stereotactic brain biopsy specimens or CSF samples.

Cerebral Infarction

As already mentioned during the discussion of demyelinating disease above, cerebral infarcts may occasionally be clinically and radiographically indistinguishable from neoplasms, edema, inflammation, or foci of demyelination (21, 22, 45, 96). This is far less likely to be the case with cerebral or spinal hemorrhages due to the different neuroimaging characteristics of blood (although hemorrhage into a tumor must also be part of the differential diagnosis).

The spectrum of cytomorphologic changes in CNS infarction will vary with the amount and severity of the tissue injury. From a practical standpoint, however, the lesions likely to mimic neoplasms radiographically are very likely to demonstrate the majority of the findings described below, and particularly the prominent presence of foamy macrophages. Since the clinical diagnosis in such cases almost invariably favors neoplasia, the pathologist will not have the advantage of being forewarned concerning the possibility of stroke (or demyelinating plaque, abscess, etc.) and must simply develop the habit of considering all of these diagnostic possibilities in every case examined.

The type and sequence of histologic changes observed in CNS infarction in the hours, days and weeks after the event are well described in many standard texts, but we have found the descriptions by Garcia and Anderson (46) and by Leestma (81) particularly lucid in this regard. These changes are briefly summarized in Table 8.5 (46). As noted in Table 8.5 neutrophils may be found in the lesion within 24 hours and can be prominent for a week or so, readily causing confusion with inflammatory or infectious

Table 8.5.
Cerebral Infarction: Microscopic Features after Single-Vessel Occlusion[a, b]

Duration of Symptoms	Neuronal Injury	Hemispheric Swelling	Swollen Axons	PMNs	Macrophages	Microvessels	Astrogliosis
3 hours	+ +	–	–	–	–	–	–
12 hours	+ + +	+	–	–	–	±	–
18 hours	+ + + +	+ + +	±	–	–	+	–
24 hours	+ + +	+ + + +	+	±	–	+	–
2 days	+ +	+ + +	+ +	+	–	+ +	–
3 days	+	+ + +	+ + +	+ +	±	+ +	–
7 days	–	+ +	+ + + +	+ +	+ +	+ +	±
16 days	–	–	+ + + +	–	+ +	+ + + +	+ +

[a] All observations are based on paraffin-embedded material stained with hematoxylin and eosin.
[b] From Garcia, J.H., and Anderson, M.L.: Circulatory disorders and their effects on the brain. Chapter 13 in: Davis, R.L., and Robertson, D.M. (Eds): Textbook of Neuropathology. Ed. 2. Williams & Wilkins, Baltimore, 1991, pp. 621-718; with permission. Data from Garcia and Kamijyo and Moossy.

diseases. Thereafter, some presence of chronic inflammatory cells in relatively modest numbers is common. Foamy macrophages make their appearance after about 3 days, are maximal during the first week or so, and often persist in smaller numbers for extended periods of months to years.

Reactive astrocytes become apparent by about 2 weeks after the infarction, and mixtures of plump reactive astrocytes and more delicate fibrillary astrocytes are generally seen at the margin of the infarction for up to several years. Binucleated astrocytes may be present, as in other reactive CNS conditions.

Cytology. As discussed in the section on demyelinating disease, an important key to the recognition of an infarction is the detection of foamy (lipid-laden) macrophages. Their cytologic characteristics are described in the section on gliosis versus glioma. Depending on the stage of evolution of the infarction, the tissue section and smear preparation may appear hypercellular due to the combination of macrophages and acute and/or chronic inflammatory cells. Careful attention to nuclear characteristics (facilitated by smears) (13, 22) will allow separation of these inflammatory cells from neoplastic cells of glial or other origin. We recommend that material for cultures be routinely sent to the microbiology laboratory in such cases even if one is reasonably confident that the lesion is an infarct, since distinction of the latter from abscess is not always possible in small samples.

CSF changes following CNS ischemic infarction are infrequently described (33, 95). The CSF is normal in approximately two-thirds of cases. In the remaining cases neutrophils may appear in the CSF in small numbers in the first few days. Later, a variety of cells—including monocytes and macrophages, plasma cells, eosinophils, and/or multinucleated giant cells—have been infrequently reported. DeReuck et al. (33) conclude that cytologic changes in the CSF are more likely to be present in cases in which the etiology of the infarction is other than thromboembolic disease (e.g., infectious or autoimmune vasculitis).

Cerebral Amyloid Angiopathy

Primary cerebral amyloid deposition in the absence of systemic amyloidosis is not uncommon. It may occur in otherwise normal brains with aging, or in association with other neuropathological disorders. The latter include cerebral arteriovenous malformations, Down's syndrome, demyelinating disease, Alzheimer's disease, radiation necrosis, chronic vasculitis, dementia pugilistica, and hereditary ataxia (19, 46, 59). Its inclusion in this chapter is based on the fact that it may present as a hemorrhagic or ischemic stroke or as a cerebral mass lesion (91) and has been diagnosed on the basis of a brain biopsy.

In addition to the cytohistologic features already described for cerebral infarctions above, the characteristic feature in most cases of cerebral amyloid angiopathy is the presence of amyloid in the tunica media and adventitia of leptomeningeal, cortical, and subcortical arteries and arterioles (46). There may be accompanying senile plaques in the adjacent neuropil, chronic inflammatory cells, and/or rare multinucleated giant cells (19). Variants include a microangiopathic form that primarily affects capillaries, and various familial forms. Ancillary methods used for the demonstration of amyloid are therefore recommended in cerebral biopsies demonstrating hyalin eosinophilic thickening of vessel walls, particularly in the presence of the other disorders listed above.

Vascular Malformations

Small vascular malformations will occasionally be difficult to distinguish from neoplasms or inflammatory lesions on neuroimaging techniques, and may thus be unintentionally biopsied. Although the diagnosis may be made on the basis of stereotactic brain biopsy in such cases (28), recent progress in neuroimaging studies is likely to make this a rare occurrence.

Chandrasoma and Apuzzo (26) list the presence of an extensively vascular lesion as a relative contraindication to elective stereotactic brain biopsy (see Chapter 6). However, the rapid development of stereotactically guided radiotherapy may soon make the latter the treatment of choice for small, deeply placed vascular malformations (63).

Infectious Diseases

General Considerations

The role of the clinical microbiology laboratory is paramount in the rapid diagnosis and management of infectious disease (50a, 96a, 101, 127). However, there are a few neurological infectious diseases in which morphologic methods applied to CNS tissue aspirates, biopsies, or CSF samples also play a significant contributory role. These include herpes simplex virus, cytomegalovirus (89a), *Nocardia asteroides*, mycobacterial infections, fungal infections (67, 72), toxoplasmosis (31), amebic infections (12), and certain helminthic infestations (Figs. 8.2 and 8.3). While a highly reliable diagnosis of nonbacterial CNS infections is possible, selected confirmatory tests (e.g., cultures, immunostains, PCR techniques, electron microscopy) are indicated not only for verification of the cytologic diagnosis but to minimize the frequency with which multiple simultaneous infections might be missed.

In recent years, modern treatment methods for neoplastic and other diseases, organ transplantation procedures, and diseases such as the acquired immune deficiency syndrome (AIDS) have resulted in an increasing population of immunologically compromised patients, susceptible not only to the usual pathogens but also to a remarkable variety of opportunistic infections. This has created new challenges in laboratory safety issues (27a) as well as in the rapid diagnosis and treatment of hosts whose hematologic and systemic signs and symptoms in response to invasion by organisms is altered in unpredictable fashion and/or suppressed to varying degree. For example, Elovaara et al. (37) reported CSF protein and cellular profiles in 28 HIV-infected patients. CSF leukocytes were found to be increased in the early stages of the disease, but later the cellular reaction subsided. The CSF/serum albumin ratio was slightly increased in patients with neurological deficits, but this ratio showed no association with other clinical factors analyzed. More recently, Chalmers et al. (25) have described CSF abnormalities in asymptomatic patients seropositive for HIV infection.

CSF cellular changes observed in a variety of CSF infections have already been reviewed in Chapters 3 and 4, and some of the basic features are summarized in Tables 8.6 and 8.7. While generally nonspecific, such changes do alert the clinician to the need for further exploration of infectious and/or inflammatory disorders. They may also yield neoplastic cells in, for example, cases in which the increased incidence of neoplasia seen in immunosuppressed patients is manifested by primary or secondary CNS neoplasms (e.g., primary CNS lymphoma in AIDS; see also Radiation and Chemotherapeutic Effects in Chapter 7).

Attempts to define preliminary CSF parameters that will lead to more cost-effective utilization of specialized laboratory studies, such as cultures and immunostains, have thus far been confounded by the variety of factors that may influence CSF results in the presence of infections (10, 17, 58, 74, 86, 98). We conclude that the clinician remains the most appropriate individual to determine whether or not cultures or other special studies are indicated on CSF samples with minimal or no abnormality on routine screening studies. The role of the pathologist (until more specific, sensitive, and rapid tests become available for microbes in the CSF) may more appropriately be to suggest that cultures and/or repeat CSF studies be performed in instances when initial CSF results are unremarkable but when the clinical situation remains very suspicious for meningitis (58).

CSF wet mounts (e.g., amebic meningitis) and CSF and/or tissue special stains may facilitate organism identification; e.g., Gram stain for bacteria and *Aspergillus*, Ziehl-Neelsen stain for acid-fast organisms, a modified acid-fast stain (Fite) for *Nocardia*, phase contrast and/or potassium hydroxide methods for fungi, India ink preparations for *Cryptococcus*, Giemsa stain for amebas (12) and for toxoplasmosis (31), and Auramine-Rhodamine stain for non-viable AFB (to be followed by acid-fast stains if positive). Always to be kept in mind, particularly in immunocompromised patients, is the possibility of simultaneous and/or sequential infections with multiple infectious agents. The pathologist should also be aware of the confusing effects of the Splendori-Hoeppli phenomenon, which can produce conspicuous stellate, radiating eosinophilic deposits or thick, ring-like structures around a variety of organisms in tissue sections (70).

Cytologic features of the more common CNS infectious agents are well illustrated in a number of infectious disease and neuropathology references, examples of which are included in the references for this chapter (2, 15, 30, 40, 60, 61, 124, 129). Data more specific to immunosuppressed patient populations are also widely available (5, 30a, 34, 50, 54, 63a, 88, 110, 123, 124a, 126, 127, 138).

Incidence patterns of various infections will vary with a number of factors such as patient age, associated diseases, immunologic status, and geographical area. Familiarity with geographic variations is particularly important for the pathologist or clinician who relocates (23).

Herpes simplex virus (HSV) encephalitis has, in recent years, provoked a lively debate concerning the need for brain biopsy as a means of confirming the diagnosis (8, 41, 55, 128). Recent articles seem to indicate an evolving consensus that favors brain biopsy not only to confirm a suspected diagnosis of HSV encephalitis but also to determine the presence (and allow appropriate treatment) of diseases that mimic HSV encephalitis (77, 112, 133). Less controversial is the important role the cytopathologist may play in the rapid and accurate diagnosis of several of the diseases that are found in such biopsies. These include not only HSV but also bacterial abscesses, tuberculosis, fungal infections, primary and secondary neoplasms, subdural hematoma, systemic lupus erythematosus, stroke, toxic encephalopathy, Reye's syndrome, and viral encephalitides other than HSV such as subacute sclerosing panencephalitis (133).

Cerebral Abscess

Cerebral abscess (and progressive multifocal leukoencephalopathy, in the following

Table 8.6.
Neurocytologic Features of Selected CNS Infections[a]

Microorganism	Type of Specimen	Frequency	Morphologic Features	Confirmatory Tests
Bacterial				
Usual pathogens	CSF Smears Sections	Common	Cocci, rods, etc. Associated: increased neutrophils	Culture
Mycobacteria	Same		Acid-fast bacilli	Culture
Nocardia	Same		Gram +, acid-fast bacilli	Culture
Fungal				
Cryptococcus	CSF	Common	Round (5-10μm) yeast forms: Thin-neck buds Mucopolysaccharide capsule (mucicarmine +) Neutrophils Lymphocytes	Culture Serology (antigen detection by radioimmunoassay)
Candida	Smears Sections	Common	GMS and PAS budding spores and pseudohyphal branching fungi	Culture Serology
Aspergillus	Smears Sections	Common	GMS and branching fungi with septal hyphae	Culture Serology
Protozoan				
Toxoplasma	Smears Sections	Common	Trophozoites of pseudocysts	Serology E.M.
Viral				
CMV	CSF Smears Sections	Rare	Nuclear inclusions in cells	Serology Immunostain E.M.
Herpes (HSV)	CSF Smears Sections	Most common sporadic viral encephalitis in U.S.	Nuclear inclusions	Serology Immunostain E.M. Culture
Varicella-zoster (VZV)	Dorsal root ganglia sections, smears		Intranuclear inclusions (usually in satellite, not ganglion cells)	Serology Culture
PML	Smears Sections		Enlarged oligodendrocyte nuclei. Clumped & smudged chromatin resembles polyomavirus as seen in urine	E.M. - papavavirus particles Culture Immunostains In situ hybridization
AIDS	CSF Smear Sections	Increasingly common	"Indicator" diseases: *Cryptococcus, Toxoplasma,* lymphoma, PML, etc. Multinucleated histiocytes may be a helpful clue	Serology In situ hybridization, Other (82)

[a] Modified from Walker, R.C.: The role of the clinical microbiology laboratory in transplantation. Arch. Pathol. Lab. Med. 115:299-305, 1991; with permission.

Table 8.7.
CSF Findings in Patients with Infectious Diseases[a]

Condition	Cell Count *µl*	Protein *mg%*	CSF Glucose / Serum Glucose	Other
Normal	<8	15-45	0.5	—
Bacterial meningitis	↑ ↑	↑	↓ ↓	Gram stain usually positive Polymorphonuclear leukocytes predominant on cell count
Viral meningitis	↑	↑	→	Lymphocytes predominant on cell count
Tuberculous meningitis	↑	↑	↓	Lymphocytes and/or monocytes predominant on cell count
Fungal meningitis	↑	↑	↓	India ink may be positive if *Cryptococcus* is present
Syphilis	→ to ↑	→ to ↑	→	May vary depending on stage of disease; serology positive
Leptospirosis	↑	↑	→	Lymphocytes predominant
Viral encephalitis	↑	→ to ↑	→	Early response is polymorphonuclear leucocytes, lymphocytes, later lymphocytes predominant
Brain abscess	↑	→ to ↑	→	Early response is polymorphonuclear; later lymphocytes predominant
Amebic meningitis	↑	↑	↓	Wet preparation using prewarmed slide to look for motile amebae

[a] ↑ - increased; ↓ - decreased; → - normal; ↓ ↓ - markedly decreased.

section) is discussed separately because its cytohistologic features raise a number of issues beyond that of identification of the responsible organism. Depending on factors such as the nature of the organism, the stage of evolution of the process, and host response, *cytologic features* may be quite different from case to case. For example, the inflammatory cell component may quantitatively vary from nil to florid, and the qualitative aspects may demonstrate varying elevations and combinations of leukocytes, histiocytes, and reactive glial components. Further, the zonal or laminated character of the abscess wall may give rise to sampling error in small biopsy specimens. The following description will focus on the typical characteristics of a pyogenic abscess in a host capable of marshaling a normal inflammatory response, with the caution that variations in any of the clinical parameters previously discussed may alter this classic pattern.

Initially, the infected brain tissue becomes hyperemic with congested and necrotic blood vessels, extravasated erythrocytes, edema, and infiltration by neutrophils (i.e., cerebritis). Special stains may reveal bacteria. There follows central liquefaction, fibroblastic proliferation and collagen production, accumulation of lipid-laden macrophages, the appearance of mononuclear inflammatory cells, and proliferation of capillaries and reactive astrocytes (i.e., encapsulation) (22, 57, 75). From within outward, then, one may encounter fibrinopurulent and necrotic debris with varying numbers of foamy macrophages; a zone of prominent foamy macrophages and chronic greater than acute inflammatory cells, fibrosis, and capillary proliferation (i.e., granulation tissue); and varying degrees of gemistocytic and/or fibrillar gliosis and edema in the surrounding neural tissue. The latter may cause confusion with astrocytomas (see Gliosis versus Glioma section of this chapter).

Ependymal proliferation and formation

of ependymal rosettes and canals may occur in response to inflammatory conditions adjacent to the ventricular system and could potentially lead to confusion with ependymal neoplasms in small biopsies (113).

The course of an abscess may be complicated by rupture, hemorrhage (rare), or mass effects. Biopsy diagnosis of abscesses is further discussed by Scheithauer (113), and many of the principles learned in aspiration cytology studies of non-neural inflammatory masses are also directly applicable to CNS abscess aspirates (18).

The inability to invariably distinguish, clinically or radiographically, between neoplasia, abscess, demyelination, or infarction is discussed elsewhere in this chapter. The comments under these various topics are also applicable here. In addition, we would stress that the necrosis and inflammation occasionally associated with rapidly growing neoplasms may be cytologically indistinguishable from that seen in an abscess cavity. If this question arises in the intraoperative situation, knowledge of the clinical and radiological aspects of the case and discussion with the neurosurgeon concerning differential diagnostic possibilities will enhance the possibility of obtaining representative and diagnostic material from a more peripherally situated area of the lesion.

Progressive Multifocal Leukoencephalopathy (PML)

This condition is separately discussed in this section because it is the only viral infection likely to be confused with a glioma (113). Further, it may come to the attention of the surgical pathologist in the form of a brain biopsy specimen, since it may present with features of a mass lesion. Microscopically, the most characteristic findings are multiple areas of myelin loss with low cellularity, intranuclear inclusions in enlarged (up to 15 μm in diameter) oligodendrocyte nuclei (100) (Fig. 8.3**E**) and the presence of scattered bizarre, giant (up to 60 μm in diameter) and/or multinucleated astrocytes (100) (Fig. 8.3**F**). The usual forms of reactive gemistocytic and/or fibrillar astrocytes are also present. The inclusion-bearing oligodendrocytes (and rarely astrocytes with inclusions) are more likely to be found in the margin of the demyelinated zone. The atypical astrocytes may also demonstrate abnormal mitotic figures, further suggesting the possibility of an astrocytic neoplasm.

The distinction between PML and an astrocytoma is usually apparent if one gives careful attention to the associated findings, which include hypocellularity and an absence of microvascular proliferation, palisading necrosis, and Scherer's secondary structures (113). In questionable cases or with small samples, ancillary studies that may be helpful include electron microscopy (demonstrating paracrystalline arrays of papovavirus virions), immunocytochemical staining for JC viral antigens, and/or in-situ hybridization techniques (82, 115).

The microscopic differential diagnosis also includes subacute sclerosing panencephalitis, adrenoleukodystrophy, radiation cerebritis, and other white matter diseases. Perivascular chronic inflammatory infiltrates are rare, an additional feature aiding in the distinction of PML from multiple sclerosis (100).

Cytology of Infectious Diseases. Major cytologic features of various infectious diseases are referenced in the appropriate sections above, and selected examples are illustrated in Figs. 8.2 and 8.3. For the reader's convenience, illustrations of cytologic features of tissue and/or CSF samples from several infectious conditions are also included in the following references: bacterial meningitis (13, 32, 61, 76, 78, 95); brain abscess (13, 26, 38, 78, 95, 107, 113); tuberculoma (3); syphilis (95); cryptococcus and other fungi (13, 26, 61, 76, 107); viral meningoencephalitis (3, 13, 26, 32, 38, 61, 76, 95); toxoplasmosis (3); amebic abscess (87); cysticercal cyst (26); HIV encephalopathy, and PML (93).

Inflammatory Disorders

Inflammatory conditions involving the CNS are usually described as acute, subacute, or chronic. Most CSF cytopathology laboratories report the type of inflammatory cell population and assess the degree of inflammation using semi-quantitative terms such as mild, moderate, or marked. One must be able to accurately identify neutrophils, lymphocytes (normal, reactive, and atypical forms), monocytes (normal, reactive, and atypical forms), eosinophils, plasma cells, histiocytes/macrophages, and epithelioid cells. The reader is referred to Chapter 3 for descriptions of cellular alterations found in the CSF and their disease associations (Table 3.6). Most cytopathology laboratories have found the use of both the Papanicolaou and Wright's/Diff-Quik stains valuable in identifying hematopoietic and lymphoid cell populations, and relatively easy to correlate with morphologic features demonstrated in H&E-stained sections and smears.

Inflammatory patterns found in CSF and brain tissue are generally nonspecific but represent important associated morphological findings. Searching for an etiologic agent stimulating the inflammation is appropriate even if it is considered clinically unlikely. That having been accomplished, the role of the cytopathologist in further defining the nature of inflammatory disorders involving the nervous system (and not already discussed elsewhere in this chapter) are quite limited. Most of the remaining disorders consist of nervous system manifestations of systemic disease (e.g., paraneoplastic inflammatory disorders [see Chapter 7]; sarcoidosis [14, 24]; collagen vascular disease) (111) or rare disorders (e.g., CNS malakoplakia) (16) that infrequently lead to CNS biopsy. CNS manifestations of many of these conditions have been alluded to in Chapter 3 (Table 3.6).

Non-Neoplastic Disorders of the Eye and Orbit

Several non-neoplastic neuropathological disorders may involve the eye and/or orbit. To date, cytologic methods in this anatomic area have almost exclusively been limited to neoplasms (106) (see Chapter 7). Aside from the infectious agents (e.g., in AIDS patients) (31a) that may be encountered in cytologic preparations of vitreous or aqueous aspirates or conjunctival or corneal scrapings, the literature on ocular cytology that may have neuropathological relevance describes only a few non-neoplastic conditions in which cytologic methods may have played a diagnostic role. These include sarcoidosis and other granulomatous diseases, benign cysts, amyloidosis (36), and a cited case of ocular involvement by Whipple's disease (which may involve the CNS in association with systemic manifestations of the disease, or present with exclusive CNS involvement) (4, 75, 118, 120). Zajdela et al. (139) encountered only two non-neoplastic cases (one lymphoid hyperplasia and one nonspecific inflammation) in a fine-needle aspiration cytologic study of 292 palpable orbital and eyelid tumors.

Conjunctival biopsies have proved useful, however, in the diagnosis of neuroaxonal dystrophy (39) and of several metabolic disorders that may also affect the CNS, including ceroid lipofuscinosis and several of the lysosomal storage diseases (e.g., GM2 gangliosidosis, Fabry's disease) (11). In the conjunctivae, as well as in other anatomic sites sampled for a suspected diagnosis of metabolic disease, it is important to remember that light microscopy alone will rarely allow more than a suspicion of a metabolic disorder and possibly its general category (e.g., vacuolated fibroblasts with certain histochemical and/or immunochemical staining characteristics). Definitive diagnosis is more often dependent on ultrastructural and/or biochemical study, and the handling of biopsy tissue should be planned with these priorities in mind (121, 137).

Miscellaneous Conditions

Fetal Neural Tube Defects

In the past, fetal neural tube defects have been studied by cytologic examination of the amniotic fluid (27, 76). Findings have included the presence of small, dark-staining cells of presumed neural origin and cells that demonstrate immunostaining for S-100 or for glial fibrillary acidic protein (GFAP). However, the trend is now away from cytologic methods for the diagnosis of fetal neural tube defects, and emphasis is currently being placed on the combined use of amniotic fluid α-fetoprotein and acetylcholinesterase assays and ultrasonography (9, 64, 76, 83, 84, 132).

Extramedullary Hematopoiesis

Extramedullary hematopoiesis (in the form of erythropoiesis) has been previously discussed in the context of the capillary hemangioblastoma (see Chapter 7). This tumor, as well as a few others, may occasionally produce an erythropoietin-like substance causing peripheral blood polycythemia, and hemangioblastomas may demonstrate intratumoral extramedullary erythropoiesis.

Extramedullary hematopoiesis may also occur in a variety of hematologic diseases, often in response to chronic severe anemia, and may be found in unusual sites, which may include peripheral nerves, cranial dura, and the spinal epidural space. In the latter site, the hematopoietic tissue may rarely form highly vascular, purplish-red tumors, which can cause clinical symptoms of spinal cord compression sufficient to precipitate surgical decompression (122). Since the spinal epidural space is a potential needle biopsy target (78a), this rare condition is mentioned here as an additional cause of spinal epidural tumors that could be encountered in a relatively restricted clinical setting.

Benign Lymphoproliferative Disorders

Neurological manifestations may occur during the course of several benign lymphoproliferative disorders. Infrequently, CNS manifestations are the initial or sole manifestation of the disease. Foucar et al. (42) discuss several lymphoproliferative disorders in this unique category. Sinus histiocytosis with massive lymphadenopathy may produce infiltrative and mass lesions capable of causing vertebral body destruction, epidural or subdural cranial or spinal lesions, or even invasion of CNS parenchyma and death. Fibrosis is often associated with dural involvement. Other "benign" lymphoproliferative conditions that may involve the nervous system include plasma cell granuloma, angioimmunoblastic lymphadenopathy, and possibly nonspecific benign "pseudolymphoma." The diagnosis of these disorders in extranodal sites is difficult and will generally require ancillary studies (e.g., lymphoid markers, etc.). The differential diagnosis includes Hodgkin's disease, malignant histiocytosis, histiocytic lymphoma, monocytic leukemia, and histiocytosis X (42).

It is clear that these benign disorders may express their potential for producing destructive and/or mass lesions in vertebral column or cranial sites (potential targets for fine-needle aspiration biopsy), or may gain access to CSF spaces. Therefore, the cytopathologist must add this special subgroup of histologically distinctive, idiopathic, benign lymphoproliferative disorders to an already extensive list of reactive and neoplastic conditions to be considered when a lymphohistiocytic cell population is found in tissue aspirates or CSF samples.

Cytologic Manifestations of Ballistic Injury

Nichols and Sens (92) have recently described cytologic findings in tissue residue on bullet fragments that have traversed a variety of human tissues, including CNS tissue. In the latter cases fragments of vasculature, meninges, ependyma, choroid plexus, and epidural tissues (i.e., scalp, muscle, fibrofatty tissue, and bone chips) were disproportionately represented in the material adhering to the projectile in comparison to neural parenchyma, given the distance traveled in each of these structures by the projectile. Assessment of the possible implications of such findings for application of cytologic techniques in forensic pathology or for the elucidation of the pathophysiology of acute ballistic trauma would be premature at the time of this writing.

References

1. Aarli, J.A., Mork, S.J., Myrseth, E., and Larsen, J.L.: Glioblastoma associated with multiple sclerosis; coincidence or induction? Eur. Neurol. 29:312–316, 1989.
2. Adams, J.H., Corsellis, J.A.N., and Duchen, L.W.: Greenfield's Neuropathology. Ed. 4. John Wiley and Sons, New York, 1984.
3. Adams, J.H., Graham, D.I., and Doyle, D.: Brain Biopsy. The Smear Technique for Neurosurgical Biopsies. J.B. Lippincott, Philadelphia, 1981.
4. Adams, M., Rhyner, P.A., Day, J., DeArmond, S., and Smuckler, E.A.: Whipple's disease confined to the central nervous system. Ann. Neurol. 21:104–108, 1987.
5. AIDS Bibliography (monthly). A National Library of Medicine Publication. U.S. Government Printing Office, Washington, D.C.
6. Allen, I.V.: Demyelinating diseases. Chapter 9 in: Adams, J.H., Corsellis, J.A.N., and Duchen, L.W. (Eds.): Greenfield's Neuropathology. Ed. 4. John Wiley and Sons, New York, 1984. pp. 338–384.
7. Antonen, J., Syrjala, P., Oikarinen, R., Frey, H., and Krohn, K.: Acute multiple sclerosis exacerbations are characterized by low cerebrospinal fluid suppressor/cytotoxic T cells. Acta Neurol. Scand. 75:156–160, 1987.
8. Arvin, A.M., Johnson, R.T., Whitley, R.T., Nelson, J.D., and McCracken, G.H. Jr.: Consensus: Management of the patient with herpes simplex encephalitis. Pediatr. Infect. Dis. J. 6:2–5, 1987.
9. Ashwood, E.R., Cheng, E., Luthy, D.A.: Maternal serum alpha-fetoprotein and fetal trisomy-21 in women 35 years and older: Implications for alpha-fetoprotein screening programs. Am. J. Med. Genet. 26:531–539, 1987.
10. Baker, R.C., and Lenane, A.M.: The predictive value of cerebrospinal fluid differential cytology in meningitis. Pediatr. Infect. Dis. J. 8:329–330, 1989.
11. Becker, L.E., and Yates, A.J.: Inherited metabolic disease. Chapter 9 in: Davis, R.L. and Robertson, D.M. (Eds.): Textbook of Neuropathology. Ed. 2. Williams & Wilkins, Baltimore, 1991, pp. 331–427.
12. Benson, R.L., Ansbacher, L., Hutchison, R.E., and Rogers, W.: Cerebrospinal fluid centrifuge analysis in primary amebic meningoencephalitis due to *Naegleria fowleri*. Arch. Pathol. Lab. Med. 109:668–671, 1985.
13. Bigner, S.H., and Johnston, W.W.: Cytopathology of the central nervous system. In: Johnston, W.W. (Ed.): Monographs in Diagnostic Cytopathology, Vol. 3. Masson Publishing U.S.A., Inc, New York, 1983.
14. Bigner, S.H., Elmore, P.D., Dee, A.L., Hoffman, M., and Johnston, W.W.: Unusual presentations of inflammatory conditions in cerebrospinal fluid. Acta Cytol. 29:291–296, 1985.
15. Binford, C.H., and Connor, D.H. (Eds.): Pathology of Tropical and Extraordinary Diseases (in two volumes). Armed Forces Institute of Pathology, Washington, D.C., 1976.
16. Blumbergs, P.C., Hallpike, J.F., and McClure, J.: Cerebral malakoplakia. J. Clin. Pathol. 34:875–878, 1981.
17. Bonadio, W.A.: Bacterial meningitis in children whose cerebrospinal fluid contains polymorphonuclear leukocytes without pleocytosis. Clin. Pediatr. 27:198–200, 1988.
18. Bottles, K., Miller, T.R., Jeffrey, R.B., Cohen, M.B., Stoloff, A., Hales, M., Ljung, B-M., and Donegan, E.: Aspiration cytology characterization of inflammatory masses. West. J. Med. 144:695–699, 1986.

19. Briceno, C.E., Resch, L., and Bernstein, M.: Cerebral amyloid angiopathy presenting as a mass lesion. Stroke 18:234–239, 1987.
20. Brownell, B., and Tomlinson, A.H.: Virus diseases of the nervous system. Chapter 7 in: Adams, J.H., Corsellis, J.A.N., and Duchen, L.W. (Eds.): Greenfield's Neuropathology. Ed. 4. John Wiley and Sons, New York, 1984, pp. 260–303.
21. Burger, P.C., and Bigner, S.H.: Short course. Practical approaches to the diagnosis of central nervous system tumors. Mod. Pathol. 1:493–511, 1988.
22. Burger, P.C., Scheithauer, B.W., and Vogel, F.S.: Surgical Pathology of the Nervous System and Its Coverings. Ed. 3. Churchill Livingstone, New York, 1991.
23. Burns, D.K., Risser, R.C., and White, C.L. III: The neuropathology of human immunodeficiency virus infection. The Dallas, Texas, experience. Arch. Pathol. Lab. Med. 115:1112–1124, 1991.
24. Case records of the Massachusetts General Hospital (Case 10-1991). N. Engl. J. Med. 324:677–687, 1991.
25. Chalmers, A.C., Aprill, B.S., and Shepard, H.: Cerebrospinal fluid and human immunodeficiency virus. Findings in healthy, asymptomatic, seropositive men. Arch. Intern. Med. 150:1538–1540, 1990.
26. Chandrasoma, P.T., and Apuzzo, M.L.J.: Stereotactic Brain Biopsy. Igaku-Shoin, New York, 1989.
27. Chapman, P.A., Blenkinsopp, W.K., and Lewis, B.V.: The detection of neural tube closure defects by exfoliative cytology of amniotic fluid. Acta Cytol. 25:367–372, 1981.
27a. Cohen, M.B., Zaleski, M.S., and Wenzel, R.P.: AIDS-related safety issues for the cytology laboratory. Diagn. Cytopathol. 7:543–545, 1991.
28. Daumas-Duport, C., Mann, M., Munari, C., Blond, S., Musolino, A., Monsaingeon, V., and Chodkiewiczy, L.P.: Cryptic vascular malformations diagnosed by stereotactic biopsies—a preliminary study. Appl. Neurophysiol. 48: 440–443, 1985.
29. Daumas-Duport, C., Sheithauer, B.W., and Kelly, P.J.: A histologic and cytologic method for the spatial definition of gliomas. Mayo Clin. Proc. 62:435–449, 1987.
30. Davis, R.L., and Robertson, D.M. (Eds.): Textbook of Neuropathology, Ed. 2. Williams & Wilkins, Baltimore, 1991.
30a. De Girolami, U., Smith, T.W., Hénin, D., and Hauw, J.-J.: Neuropathology and Ophthalmologic Pathology of the Acquired Immunodeficiency Syndrome: A Color Atlas. Butterworth-Heineman, Stoneham, MA, 1992.
31. DeMent, S.H., Cox, M.C., and Gupta, P.K.: Diagnosis of central nervous system *Toxoplasma gondii* from the cerebrospinal fluid in a patient with acquired immunodeficiency syndrome. Diagn. Cytopathol. 3:148–151, 1987.
31a. de Smet, M.D., and Nussenbatt, R.B.: Ocular manifestations of AIDS. JAMA 266:3019–3022, 1991.
32. den Hartog Jager, W.A.: Color Atlas of C.S.F. Cytopathology. J.B. Lippincott, Philadelphia, 1980.
33. DeRueck, J., DeCoster, W., and Vander Eecken, H.: Cerebrospinal fluid cytology in acute ischemic stroke. Acta Neurol. Belg. 85:133–136, 1985.
34. Dickson, D.W., Belman, A.L., Park, Y.D., Wiley, C., Horoupian, D.S., Llena, J., Kure, K., Lyman, W.D., Morecki, R., Mitsudo S., and Cho, S.: Central nervous system pathology in pediatric AIDS: an autopsy study. APMIS Suppl. 8:40–57, 1989.
35. Duchen, L.W.: General pathology of neurons and neuroglia. Chapter 1 in: Adams, J.H., Corsellis, J.A.N., and Duchen, L.W. (Eds.): Greenfield's Neuropathology. Ed. 4. John Wiley and Sons, New York, 1984, pp. 1–52.
36. Eagle, R.C. Jr., and Yanoff, M.: The Eye. Chapter 51 in: Silverberg, S.G. (Ed.): Principles and Practice of Surgical Pathology. John Wiley and Sons, New York, 1983, 2:1547–1578.
37. Elovaara, I., Iivanainen, M., Valle, S-L., Suni, J., Tervo, T., and Lähdevirta, J.: CSF protein and cellular profiles in various stages of HIV infection related to neurological manifestations. J. Neurol. Sci. 78:331–342, 1987.
37a. Epstein, M.A., Zimmerman, R.A., Rorke, L.B., and Sladky, J.T.: Late-onset globoid cell leukodystrophy mimicking an infiltrating glioma. Pediatr. Radiol. 21:131–132, 1991.
38. Esiri, M.M., and Oppenheimer, D.R.: Diagnostic Neuropathology. A Practical Manual. Blackwell Scientific Publications, Oxford, 1989.
39. Ferrer, I., Fabregues, I., Pineda, M., Fernandez Alvarez, E., Cusi, V., and Vila, J.: Diagnosis of infantile neuro-axonal dystrophy by conjunctival biopsy. Neuropediatrics 14:53–55, 1983.
40. Fetter, B.F., Klintworth, G.K., and Hendry, W.S.: Mycoses of the Central Nervous System. Williams & Wilkins, Baltimore, 1967.
41. Fishman, R.A.: No, brain biopsy need not be done in every patient suspected of having herpes simplex encephalitis. Arch. Neurol. 44:1291–1292, 1987.
42. Foucar, E., Rosai, J., Dorfman, R.F. and Brynes, R.K.: The neurologic manifestation of sinus histiocytosis with massive lymphadenopathy. Neurology 32:365–371, 1982.
43. Fredrikson, S., Ernerudh, J., Olsson, T.K., Forsberg, P., and Link, H.: Mononuclear cell types in cerebrospinal fluid and blood of patients

with multiple sclerosis. Quantitation by immunoenzyme microassay with panel of monoclonal antibodies. Arch. Neurol. 46:372–375, 1989.
44. Friede, R.L.: Developmental Neuropathology. Ed. 2, Springer-Verlag, New York, 1989.
45. Friedman, W.A., Sceats, D.J. Jr., Nestok, B.R., and Ballinger, W.E. Jr.: The incidence of unexpected pathological findings in an image-guided biopsy series: a review of 100 consecutive cases. Neurosurgery, 25:180–184, 1989.
46. Garcia, J.H., and Anderson, M.L.: Circulatory disorders and their effects on the brain. Chapter 13 in: Davis, R.L., and Robertson, D.M. (Eds.): Textbook of Neuropathology. Ed. 2. Williams & Wilkins, Baltimore, 1991, pp. 621–718.
46a. Garcia, J.H., and Cervós-Navarro, J.: Brain biopsy. Chapter 6 in: Garcia, J.H., Escalona-Zapata, J., Sandbank, U., and Cervós-Navarro, J. (Eds.): Diagnostic Neuropathology. Field and Wood Medical Publishers, New York, 1990, 2:47–122.
47. Gibb, W.R.G.: Idiopathic Parkinson's disease and the Lewy body disorders. Neuropathol. Appl. Neurobiol. 12:223–234, 1986.
48. Goebel, H.H.: Neuropathological diagnosis of childhood neurodegenerative disorders by biopsy: invited topic. Turk. J. Pediatr. 30:193–211, 1988.
49. Goetz, C.G., Klawans, H.L., and Cohen, M.M.: Neurotoxic agents. Chapter 20 in: Joynt, R.J. (Ed.): Clinical Neurology. J.B. Lippincott, Philadelphia, 1988, Vol. 2, pp. 1–84.
50. Gray, F., Gherardi, R., and Scaravilli, F.: The neuropathology of the acquired immune deficiency syndrome (AIDS). Brain 111:245–266, 1988.
50a. Greenlee, J.E.: Approach to diagnosis of meningitis. Cerebrospinal fluid evaluation. Inf. Dis. Clin. North Am. 4:583–598, 1990.
51. Griffin, D.E., Moser, H.W., Mendoza, Q., Moench, T.R., O'Toole, S., and Moser, A.B.: Identification of the inflammatory cells in the central nervous system of patients with adrenoleukodystrophy. Ann. Neurol. 18:660–664, 1985.
52. Hafler, D.A., Duby, A.D., Lee, S.J., Benjamin, D., Seidman, J.G., and Weiner, H.L.: Oligoclonal T lymphocytes in the cerebrospinal fluid of patients with multiple sclerosis. J. Exp. Med. 167:1313–1322, 1988.
53. Hafler, D.A., and Weiner, H.L.: In-vivo labeling of blood T cells: rapid traffic into cerebrospinal fluid in multiple sclerosis. Ann. Neurol. 22:89–93, 1987.
54. Hall, W.A., Martinez, A.J., Dummer, J.S., Griffith, B.P., Hardesty, R.L., Bahnson, H.T., and Lunsford, L.D.: Central nervous system infections in heart and heart-lung transplant recipients. Arch. Neurol. 46:173–177, 1989.
55. Hanley, D.F., Johnson, R.T., and Whitley, R.J.: Yes, brain biopsy should be a prerequisite for herpes simplex encephalitis treatment. Arch. Neurol. 44:1289–1290, 1987.
56. Harper, C., Halliday, G., Pamphlett, R., McCann, H., and Broc, G.: Problems with using the Khachaturian criteria for the diagnosis of Alzheimer's disease (AD). J. Neuropathol. Exp. Neurol. 50:299, 1991.
57. Harriman, D.G.F.: Bacterial infections of the central nervous system. Chapter 6 in: Adams, J.H., Corsellis, J.A.N., and Duchen, L.W. (Eds.): Greenfield's Neuropathology. Ed. 4. John Wiley and Sons, New York, 1984, pp. 236–259.
58. Hegenbarth, M.A., Green, M., Rowley, A.H., and Chadwic, E.G.: Absent or minimal cerebrospinal fluid abnormalities in *Haemophilus influenzae* meningitis. Pediatr. Emerg. Care 6:191–194, 1990.
59. Hendricks, J.T., Franke, C.L., and Tehunissen, P.H.M.H.: Cerebral amyloid angiopathy: diagnosis by MRI and brain biopsy. Neurology 40:1308–1310, 1990.
60. Henry, J.B.(Ed.): Clinical Diagnosis and Management by Laboratory Methods. W.B. Saunders, Philadelphia, 1991.
61. Herndon, R.M., and Brumback, R.A. (Eds.): The Cerebrospinal Fluid. Kluwer Academic Publishers, Boston, 1989.
62. Hirano, A.: Neurons and astrocytes. Chapter 1 in: Davis, R.L. and Robertson, D.M. (Eds.): Textbook of Neuropathology. Ed. 2. Williams & Wilkins, Baltimore, 1991, pp. 1–94.
63. Hirschfeld, A.: Stereotectic techniques in the management of cerebral neoplasms. Oncology 3:25–32, 1989.
63a. Ho, K.-L., Gottlieb, C., and Zarbo, R.J.: Cytomegalovirus infection of cerebral astrocytoma in an AIDS patient. Clin. Neuropathol. 10:127–133, 1991.
64. Hobbins, J.C.: Diagnosis and management of neural tube defects today. N. Engl. J. Med. 324:690–691, 1991.
65. Hori, A., Weiss, R., and Schaake, T.: Ganglioglioma containing osseous tissue and neurofibrillary tangles. Arch. Pathol. Lab. Med. 112:653–655, 1988.
66. Hunter, S.B., Ballinger, W.E. Jr., and Rubin, J.J.: Multiple sclerosis mimicking primary brain tumor. Arch. Pathol. Lab. Med. 111:464–468, 1987.
67. Ioachim, H.L.: Biopsy diagnosis in human immunodeficiency virus infection and acquired immunodeficiency syndrome. Arch. Pathol. Lab. Med. 114:284–294, 1990.
68. Jane, J.A., and Yashon, D.: Cytology of Tumors Affecting the Nervous System. Charles C. Thomas, Springfield, Ill., 1969.

69. Johnson, P.C.: Peripheral nerve. Chapter 18 in: Davis, R.L., and Robertson, D.M. (Eds.): Textbook of Neuropathology. Ed. 2. Williams & Wilkins, Baltimore, 1991, pp. 1004–1007.
70. Johnston, F.B.: Splendori-Hoeppli phenomenon. Chapter 7 in: Binford, C.H., and Connor, D.H.: Pathology of Tropical and Extraordinary Diseases. Armed Forces Institute of Pathology, Washington, D.C., 1976, pp. 681–683.
71. Kato, T., Katagiri, T., Hirano, A., Sasaki, H., and Arai, S.: Sporadic lower motor neuron disease with Lewy body-like inclusions: a new subgroup? Acta Neuropathol. 76:208–211, 1988.
72. Katz, R.L., Alappattu, C., Glass, J.P., and Bruner, J.M.: Cerebrospinal fluid manifestations of the neurologic complications of human immunodeficiency virus infection. Acta Cytol. 33:233–244, 1989.
73. Khachaturian, Z.S.: Diagnosis of Alzheimer's disease. Arch. Neurol. 42:1097–1105. 1985.
74. Kilpatrick, M.E., Mikhail, I.A., and Girgis, N.I.: Negative cultures of cerebrospinal fluid in partially treated bacterial meningitis. Trop. Geogr. Med. 39:345–349, 1987.
75. Kirkpatrick, J.B.: Neurologic infections due to bacteria, fungi and parasites. Chapter 14 in: Davis, R.L., and Robertson, D.M. (Eds.): Textbook of Neuropathology. Ed. 2. Williams & Wilkins, Baltimore, 1991, pp. 719–803.
76. Kjeldsberg, C.R., and Knight, J.A.: Body Fluids. Laboratory Examination of Amniotic, Cerebrospinal, Seminal, Serous and Synovial Fluids: A Textbook Atlas. Ed. 2. American Society of Clinical Pathologists Press, Chicago, 1986.
77. Kohl, S.: Brain biopsy for suspected herpes encephalitis. J. Pediatr. 114:335, 1989.
78. Kolmel, H.W.: Atlas of Cerebrospinal Fluid Cells. Ed. 2. Springer-Verlag, New York, 1977.
78a. Kumar, P.V., Sotoodeh, M., and Beddayat, G.R.: Aspiration findings of extramedullary hematopoiesis presenting as an epidural mass. Acta Cytol. 35:146–147, 1991.
79. Lake, B.D.: Lysosomal enzyme deficiencies. Chapter 12 in: Adams, J.H., Corsellis, J.A.N., and Duchen, L.W. (Eds.): Greenfield's Neuropathology. Ed. 4. John Wiley and Sons, New York, 1984, pp. 491–572.
80. Lantos, P.L.: Histological and cytological reactions. Chapter 2 in: Weller, R.O. (Ed.): Nervous System, Muscle and Eyes. Vol. 4 in: Symmers, W. St. C. (Ed.) Systemic Pathology. Ed. 3. Churchill Livingstone, New York, 1989, pp. 36–63.
81. Leestma, J.E.: Forensic Neuropathology. Raven Press, New York, 1988.
82. Leestma, J.E.: Viral infections of the nervous system. Chapter 15 in: Davis, R.L., and Robertson, D.M. (Eds.): Textbook of Neuropathology, Ed. 2. Williams & Wilkins, Baltimore, 1991, pp. 804–903.
83. Lenke, R.R., and Ashwood, E.R.: Use of maternal serum alpha-fetoprotein as an early pregnancy screen. The Female Patient, 12:18–26, 1987.
84. Lenke, R.R., Guerrieri, J., Nemes, J.M., Kurczynski, T.W., French, B., Gray, M., Schut, H., and Ashwood, E.R.: Maternal serum alpha-fetoprotein screening: how low is high? J. Reprod. Med. 34:511–516, 1989.
85. Lindenberg, R.: Letter to the Editor. Neuropathological diagnosis of Alzheimer's disease. J. Neuropathol. Exp. Neurol. 49:535–537, 1990.
86. Lindquist, L., Linne, T., Hansson, L-O., Kalin, M., and Axelsson, G.: Value of cerebrospinal fluid analysis in the differential diagnosis of meningitis: a study in 710 patients with suspected central nervous system infection. Eur. J. Clin. Microbiol. Infect. Dis. 7:374–380, 1988.
87. Liwnicz, B.B., and Rodriquez, C.A.: The central nervous system. Chapter 16 in: Koss, L.G., Woyke, S., and Olszewski, W.: Aspiration Biopsy. Cytologic Interpretation and Histologic Bases. Igaku-Shoin, New York, 1985.
88. Lobenthal, S.W., and Hajdu, S.I.: The cytopathology of bone marrow transplantation. Acta Cytol. 34:559–566, 1990.
89. Lumsden, C.E.: The neuropathology of multiple sclerosis. Chapter 8 in: Vinkin, P.J., and Bruyn, G.W. (Eds.): Multiple Sclerosis and Other Demyelinating Diseases. Vol. 9 in: Vinkin, P.J., and Bruyn, G.W. (Eds.): Handbook of Clinical Neurology. American Elsevier Publishing Co., Inc., New York, 1970, pp. 217–309.
89a. Marmaduke, D.P., Brandt, J.T., and Theil, K.S.: Rapid diagnosis of cytomegalovirus in the cerebrospinal fluid of a patient with AIDS-associated polyradiculopathy. Arch. Pathol. Lab. Med. 115:1154–1157, 1991.
90. Martin, J.J., and Centerick, C.H.: The contribution of pathology to the study of storage disorders. Pathol. Res. Pract. 183:375–385, 1988.
91. Matsumoto, T., Tani, E., Maeda, Y., and Natsume, S.: Amyloidomas in the cerebellopontine angle and jugular foramen: case report. J. Neurosurg. 62:592–596, 1985.
91a. Nesbit, G.M., Forbes, G.S., Scheithauer, B.W., Okazaki, H., and Rodriguez, M.: Multiple sclerosis: histopathologic and MR and/or CT correlation in 37 cases at biopsy and three cases at autopsy. Radiology 180:467–474, 1991.
92. Nichols, C.A., and Sens, M.A.: Cytologic manifestations of ballistic injury. Am. J. Clin. Pathol. 95:660–669, 1991.
93. Nochomovitz, L., Sidawy, M., Silverberg, S., Jannotta, F., and Schwartz, A.: Intraoperative Consultation. A Guide to Smears, Imprints and

Frozen Sections. American Society of Clinical Pathologists Press, Chicago, 1989.
94. Norenberg, M.D., and Bruce-Gregorios, J.: Nervous system manifestations of systemic disease. Chapter 11 in: Davis, R.L., and Robertson, D.M. (Eds.): Textbook of Neuropathology. Ed. 2. Williams & Wilkins, Baltimore, 1991, pp. 461–534.
95. Oehmichen, M.: Cerebrospinal Fluid Cytology. An Introduction and Atlas. W.B. Saunders Co., Philadelphia, 1976.
96. Paty, D.W., McFarlin, D.E., and McDonald, W.I.: Editorial. Magnetic resonance imaging and laboratory aids in the diagnosis of multiple sclerosis. Ann. Neurol. 29:3–5, 1991.
96a. Phillips, S.E., and Millan, J.C.: Reassessment of microbiology protocol for cerebrospinal fluid specimens. Lab. Med. 22:619–622, 1991.
97. Polman, C.H., DeGroot, C.J.A., Koetsier, J.C., Sminia, T., and Veerman, A.J.P.: Cerebrospinal fluid cells in multiple sclerosis and other neurological diseases: an immunocytochemical study. J. Neurol. 234:19–22, 1987.
98. Portnoy, J.M., and Olsen, L.C.: Normal cerebrospinal fluid values in children: another look. Pediatrics 75:484–487, 1985.
99. Raimonde, A.J., Mullan, S., and Evans, P.E.: Human brain tumors: an electron microscopic study. J. Neurosurg. 19:731–753, 1962.
100. Raine, C.S.: Demyelinating diseases. Chapter 12 in: Davis, R.L., and Robertson, D.M. (Eds.): Textbook of Neuropathology. Ed 2. Williams & Wilkins, Baltimore, 1991, pp. 535–620.
101. Reimer, L.G.: Approach to the analysis of body fluids for the detection of infection. Clin. Lab. Med. 5:209–222, 1985.
102. Rewcastle, N.B.: Degenerative diseases of the nervous system. Chapter 16 in: Davis, R.L., and Robertson, D.M. (Eds.): Textbook of Neuropathology. Ed. 2. Williams & Wilkins, Baltimore, 1991, pp. 904–961.
103. Rieth, K.G., DiChiro, G., Cromwell, L.D., McKeave, P.E., and Pleet, A.B.: Primary demyelinating disease simulating glioma of the corpus callosum. Report of three cases. J. Neurosurg. 55:620–624, 1981.
104. Riggs, J.E., Schochet, S.S. Jr., and Nelson, J.: Asymptomatic adult Alexander's disease: entity or nosologic misconception? Neurology, 38:152–154, 1988.
105. Rosenblum, W.I.: Letter to the Editor. Neuropathological diagnosis of Alzheimer's disease. J. Neuropathol. Exp. Neurol. 49:188, 1990.
106. Rosenthal, D.L., Mandell, D.B., and Glasgow, B.J.: Eye. Chapter 19 in: Bibbo, M. (Ed.): Comprehensive Cytopathology. W.B. Saunders, Philadelphia, 1991, pp. 484–501.
107. Rosenthal, D.L.: Cytology of the Central Nervous System. Vol. 8 in: Wied, G.L. (Ed.): Monographs in Clinical Cytology. S. Karger, New York, 1984.
108. Rubinstein, L.J.: Tumors of the central nervous system. Fascicle 6, Second Series, Atlas of Tumor Pathology. Armed Forces Institute of Pathology, Washington, D.C., 1972.
109. Russell, D.S., and Rubinstein, L.J.: Pathology of Tumors of the Nervous System. Ed. 5. Williams & Wilkins, Baltimore, 1989.
110. Sale, G.E. (Ed.): The Pathology of Organ Transplantation. Butterworths, Boston, 1990.
111. Sands, M.L., Ryczak, M., and Brown, R.B.: Recurrent aseptic meningitis followed by transverse myelitis as a presentation of systemic lupus erythematosus. J. Rheumatol. 15:862–864, 1988.
112. Sawyer, J., Ellner, J., and Ransohoff, D.F.: To biopsy or not to biopsy in suspected herpes simplex encephalitis: a quantitative analysis. Med. Decis. Making 8:95–101, 1988.
113. Scheithauer, B.W.: Central nervous system and pituitary. Chapter 8 in: Silva, E.G., and Kraemer, B.B. (Eds.): Intraoperative Pathologic Diagnosis. Frozen Section and Other Techniques. Williams & Wilkins, Baltimore, 1987, pp. 167–219.
114. Scherer, H.J.: Structural development in gliomas. Am. J. Cancer 34:333–351, 1938.
115. Schlitt, M., Morawetz, R.B., Bonnin, J., Chandra-Sekar, B., Curtiss, J.J., Diethelm, A.G. Jr., Whelchel, J.D., and Whitley, R.J.: Progressive multifocal leukoencephalopathy: three patients diagnosed by brain biopsy, with prolonged survival in two. Neurosurgery 18:407–414, 1986.
116. Schmidt, R.M., Kuppe, G., Kissig, B., Ludewig, R., and Neumann, V.: Research approaches on the diagnosis of multiple sclerosis by CSF examination. Arch. Suisses Neurol. Psychiatr. 138:13–22, 1987.
117. Schochet, S.S. Jr., and Nelson, J.: Exogenous toxic-metabolic diseases including vitamin deficiency. Chapter 10 in: Davis, R.L., and Robertson, D.M. (Eds.): Textbook of Neuropathology, Ed. 2. Williams & Wilkins, Baltimore, 1991, pp. 428–460.
118. Schochet, S.S. Jr., and Lampert, P.W.: Granulomatous encephalitis in Whipple's disease. Electron microscopic observations. Acta Neuropathol. (Berl.) 13:1–11, 1969.
119. Sekuja, S., Tanaka, M., Hayashi, S., and Oyanagi, S.: Distribution of intracytoplasmic acidophilic granule-containing neurons in the human brain. Acta Neuropathol. (Berl.), 60:145–148, 1983.
120. Selsky, E.J., Knox, D.L., Maumenee, A.E., and Green, W.R.: Ocular involvement in Whipple's disease. Retina 4:103–106, 1984.
121. Sipe, J.C., and O'Brien, J.S.: Ultrastructure of

skin biopsy specimens in lysosomal storage diseases: common sources of error in diagnosis. Clin. Genet. 15:118–125, 1979.

122. Sorsdahl, O.S., Taylor, P.E., and Noyes, W.D.: Extramedullary hematopoiesis, mediastinal masses, and spinal cord compression. J.A.M.A. 189:343–347, 1964.

123. Sotrel, A.: The nervous system. Chapter 8 in: Harawi, S.J., and O'Hara, C.J. (Eds.): Pathology and Pathophysiology of AIDS and HIV-Related Diseases. C.V. Mosby, St. Louis, 1989, pp. 201–268.

124. Strickland, G.T.: Hunter's Tropical Medicine. Ed. 6. W.B. Saunders, Philadelphia, 1984.

124a. Strigle, S.M., and Gal, A.A.: Review of the central nervous system cytopathology in human immunodeficiency virus infection. Diagn. Cytopathol. 7:387–401, 1991.

125. Tourtellotte, W.W., Baumhefner, R.W., Syndulko, K., Shapshak, P., Osborne, M., Rubinstein, G., Newton, L., Ellison, G., Myers, L., Rosario, I., Thomson, R., Sloan, R., and Engelmann, S.: The long march of the cerebrospinal fluid profile indicative of clinical definite multiple sclerosis; and still marching. J. Neuroimmunol. 20:217–227, 1988.

126. Vinters, H.V., and Anders, K.H.: Neuropathology of AIDS. CRC Press, Boca Raton, Fla., 1989.

127. Walker, R.C.: The role of the clinical microbiology laboratory in transplantation. Arch. Pathol. Lab. Med. 115:299–305, 1991.

127a. Waltregny, A., Maula, A.A., and Brucher, J.M.: Contribution of stereotactic brain biopsies to the diagnosis in several cases of dementia. Acta Neurol. Belg. 89:161–167, 1989.

128. Wasiewski, W.W., and Fishman, M.A.: Herpes simplex encephalitis: the brain biopsy controversy. J. Pediatr. 113:575–578, 1988.

129. Weller, R.O. (Ed.): Nervous System, Muscle and Eyes. Vol. 4 in: Symmers, W. St. C. (Ed.): Systemic Pathology. Ed. 3. Churchill Livingstone, New York, 1990.

130. Weller, R.O.: Demyelinating diseases: multiple sclerosis. Chapter 10 in: Weller, R.O., (Ed.): Nervous System, Muscle and Eyes. Vol. 4 in: Symmers, W. St. C. (Ed.): Systemic Pathology, Ed. 3. Churchill Livingstone, New York, 1990, pp. 224–243.

131. Weller, R.O.: Developmental, neonatal and paediatric neuropathology. Chapter 12 in: Weller, R.O. (Ed.): Nervous System, Muscle and Eyes. Vol. 4 in: Symmers, W. St. C. (Ed.): Systemic Pathology, Ed. 3. Churchill Livingstone, New York, 1990, pp. 309–359.

132. Wenk, R.E., and Rosenbaum, J.M.: Analysis of amniotic fluid. Chapter 20 in: Henry, J.B. (Ed.): Clinical Diagnosis and Management by Laboratory Methods. W.B. Saunders, Philadelphia, 1991, pp. 482–496.

133. Whitley, R.J., Cobbs, C.G., Alford, C.A. Jr., Soon, S-J., Hirsch, M.S., Connor, J.D., Corey, L., Hanley, D.F., Levin, M., Powell, D.A., and the NIAID Collaborative Antiviral Study Group: Diseases that mimic herpes simplex encephalitis. Diagnosis, presentation and outcome. J.A.M.A. 262:234–239, 1989.

134. Wisniewski, H., Rabe, A., Zigman, W., and Silverman, W.: Editorial. Neuropathological diagnosis of Alzheimer's disease. J. Neuropathol. Exp. Neurol. 48:606–609, 1989.

135. Wisniewski, H.M., Rabe, A., Silverman, W., and Zigman, W.: Reply. J. Neuropathol. Exp. Neurol. 49:189–190, 1990.

136. Wisniewski, H.M., Rabe, A., Zigman, W., and Silverman, W.: Neuropathological diagnostic criteria for Alzheimer's disease: A reply to Lindenberg. J. Neuropathol. Exp. Neurol. 49:537, 1990.

137. Yamano, T., Shimada, M., Okada, S., Yutaka, T., Yabuuchi, H., and Nakao, Y.: Electron microscopic examination of skin and conjunctival biopsy specimens in neuronal storage diseases. Brain Dev. 1:16–25, 1979.

138. Young, B.: Role of stereotactic biopsy in the management of transplant patients with intracranial lesions. Neurol. Clin. 6:639–644, 1988.

139. Zajdela, A., Vielh, P., Schlienger, P., and Haye, C.: Fine-needle cytology of 292 palpable orbital and eyelid tumors. Am. J. Clin. Pathol. 93:100–104, 1991.

9 / Pitfalls in Diagnosis

Diagnostic problems and pitfalls are not unique to neuropathology. Pathologists encounter similar problems in a variety of disorders such as lymphomas (4, 6, 12, 18), borderline epithelial lesions of the breast (14), and mesenchymal tumors of the gut (2). This chapter briefly reviews potential diagnostic pitfalls in the practice of neurocytopathology. These have been gathered from our own experience and from published observations of others. We make no claim that this list is comprehensive, or that application of these principles will guarantee an accurate diagnosis in each case. Neither our own skills nor the current state of the art allows for the achievement of this desired goal. This is particularly true in situations where the pathologist must render an intraoperative diagnosis with small tissue samples, relying solely on morphologic techniques, or must draw conclusions from rare cells in a CSF sample.

There is nearly universal appreciation of these facts, and the degree of accuracy achieved by surgical pathologists and cytologists in this complex area despite current technological limitations is, to us, a remarkable testimony to the scholarship and dedication of the individuals involved. It is a curious contradiction that, simultaneous with the achievement of this previously unequaled diagnostic accuracy, physicians currently practice in a social and legal environment that is, by our perception, quite unforgiving of error. The present chapter is, for this reason, divided into two sections.

The first section, medical/legal pitfalls, reviews the currently rather limited material we have found that specifically relates to surgical pathologists and cytologists. The second part reviews potential pitfalls related to cytomorphologic features of specimens.

Many of the following points are referenced to further discussion elsewhere in the text or to relevant reports in the literature. We have arbitrarily limited the discussion of pitfalls to 100 items, in respect to space limitations and the interest of the reader.

Medical/Legal Pitfalls

1. The greatest professional liability exposure for the pathologist is the misdiagnosis or misinterpretation of anatomic specimens with or without frozen sections (13).
2. Retrospective reviews of diagnostic errors often reveal that diagnosis was based on frozen sections of suboptimal quality (17).
3. Erroneous diagnoses are not infrequently based on minimal ("flyspeck") biopsies (17).
   COMMENT: The current trend toward procedures that are less invasive and less expensive and yield smaller tissue samples has been a result of the collective attempt to benefit patients, not pathologists. The difficulties of the pathologist have been compounded by this trend, and one of the main goals of this text has been to aid the pathologist in gaining the maximum accurate immediate information for diagnostic purposes from these limited samples by the simultaneous use of smears or imprints and frozen sections. Use of additional levels cut from blocks at the time permanent sections are prepared can also be helpful in salvaging a diagnosis from apparently nondiagnostic specimens.

Intermediate (i.e., unstained) sections should also be mounted and saved for possible later use until it is clear that they will not be required.

4. Some cases are simply so difficult that they are not diagnosable at the time of the original intraoperative consultation. The pathologist must know when it is appropriate to defer diagnosis.
5. The number of disparate pathologic entities with similar morphologic features makes it essential for the pathologist to track down the many clinicians who fail to supply at least minimal clinical information, in order to avoid serious error (Chapter 1) (17).
   COMMENT: We continue to be surprised at the ease with which some of the most perplexing histologic dilemmas can be solved with a telephone call.
6. Avoidable diagnostic problems may result from poor communication or absence of intradepartmental (or outside expert) consultation, or lack of documentation thereof (17).
7. Pick your consultants carefully. You may share liability if you accept their opinions unquestioningly (17).
8. The possibility that a tissue sample may not be representative (i.e., sampling error) must always be borne in mind (17).
9. "Legally, the only slides that are considered to be actual evidence are the *original* slides" (17). It is advisable to send recuts when possible, rather than originals, should slides be sent to consultants.
10. The pathologist must be thoroughly familiar with the legal implications and appropriate means by which reports which have already left the department may be corrected.
    COMMENT: This point cannot be overemphasized. A conscientious and innocent attempt by the pathologist to correct an error or add subsequently obtained data that improves the accuracy of the original report may provide a means by which the pathologist's veracity and professional credibility can be destroyed, if the alteration or addendum is not performed in precisely the correct manner. The reader is referred to the hospital medical records administrator and medical liability carrier for the necessary details concerning this issue.

Diagnostic Pitfalls

11. Frozen sections provide an advantage in assessing cellularity and tissue architecture, but they tend to make nuclei more angular, vacuolated, and sometimes hyperchromatic (3) and they often obscure cytoplasmic and vascular detail.
12. Smear and imprint techniques provide greatly superior cytologic detail (in comparison to frozen sections) at the expense of loss of many architectural relationships.
    COMMENT: The diagnosis of some lesions depends more on the architecture and cellularity, while that of other lesions depends more on cytologic detail. This emphasizes the value of using the combined techniques whenever possible.
13. Consider meningioma and melanoma in the differential diagnosis of every tumor.
14. Lack of complete concordance between clinical data, radiological data, frozen section results, and smear/imprint (or CSF) results suggests that a differential diagnosis or deferred diagnosis may be appropriate. Permanent sections or ancillary studies may be required to resolve the disparity.
15. Nuclei are larger on air-dried than on wet-fixed smears and imprints.
16. Cells of a variety of shapes tend to become round when suspended in CSF

due to surface tension factors, and degenerative changes often ensue (Chapter 7).

17. If you make one diagnosis, look for a second. If you find a second, look for a third, and so forth, until you are satisfied that no additional diagnoses are present. This applies not only to infectious agents in immunocompromised hosts, but to every case seen.
18. Photographs of cytologic preparations in texts and atlases can demonstrate only a limited spectrum of an entire smear or CSF sample and are limited to a single plane of focus (1). These deficiencies can be remedied by the development of a teaching slide set in each laboratory (Chapter 2).
19. Small stereotactic biopsies pose sufficient potential for diagnostic error, even with combined frozen section and cytologic techniques, to justify a recommendation for traditional open biopsy of readily accessible lesions of the CNS (16) and orbit (11).
20. Astrocytes may normally develop conspicuous fibrillary processes with aging in certain CNS locations (e.g., subpial, subependymal, perivascular, inferior olivary nuclei, Ammon's horn) and lend themselves to misinterpretation as astrocytomas in small biopsies from such sites (Chapter 2).
21. Talc crystals may superficially resemble cryptococci, corpora amylacea, polyglucosan bodies, and Lafora bodies (Chapter 2).
22. Isolated binucleate glia or neurons may occur in normal brain tissue (Chapter 2).
23. Melanin occurs in several normal brain structures as well as in benign and malignant lesions (Table 2.2; Table 7.11).
24. The cell size and cellularity of the normal cerebellar granular cell layer may cause confusion with chronic inflammatory cell infiltrates or small-cell neoplasms in smear or imprint preparations (Chapter 2).
25. The cerebellar external granular layer, present during the first few months after birth, may also superficially resemble a small-cell tumor or a chronic meningitis in tissue sections (Chapter 2) (10).
26. Cytologic preparations of normal ependymal cells may bear superficial resemblance to the cohesive cell fragments with nuclear molding seen in medulloblastomas and related tumors (Chapter 2).
27. Squamous metaplasia in normal pituitary glands may cause confusion with squamous epithelium-containing neoplasms or cysts in this region (e.g., craniopharyngioma, epidermoid cyst, etc.) (Chapter 2).
28. The "dirty" background in smears from normal anterior pituitary gland is not to be confused with tumor diathesis, but rather is due to rupture of the fragile cells when smeared (Chapter 2).
29. Normal posterior pituitary tissue somewhat resembles gliosis or a fibrillary astrocytoma (Chapter 2) (Fig. 2.12**F** and **G**).
30. Glomus bodies may resemble neoplasms (Chapter 2).
31. Beware of CSF contaminants that can mimic disease (e.g., talc crystals, lying free or phagocytosed by CSF macrophages, may—like RBCs or air bubbles—resemble cryptococci; chondrocytes and hematopoietic elements may mimic atypical or malignant cells) (Table 3.6).
32. CSF granulocytes lyse more rapidly than lymphocytes in samples stored at room temperature; samples for which processing will be delayed require refrigeration or the addition of fixative (Chapter 4).
33. CSF samples with normal total cell counts may contain malignant cells (Chapter 5).
34. Saving at least one air-dried slide for subsequent Diff-Quik or special stains may

prove critical in the diagnosis of certain small-cell tumors (Chapters 6 and 7).

35. Talc powder and bone dust may resemble psammoma bodies or other tissue calcific deposits (1, 5) (Chapter 7) (also see item 21 above).
36. The appearances in cytologic preparations of many variants of common tumors (e.g., meningiomas) and many rare tumors have not yet been described in published reports. Therefore, current concepts concerning the specificity of cytologic findings for certain tumor types are best viewed with caution.
37. Astrocyte tumor grading systems in common use apply to the diffuse astrocytomas, but not as readily to the special sub-categories of astrocytic neoplasms or other neuroglial tumors (Chapter 7).
38. Neuroepithelial tumors often display marked intratumoral cytohistologic heterogeneity (Chapters 1 and 7).
39. Many neuroepithelial tumors have cells that cling to blood vessels in smears, and this pseudopapillary appearance is not to be equated with an ependymoma on low-power screening (Chapter 7).
40. Neoplastic ganglion cells in gangliogliomas must be distinguished from entrapped, normal ganglion cells (Chapter 7).
41. The classic perinuclear halos of oligodendroglioma cells are typically absent in frozen sections and smears, since they represent a fixation artifact (Chapter 7).
42. The diagnosis of ependymomas will usually be made on criteria other than the presence of blepharoplasts or true ependymal rosettes, since neither is frequently encountered in these neoplasms (Chapter 7).
43. Tanycytic ependymomas may closely mimic astrocytomas (Chapter 7).
44. Neural heterotopias and ectopias must be included in the differential diagnosis of well-differentiated neuroglial tumors (Chapter 7).
45. Medulloblastomas (in the absence of differentiation) are cytologically indistinguishable by routine methods from most small-cell undifferentiated carcinomas of pulmonary origin, retinoblastomas, pineoblastomas, ependymoblastomas, neuroblastomas, and certain other small-cell tumors (Chapter 7).
46. A tumor that looks like an oligodendroglioma and is located in the vicinity of the septum pellucidum may be a central neurocytoma (Chapter 7).
47. Ventriculoperitoneal shunts may provide a direct route from the CNS to the peritoneal cavity for neoplastic cells and for non-neoplastic cells that can mimic malignant cells (e.g., ependymal and choroid plexus epithelial cells, histiocytes, multinucleated foreign body–type giant cells) (Chapter 7).
48. Malignant rhabdoid tumor-like areas may occur in primary CNS tumors (e.g., malignant meningioma, astrocytic tumors) and may potentially cause confusion in small biopsy specimens (5a, 9, 11a, 12a).
49. The classic morphologic features of capillary hemangioblastoma as seen in paraffin sections (e.g., prominent vascular pattern, stromal cell cytoplasmic vacuoles) may be inconspicuous in frozen sections and smears. The resemblance to astrocytic neoplasms and to clear-cell carcinoma of the kidney may be striking (Chapter 7).
50. Dense reactive gliosis, with or without Rosenthal fiber formation, may occur to an extent that readily mimics an astrocytoma (Table 7.6).
51. Choroid plexus papillary fragments may be present in CSF samples in conditions other than choroid plexus papilloma (Chapter 7).
52. Granulomatous lesions in small biopsy

samples from the pineal or suprasellar area, in particular, should raise suspicion of a germinoma (Chapter 7). The differential diagnosis should include infections, sarcoidosis, and histiocytosis X.

53. Syncytiotrophoblasts in a germinoma, in the absence of cytotrophoblastic and/or intermediate trophoblastic cellular components, do not warrant a diagnosis of mixed germ cell tumor (Chapter 7).
54. Multinucleation and nuclear pleomorphism are common in benign pituitary adenomas and are not synonymous with malignancy.
55. Enlarged, bizarre, hyperchromatic nuclei occur in several types of neural tumors, and in the absence of mitotic figures and/or hypercellularity or other ominous features are not necessarily indicators of malignancy (e.g., meningioma, subependymal giant cell astrocytoma, schwannoma) (Chapter 7).
56. Metaplastic features (e.g., cartilage) are more commonly encountered in malignant peripheral nerve sheath tumors than in any other spindle-cell sarcoma.
57. No type of rosette (i.e., Flexner-Wintersteiner, Homer Wright, perivascular pseudorosette) or fleurette is pathognomonic for a single tumor type (Table 7.9).
58. Primary CNS tumors may occasionally demonstrate extraneural spread to lymph nodes, bone, lung, and other sites in the absence of prior surgery (Chapter 7).
59. Occasional extraneural tumors metastatic to the subarachnoid space will present primarily or exclusively as single tumor cells rather than cell fragments in CSF samples, rendering diagnosis more difficult (Chapter 7).
60. Marker studies are often required to distinguish reactive from neoplastic CSF lymphoid populations (14a) (Chapter 7).
61. Blast-like cells may rarely be seen in childhood CSF samples in the absence of malignancy (Chapter 7).
62. Ocular lesions, including melanocytic lesions, present a number of unique features that require specialized ophthalmic pathology training for proper interpretation (Chapter 7).
63. The differential diagnosis of retinoblastomas includes at least two benign conditions: retinal dysplasia and retinocytoma (Chapter 7).
64. In children, the most common orbital tumor is primary; in adults it is metastatic (Chapter 7).
65. Radiation cerebritis may clinically and pathologically closely mimic tumor recurrence (Chapter 7).
66. Development of a second neoplasm differing from the original tumor type is being seen with increased frequency as modern treatment measures improve survival (Chapter 7).
67. A number of paraneoplastic syndromes may mimic tumor metastasis or recurrence (Chapter 7).
68. Giant cells are not pathognomonic for a specific neural tumor type (Table 7.3).
69. Cystic change occurs in a wide variety of neural tumors (Table 7.4).
70. Vascular and endothelial hyperplasia is displayed by a number of tumors other than glioblastomas, both primary and secondary (Table 7.5).
71. Rosenthal fibers occur in a variety of neoplastic and non-neoplastic disorders (Table 7.6).
72. Xanthomatous cells occur in neural tissue in a variety of neoplastic and nonneoplastic conditions (Table 7.7).
73. Calcification, although commonly associated with oligodendrogliomas, occurs in a wide variety of settings (Table 7.8).
74. Ganglion cells may occur in a variety of neural tumors (Table 7.10).
75. Many neural tumors, upon infiltration

of the dura or leptomeninges, elicit a prominent desmoplastic response that can mimic meningiomas, metastatic carcinomas, or sarcomas (Table 7.15) (10, 15).

76. Metastases from extraneural systemic tumors may occasionally occur into an existing primary cerebral tumor (Table 7.18).
77. Cellular whorls resembling those of meningiomas may occasionally be seen in other situations such as in normal pia-arachnoid, schwannomas, metastatic squamous cell carcinomas, and melanomas (Chapter 7).
78. Both capillary hemangioblastomas and renal cell carcinomas occur with increased frequency in von Hippel-Lindau disease, can be found in cerebellum, can produce an erythropoietin-like substance, may contain glycogen, and may closely resemble one another in frozen sections, smears, and permanent sections (Chapter 8).
79. Inflammatory cell infiltrates in primary brain tumors may, in small biopsies, resemble infectious/inflammatory lesions (Chapter 7).
80. Occult tumor is occasionally found in intracerebral or subdural hemorrhage specimens (Chapter 7).

COMMENT: Pitfalls No. 81-91 include some notorious ''look-alikes'' in neuropathology (7, 9, 19).

81. Ependymoma versus protoplasmic astrocytoma versus oligodendroglioma versus pituitary adenoma.
82. Ependymoma versus fibrillary astrocytoma (Chapter 7) (also see item 43 above).
83. Polar spongioblastoma versus schwannoma.
84. Papillary ependymoma versus choroid plexus papilloma or carcinoma versus metastatic papillary carcinoma.
85. Mucinous adenocarcinoma versus myxopapillary ependymoma versus chordoma versus meningioma.
86. Primary sarcoma versus metastatic sarcoma versus gliosarcoma (Chapter 7).
87. Epithelioid and other variants of glioblastoma versus metastatic carcinoma.
88. Astroblastoma versus ependymoma versus oligodendroglioma (Chapter 7).
89. Pleomorphic xanthoastrocytoma versus glioblastoma.
90. Anaplastic (malignant) oligodendroglioma increasingly resembles the cytologic features of an astrocytoma (Chapter 7).
91. Dural hemangiopericytoma versus cellular meningioma (Chapter 7).
92. Highly vascular, low-grade gliomas versus vascular malformations (11b, 15).
93. Neuro-imaging techniques will occasionally be unable to distinguish between (*a*) neoplasia, radiation cerebritis, abscess, infarction, and demyelinating disease (Chapters 7, 8); and (*b*) multicentric gliomas, metastatic tumors, lymphomas, and multiple cerebral abscesses (8).
94. Gliosis may closely resemble glioma (Chapter 8).
95. Bacterial meningitis may occur in the presence of a normal CSF cell count (Chapter 8).
96. Progressive multifocal leukoencephalopathy is the one viral infection that may mimic a glioma (Chapter 8).
97. Bizarre, multinucleated astrocytes may rarely occur in multiple sclerosis plaques (Chapter 8).
98. Malakoplakia, amyloidoma, and endometriosis are among the diseases whose rare presence in the nervous system can cause considerable confusion (Chapters 7 and 8).
99. Extramedullary hematopoiesis may rarely cause spinal extradural mass lesions necessitating surgical decompression (Chapter 8).
100. Benign lymphoproliferative disorders

(e.g., sinus histiocytosis with massive lymphadenopathy) may rarely cause destructive bone lesions, mass lesions, and cerebral parenchymatous infiltration and death (Chapter 8).

Final Comments

At the conclusion of this list of pitfalls, we wish to emphasize certain points.

First, a similar list can be compiled for virtually every other discipline in pathology and cytopathology. We regard neuropathology as no more, and no less, difficult than other subspecialties.

Second, the common disorders are relatively few and relatively quickly mastered, which saves us all from more frequent embarrassment. As Adams et al. point out (in the context of the use of smear techniques alone in intraoperative neuropathology), "it is not difficult for a general pathologist to achieve a correct diagnosis in some 75% to 80% of smears after only limited experience with the technique"(1). We believe that simultaneous use of frozen sections and smears can substantially improve this figure (see Chapter 6).

Third, we suggest that this list can stimulate the recall of previously learned but infrequently needed facts. At times, cytohistologic features in a given case do not seem *exactly* right for the suspected diagnosis in a manner the pathologist can sense, but perhaps not precisely define at the moment. Our intent is that this list of pitfalls may be of practical value to the reader when used in this manner.

References

1. Adams, J.H., Graham, D.I., and Doyle, D.: Brain Biopsy. The Smear Technique for Neurosurgical Biopsies. J.B. Lippincott Co., Philadelphia, 1981.
2. Appelman, H.D.: Mesenchymal tumors of the gut: historical perspectives, new approaches, new results, and does it make any difference? Chapter 6 in: Goldman, H., Appelman, H.D., and Kaufman, N. (Eds.): Gastrointestinal Pathology. Williams & Wilkins, Baltimore, 1990, pp. 220–246.
3. Burger, P.C.: Use of cytologic preparations in the frozen section diagnosis of central nervous system neoplasia. Am. J. Surg. Pathol. 9:344–354, 1985.
4. Burns, B.F., Comrie, W., Willan, A.R., and McCaughey, W.T.E.: Observer variation in the pathologic diagnosis of malignant lymphoma in Canada. Cancer 62:314–318, 1988.
5. Chandrasoma, P.T., and Apuzzo, M.L.J.: Stereotactic Brain Biopsy. Igaku-Shoin, New York, 1989.

5a. Chou, S.M., and Anderson, J.S.: Primary CNS malignant rhabdoid tumor (MRT): report of two cases and review of the literature. Clin. Neuropathol. 10:1–10, 1991.

6. Dardick, I., and Caldwell, D.R.: Follicular center cell lymphoma. Morphologic data relating to observer reproducibility. Cancer 58:2477–2484, 1986.
7. Hardman, J.M., and Yang, H-Y.: The central nervous system. Chapter 52 in: Silverberg, S.G. (Ed.): Principles and Practice of Surgical Pathology. John Wiley and Sons, New York, 1983. Vol. 2:1579–1656.
8. Kalyan-Raman, U.P., Kimm, J., Kalyan-Raman, K., and Wright, R.: Multicentric glioma (MCG) manifesting as multiple brain lesions: clinicopathologic and radiologic study of four cases. J. Neuropathol. Exp. Neurol. 50:365, 1991.
9. Kepes, J.J., and Moral, L.A.: Malignant rhabdoid tumors (MRT-S) of the central nervous system (CNS) and their morphological features seen in other CNS neoplasms. J. Neuropathol. Exp. Neurol. 50:362, 1991.
10. Kepes, J.J.: Differential diagnostic problems in brain tumors. Chapter 164 in: Minckler, J. (Ed.): Pathology of the Nervous System. McGraw-Hill, New York, 1971, Vol. 2:2219–2237.
11. Krohel, G.B., Tobin, D.R., and Chavis, R.M.: Inaccuracy of fine needle aspiration biopsy. Ophthalmology 92:666–670, 1985.

11a. Layfield, L.J., and Glasgow, B.J.: Rhabdomyosarcomatous differentiation in a neuroblastoma: a potential pitfall in the cytologic diagnosis of small round-cell tumors of childhood. Diagn. Cytopathol. 7:193–197, 1991.

11b. Lombardi, D., Scheithauer, B.W., Piepgras, D., Meyer, F.B., and Forbes, G.S.: "Angioglioma" and the arteriovenous malformation-glioma association. J. Neurosurg. 75:589–596, 1991.

12. NCI Non-Hodgkin's Classification Project Writing Committee: Classification of non-Hodgkin's lymphomas. Reproducibility of major classification systems. Cancer 55:91–95, 1985.

12a. Perilongo, G., Sutton, L., Czaykowski, D., Gusnard, D., and Biegel, J.: Rhabdoid tumor of the central nervous system. Med. Pediatr Oncol. 19:310–317, 1991.
13. Professional Affairs Committee: Professional Relations Manual. Ed. 9. College of American Pathologists, Skokie, IL, 1988, p. 122.
14. Rosai, J.: Borderline epithelial lesions of the breast. Am. J. Surg. Pathol. 15:209–221, 1991.
14a. Ross, J.S., Magro, C., Szyfelbein, W., and Sorensen, S.: Cerebrospinal fluid pleocytosis in aseptic meningitis: cytomorphic and immunocytochemical features. Diagn. Cytopathol. 7:532–596, 1991.
15. Scheithauer, B.W.: Central nervous system and pituitary. Chapter 8 in: Silva, E.G., and Kraemer, B.B.: Intraoperative Pathologic Diagnosis. Frozen Section and Other Techniques. Williams & Wilkins, Baltimore, 1987, pp. 167–219.
16. Sugita, Y., and Kepes, J.J.: Potential diagnostic pitfalls in stereotactic needle biopsies of the central nervous system. J. Neuropathol. Exp. Neurol. 49:273, 1990.
17. The Doctors' Company: Loss Prevention and Risk Management in Pathology. Available through The Doctors' Company, Risk Management Dept., 1127 First Street, Napa, CA, 94558.
18. Vélez-Garcia, E., Durant, J., Gams, R., and Bartolucci, A.: Results of a uniform histopathologic review system of lymphoma cases. A ten-year study from the Southeastern Cancer Study Group. Cancer 52:675–679, 1983.
19. Vogel, F.S.: Short course. Diagnostic surgical neuropathology. Mod. Pathol. 4:396–415, 1991.

10 / Future Trends

Neurocytopathology is a practical and proven method for establishing an accurate diagnosis of brain smears, aspirates, and CSF materials. As cytologic methods are continually being evaluated and improved, new information regarding neurocytopathology will have been reported even as this textbook is being published.

New cytologic concepts, applications, and trends in diagnostic pathology will undoubtedly influence this rapidly evolving field of neurocytopathology (24, 44, 86). These include immunocytochemical markers, flow cytometry, polymerase chain reaction (PCR), computer-assisted image analysis, and biochemical studies (Table 10.1). Many of these techniques to be described are currently being used in clinical diagnosis and patient management, but have not been routinely applied to neurocytopathology (8, 50) (Table 10.1). Readers are encouraged to read the excellent review articles by Wied (85) and by Bigner and Cohen (7a) to gain a greater appreciation of advances in diagnostic cytology.

Certain laboratories are already implementing some of these methods in their diagnostic routine and are at the forefront of research and development in the area of neurocytopathology. Some techniques are at an early stage of development and should be considered investigational rather than for routine diagnostic purposes. For the vast majority of medical laboratories, however, budgetary and personnel limitations will require a clear demonstration that such methods provide significant advantages over current practice standards in neurocytopathology before they are likely to receive widespread clinical acceptance and utility (4, 85).

Because the general hospital environment has been the focus of this textbook, we have attempted to provide useful and practical guidelines for surgical pathologists and cytopathologists in community hospitals and private laboratories presented with an occasional case for which neurocytopathology methods may be of value. The combined cytology and frozen section technique for neural tissue is a practice standard that requires a minimum of reagents, equipment, and technical time, and thus should be universally available. The previous chapters have outlined practical methods for improved cell recovery in CSF; i.e., membrane filtration and cytocentrifugation. Most of the laboratory supplies, equipment, and stains (H&E, Papanicolaou, and Wright's) are readily available in the general cytology or medical laboratory facilities. We suggest, however, that the reader monitor progress in the new technologies discussed below since we believe they have potential for a significant impact on neurocytopathologic diagnosis in the next few years. Brief statements and selected references, including more comprehensive reviews of these topics, follow.

Immunocytochemical Markers

Immunocytochemical markers are continually being developed for various cell types found in the CNS (Table 10.2). Glial fibrillary acidic protein (GFAP) positivity has been reported, for example, with several types of brain tumors (Table 10.3). Currently some pathology laboratories utilize

Table 10.1.
Potential Clinical Application of New Laboratory Techniques

IMMUNOCYTOCHEMISTRY (60, 65, 75, 79, 88)	
Aim:	Determine cell lineage of a poorly differentiated tumor. Assess cell surface markers (receptors) and cytoplasmic intermediate filaments, oncoproteins, and other antigens.
Methods:	Monoclonal antibodies (3, 9, 16, 20, 21, 27, 31, 34, 35, 40, 43, 47, 53, 64, 74, 76) In situ hybridization Steroid receptor assays Flow cytometry (18, 19, 38, 42, 52, 59, 68, 78, 87) Computer-assisted image analysis (28, 34, 82)
MOLECULAR GENETICS AND BIOLOGY (23, 62)	
Aim:	Elucidate the genetic nature of cancer at the DNA level (70). Activate and inactivate oncogenes and tumor suppressor genes (13, 62). Determine biological grade (45) and molecular staging of tumors. Identify individuals who are genetically predisposed to certain diseases. Design new chemotherapeutic agents to regulate tumor cell growth (33).
Methods:	In-situ hybridization PCR (41, 46, 72) Biochemistry
DNA PLOIDY AND CELL CYCLE ANALYSIS (25, 62, 77)	
Aim:	Determine DNA content and abnormal amounts of DNA (aneuploidy) (14, 15). Assess tumor cell proliferation indices (25). Determine biological grade of tumor (25). Monitor therapeutic response and design more effective treatment strategies.
Methods:	Monoclonal antibodies—Ki-67 (12, 56, 57, 69); PCNA/cyclin Flow cytometry (18, 19, 38, 42, 52, 59, 68, 78, 87) Computer-assisted image analysis (28, 36)

Table 10.2.
Immunocytochemical Markers in CNS[a]

Cell Type	Markers
Neuron	Neuron-specific enolase Neurofilament
Astrocyte	Glial fibrillary acidic protein (GFAP) Glutamine synthetase
Oligodendrocyte	Carbonic anhydrase II Myelin basic protein
Ependyma	None
Choroid plexus	Carbonic anhydrase II
Microglia	α_1-Antitrypsin α_1-Antichymotrypsin Fc receptor Lysozyme
Endothelium	Factor U111-related antigen
Leptomeningeal cells	Fibronectin Vimentin Desmoplakin

[a] Modified from Weller, R.O. Nervous System, Muscle and Eyes. Vol. 4 in: Symmers, W. St C. (Ed.): Systemic Pathology, 3rd ed. Churchill Livingstone, New York, 1990.

antibody panels such as outlined in Table 10.4 (7). Vick et al. (79) describe a panel of monoclonal antibodies used to differentiate among primary brain tumors, metastases, leukemia, and lymphoma. They recommend: (*a*) a monoclonal antibody cocktail composed of three antiglial fibrillary acidic protein antibodies (α-GFAP); (*b*) UJ 13A, a pan-neuroectodermal antibody; (*c*) B72.3, which recognizes a carcinoma-distinctive tumor-associated glycoprotein complex; and (*d*) 2D1, a pan-leukocytic antibody. Although no single antibody was diagnostic of a specific tumor type, this panel accurately differentiated among most primary brain tumors, metastases, and leukemia and has been applied in the examination of CSF for detecting subarachnoid dissemination of neoplastic cells.

This area of applied research and development will almost certainly find widespread use as markers become more efficient and cost-effective. As new antibodies become available the diagnostic precision of cytopathology will become greatly enhanced, especially in patients with no prior

Table 10.3.
Positive Immunostaining with Glial Fibrillary Acidic Protein (GFAP) (25, 60, 67, 75, 87a)

Astrocytoma
Choroid plexus tumors
Ependymoma
Ganglioglioma
Glioblastoma
Hemangioblastoma
Medulloblastoma
Oligodendroglioma
Subependymoma
Other neoplastic and non-neoplastic cells (see references)

documentation of CNS disease. Immunocytochemical study users are cautioned that adequate controls and objective laboratory observations are essential for quality differential diagnosis (55). For example, GFAP is widely used as a marker for astrocytic tumors (76), but results may be positive in a variety of other conditions (Table 10.3) (63, 87a).

Special lymphocyte immunocytochemical markers already have an established role in the diagnostic phase of lymphoproliferative CNS disorders (7, 16, 41, 47). In the case of meningeal carcinomatosis, it is not yet clear that currently available immunocytochemical marker technology provides any clear superiority in diagnostic sensitivity and specificity compared with routine CSF cytologic methods (16, 34), but we consider it probable that the rapidly evolving marker techniques will alter this equilibrium in the near future. The following are important areas of study designed to obtain the optimal utilization of immunocytochemical markers as applied to neurocytopathology:

1. Improved methods of cellular preservation, including storage and transportation of clinical material, are essential for optimal cytodiagnosis (2).
2. Cell-recovery enhancement techniques and improved technical methods that eliminate confounding background material are needed. Currently, we discourage smears of cytologic material (CSF, aspirates) for marker studies, because of such problems as cell population variance, background proteins, and artifacts. We believe that cell blocks provide the best compromise for immunocytochemical marker studies. Cytocentrifugation can now be used to produce cell blocks.
3. Additional immunocytochemical markers are being developed to enhance morphological information and to subtype spindle and small round-cell lesions.
4. Functional markers such as Ki-67, PCNA/cyclin will be increasingly utilized to monitor progression, regression, and recurrence of neoplastic conditions. Determination of markers for drug resistance (6, 49a, 83, 84), oncogene expression and cell kinetics will also likely become a part of cellular monitoring and find valuable application in new therapeutic protocols.

The recent review by Miller (54) of immunohistochemistry in the community practice of pathology provides a discussion of methods and lists of reagents and vendors for those initiating such procedures in their laboratory. This article could serve as an aid to a laboratory that is experiencing problems with immunohistochemistry. Russell and Rubinstein (63) provide valuable insights regarding this technology and caution us regarding the current nonspecificity of this technology in neural tumors. In time, improvements in the methodologies should allow greater confidence in results. Daily use of immunocytological markers will be commonplace for the diagnostic practitioner and a standard part of the delivery of health care (29).

Flow Cytometry

The clinical application of flow cytometry to neural specimens poses some technical

Table 10.4.
Antibodies Useful in Distinguishing Among Lymphoma/Leukemia, Metastatic Carcinoma, Melanoma, and Primary Brain Tumors[a]

	Anticytokeratin	B72.3	S-100	Mel-14	UJ13A[b]	GFAP[c]	2D1
Carcinoma	+	+	−/+	−	−	−	−
Melanoma	−	−	+	+	−	−	−
Lymphoma/ leukemia	−	−	−	−	−	−	+
Glioblastoma	−	−	+	+	+	+	−
Medullo- blastoma	−	−	+	+	+	−	−

[a] Modified from Bigner, S.H.: Central nervous system. Chapter 18 in: Bibbo, M. (Ed.): Comprehensive Cytopathology. W.B. Saunders, Philadelphia, 1991, pp. 473-478.
[b] UJ13A is a panneuroectodermal antigen.
[c] GFAP, glial fibrillary acidic protein.

and logistical problems, which primarily relate to the cellularity of the specimen (38, 44). For example, immunofluorescent cell markers may be satisfactorily studied on as few as 100 cells, but a reliable result is more likely with 1,000 or more cells. DNA and cell-cycle studies currently require specimens in the range of 10,000 cells for reliable results. This volume requirement is not an insurmountable problem, as recent experimental studies indicate (14, 38, 59), but the relative cellularity of many CSF specimens and resultant volumes of CSF required currently preclude the routine application of flow cytometry in CSF analysis.

Future developments of flow cytometry are likely to include cell sorting, karyotyping, in-situ hybridization, and the analysis of the effects of chemotherapeutic agents on tumor cells. These aspects are now being utilized for research purposes, but are yet to be of demonstrated advantage for routine clinical use (78).

Polymerase Chain Reaction (PCR)

This recently developed method, utilizing gene amplification techniques, appears to be capable of detecting as few as one or two copies of abnormal gene rearrangements (87b). It is already being applied to such problems as the diagnosis of human genetic diseases (23, 61), the demonstration of viral-coded proteins in paraffin-embedded human tumor material (77), and the detection of diagnostic abnormal gene rearrangements in lymphomas and leukemias (71). Recently, Kunishio et al. (46) reported findings suggesting that the immunostaining of DNA polymerase α is a convenient and important new method by which to estimate the cellular proliferation rate of brain tumors. Polymerase α scores may be closer to the growth fraction of the individual tumor than the MAP Ki-67 or other scores. In 1990 Shibata et al. (71) reported a rare case of secondary CNS involvement by a follicular small cleaved lymphoma. The CNS involvement was difficult to document by conventional morphologic techniques, but was readily detected by molecular genetic analysis after in vitro DNA amplification by PCR. Since the PCR exponentially increases in vitro the number of original DNA copies, the PCR is suitable for the molecular genetic analysis of specimens with very small cell numbers such as the CSF. Hopefully, many markers of neoplasia will soon be analyzed with PCR. Characterization of the initial tumor for the presence of these markers may, for example, allow the detection of subclinical persistent or recurrent disease, and thus be useful in monitoring response to therapy.

Computer-Assisted Image Analysis

Morphometry is a growing technology with the potential to provide visual enhancement and precise measurements of fine cellular detail (86). However, its practical application to neurocytopathology remains to be seen (85). In other areas of diagnostic cytopathology, computer-assisted image analysis is receiving increasing acceptance as a rapid, objective tool to analyze and confirm subjective cytomorphologic interpretations (1, 10, 28, 36, 49, 81). Its potential diagnostic value is increased when combined with DNA ploidy determinations and immunocytochemical markers and probes (15). Distinct advantages over flow cytometry are that fewer cells are required, it is complementary to conventional light microscopy, and it allows a selection of individual cells to be analyzed. It may also provide a reliable and rapid method for cell counts and further characterization of mononuclear cells. At the present there is no accurate, cost-effective, automated imaging system similar to that used in the clinical hematology laboratory that would provide an objective analysis of CSF or brain tissue cytologic material. Our current opinion is that computer-assisted image cytometry is more likely to find a role as a confirmatory, prognostic or quality control tool, but it is less likely to assist in the initial diagnostic workup of specimens from neural lesions. The latter will still require the use of binocular light microscopy by trained personnel. Standard textbooks on the topic of image analysis (1, 28) and videomicroscopy (36) are available.

Biochemical Studies

Many biochemical techniques have been applied to the noncellular components of CSF, but few are employed on a routine basis in clinical practice. There are studies attempting to identify chemical (37, 67) or immunologic (27) markers or selected drug level-monitoring procedures (30, 31) that will provide diagnostic or therapeutic advantages over current methods. Biochemical techniques may be combined with cytologic analysis to yield greater information on neurocytopathology. However, more correlative studies are needed.

Miscellaneous Techniques

Tissue culture (63) and electron microscopy (32) are currently utilized primarily as research tools in neurocytopathology. If the size of the specimen permits, and initial frozen section and smear preparations indicate one is dealing with tumors of certain types (e.g., small round-cell tumors, spindle-cell tumors), setting aside some tissue in a glutaraldehyde-based fixative for subsequent ultrastructural study may allow further refinement of the classification of certain light-microscopically similar tumors. As noted in Chapter 6, saving frozen tissue and the preparation and storage of additional frozen sections and air-dried smears may also prove very useful under these circumstances. Such material can be periodically purged to conserve storage space, if subsequent permanent sections and stains that can be applied to paraffin-embedded tissue prove adequate to guide the necessary treatment decisions.

Quality Assurance and Improvement

As in all other areas of laboratory practice, quality assurance and quality improvement are necessary in neurocytopathology to maximize its potential in the clinical diagnosis and management of patients. Several textbooks and continuing education activities on quality control and assurance are available in the clinical laboratory, but few are specifically targeted for anatomic pathology or its subspecialties (e.g., neurocytopathology) (39, 73).

Personal computers close to the pathologist and microscopist's workstation (85) can aid in the transmitting of anatomic pathology laboratory results and facilitate their comparison with pertinent clinical and other types of pathologic findings (58, 66). We agree with Wied's statement that current centralized large hospital or university-wide systems are economically inefficient and are unable to respond to the need of laboratories on a day-to-day basis (85). Microcomputer systems, which decentralize the data collection procedure, will likely be the data management system of the future. Correlative analysis and more powerful data management systems will improve the quality of neurocytopathology as well as other areas of diagnostic cytopathology. Telepathology will likely become more integral in providing diagnostic services to rural and regional clinical settings as cost efficiency and the resolution of transmitted images improve.

Interactive computerization programs using laser videodisc or CD-ROM (compact disc read-only memory) will provide the pathologist and cytologist access to expert system information in a matter of seconds (17, 26, 48, 89). Visual images, descriptions of morphologic criteria, and literature updates will be readily available to the pathology laboratory through this state-of-the-art technology. Wied (85) describes a variety of applications of expert systems for diagnostic cytopathology (Table 10.5).

Medical informatics, a growing new subspecialty of medicine, is playing a critical role in the development and use of these expert systems applications. Subspecialty journals are now becoming available that allow convenient access to developments in this area (e.g., M.D. Computing) (51).

Table 10.5.
Applications of Expert Systems[a]

Cytohistologic correlation of cytometric data
Sequential and comparative assessment data
Prognostic criteria data
Therapeutic response data
Data to expand differential diagnosis
Data to support or confirm diagnosis
Data to check quality control measurements (e.g., optimal staining, fixatives, use of filters for fluorochromes, etc.)

[a] Modified from Wied, G.L. Clinical cytology: past, present and future. Beitr. Onkol. 38:1–58, 1990.

Laser disc technology (and the newer compact disc technology) also have the potential to become a practical method for professional self-assessment and review and proficiency testing. In the future, numerous morphologic images will be stored on disc and readily available for the student, educator, and medical practitioner. Rapid comparisons of cytologic features in neural tissue, for example, can be performed using this technology. Artificial intelligence will not lead to the replacement of cytotechnologists or pathologists, but will rather increase our knowledge base, objectivity, reproducibility, and accuracy.

Conclusion

This textbook has attempted to provide the reader with an overview of the current state of the art and science of neurocytopathology as it relates to brain aspirates and smears and CSF. Previous chapters have provided a review of concepts, methods, and morphologic features of normal and pathologic states of the nervous system. While traditional hematoxylin and eosin-stained slides continue to be the primary tool for histopathological diagnoses, there is growing appreciation that this is no longer sufficient for the diagnosis and treatment of many patients (11, 50, 80). The contemporary pathologist is faced with the challenge of using highly sophisticated techniques to obtain maximum information from increasingly small samples. This final chapter is intended to provide a brief discussion and prediction of new and important laboratory methodologies that the reader is encouraged to follow as they relate to the field of neurocytopathology. Gene rearrangement studies represent an example for new and impressive achievements that will clearly play a role in our understanding of the pathogenesis of neural disease, although their present application and use are limited in the daily clinical practice of surgical pathology and cytopathology. Banks (5) states that morphology is important, but increasingly it is only the starting point. Pathologists must, with increasing frequency, go beyond morphology to explore and appropriately apply ancillary methods. "If we don't, someone else will" (5).

In summary, the cornerstone of diagnostic cytopathology remains the accurate microscopic assessment of morphologic information found in tissue and cells of the nervous system. The first nine chapters are intended to provide a "core of knowledge" from which to build a firm foundation for the implementation of future relevant advances. Conceptual flexibility will be required in the rapid application of many of these new techniques. Prerequisites for their medical laboratory acceptance will be safety, simplicity, reproducibility, cost reduction, and/or improved diagnostic and clinical monitoring information, in comparison to the methods presently in common use.

References

1. Aherne W.A., Dunnill M.S.: Morphometry. Edward Arnold, Baltimore, 1982.
2. Albright, R.E., Christenson R.H., Habig R.L., et al.: Cerebrospinal fluid (CSF) trap. A method to improve CSF laboratory efficiency. Am. J. Clin. Pathol. 90;707–710, 1988.
3. Andrew S.M., and Gradwell E.: Immunoperoxidase labelled antibody staining in differential diagnosis of central nervous system haemangioblastomas and central nervous system metastases of renal carcinomas. J. Clin. Pathol. 39:917–919, 1986.
4. Appelman H.D.: Mesenchymal tumors of the gut: historical perspectives, new approaches, new results, and does it make any difference? Chapter 6 in: Goldman, H., Appelman, H.D., and Kaufman, N. (Eds.): Gastrointestinal Pathology. Williams & Wilkins, Baltimore, 1990, pp. 220–246.
5. Banks, P.M.: When morphology is not enough. Am. J. Clin. Pathol. 93:153–154, 1990.
6. Bates S.E., Micley L.A., Chen Y-N., Richert N., Rudick J., Biedler, J.L., and Fojo, A.T.: Expression of a drug resistance gene in human neuroblastoma cell lines: modulation by retinoic acid-induced differentiation. Mol. Cell. Biol. 9:4337–4344, 1989.
7. Bigner, S.: Central nervous system. Chapter 18 in: Bibbo, M. (Ed.): Comprehensive Cytopathology. W.B. Saunders, Philadelphia, pp. 473–478, 1990.
7a. Bigner, S.H., and Cohen, C.G.: Cytopathology during the 1980s. Am. J. Clin. Pathol. 96(Suppl. 1):S15–S19, 1991.
8. Black, P.M.: Brain tumors. N. Engl. J. Med. 324:1471–1476, 1991.
9. Boogerd, W., Vroom, T.H.M., Van Heerde, P., et al.: CSF cytology versus immunocytochemistry in meningeal carcinomatosis. J. Neurol. Neurosurg. Psychiatry 51:142–145, 1988.
10. Braendgaard, H., and Gundersen, H.J.: The impact of recent stereological advances on quantitative studies of the nervous system. J. Neurosci. Methods 18:39–78, 1986.
11. Burger, P.C.: Morphologic correlates in gliomas: where do we stand? Monogr. Pathol. 32:16–29, 1990.
12. Burger, P.C., Shibata, T., and Kleihues, P.: The use of the monoclonal antibody Ki-67 in the identification of proliferating cells: application to surgical neuropathology. Am. J. Surg. Pathol. 10:611–717, 1986.
13. Chofflon, M., Weiner, H.L., Morimoto, C., et al.: Decrease of supressor inducer (CD4+,2H4+) T cells in multiple sclerosis cerebrospinal fluid. Ann. Neurol. 25:484–499, 1989.
14. Cibas, E.S., Malkin, M.G., Posner, J.B. et al.: Detection of DNA abnormalities by flow cytometry in cells from cerebrospinal fluid. Am. J. Clin. Pathol. 88:570–577, 1987.
15. Claud, R.D., Weinstein, R.S., Howeedy, A., et al.: Comparison of image analysis of imprints with flow cytometry for DNA analysis of solid tumors. Mod. Pathol. 2:463–466, 1989.
16. Coakman, H.B., Brownell, B., Harper, E.I., et al.: Use of monoclonal antibody panel to identify malignant cells in cerebrospinal fluid. Lancet 1:1095–1098, 1984.
17. Connelly, D.P.: Embedding expert systems in laboratory information systems. Am. J. Clin. Pathol. 94(Suppl. 1):S7-S14, 1990.

18. Coon, J.S., and Weinstein, R.S. (Eds.): Diagnostic Flow Cytometry. Williams & Wilkins, Baltimore, 1991.
19. Darzynkiewicz, Z.: Flow cytometry in cytopathology. Overview and perspectives. Anal. Quant. Cytol. Histol. 10:459–461, 1988.
20. de la Monte, S.M.: Immunohistochemical diagnosis of nervous system neoplasms. Tumor markers in diagnostic pathology. Clin. Lab. Med. 10:151–178, 1991.
21. Edwards, M.S.B., Davis, R.L., and Laurent, J.P.: Tumor markers and cytologic features of cerebrospinal fluid. Cancer 56:1773–1777, 1985.
22. Esiri, M.M., and Oppenheimer, D.R.: Diagnostic Neuropathology. A Practical Manual. Blackwell Scientific Publications, Boston, 1989.
23. Fenoglio-Preiser, C.M., and Willmans, C.L. (Eds.): Molecular Diagnostics in Pathology (No. 3, Techniques in Diagnostic Pathology). Williams & Wilkins, Baltimore, 1990.
24. Frable, W.J.: Needle aspiration biopsy: past, present and future. Hum. Pathol. 20:504–517, 1989.
25. Franzini, A., Broggi, G., Giorgi, C., Caiola, L., and Allegranza, A.: Predictive accuracy of cell kinetics data in glial tumors investigated by serial stereotactic biopsy. J. Neurosurg. Sci. 33:43–45, 1989.
26. Friedman, B.A.: Informatics as a separate section within a department of pathology. Am. J. Clin. Pathol. 94 (Suppl. 1):S2-S6, 1990.
27. Graus, F., Segurado, O.G., Tolosa, E.: Selective concentration of anti-Purkinje cell antibody in the CSF of two patients with paraneoplastic cerebellar degeneration. Acta Neurol. Scand. 78:210–213, 1988.
28. Greenberg, S.D.: Computer-Assisted Image Analysis Cytology. S. Karger, New York, 1984.
29. Hansen, C.A.: Editorial. Immunophenotyping of hematologic malignant conditions: to flow or not to flow? Am. J. Clin. Pathol. 96:295–298, 1991.
30. Heideman, R.L., Cole, D.E., Balis, F., et al.: Phase I and pharmacokinetic evaluation of thiotepa in the cerebrospinal fluid and plasma of pediatric patients: evidence for dose-dependent plasma clearance of thiotepa. Cancer Res. 49:736–741, 1989.
31. Herbert, J., Cavallaro, T., and Dwork, A.J.: A marker for primary choroid plexus neoplasms. Am. J. Pathol. 136:1317–1325, 1990.
32. Herndon R.M., and Brumback R.A.: The cytology of cerebrospinal fluid: methods and normal constituents. Chapter 10 in: Herndon, R.M., and Brumback, R.A. (Eds.): The Cerebrospinal Fluid. Kluwer Academic Publishers, Boston, 1989, pp. 245–260.
33. Hormans, A.C., Barker, B.E., Forman, E.N., et al.: Immunophenotypic characteristics of cerebrospinal fluid in children with acute lymphoblastic leukemia at diagnosis. Blood 76:1807–1811, 1990.
34. Hormans, A.C., Forman, E.N., and Barker, B.E.: Use of monoclonal antibodies to identify cerebrospinal fluid lymphoblasts in children with acute lymphoblastic leukemia. Blood 66:1321–1325, 1985.
35. Hovestadt, A., Henzen-Logmans, S.C., and Vecht, C.J.: Immunohistochemical analysis of the cerebrospinal fluid for carcinomatous and lymphomatous leptomeningitis. Br. J. Cancer 62:653–654, 1990.
36. Inoue, S.: Video Microscopy. Plenum Press, New York, 1986.
37. Jaeckle, K.A.: Assessment of tumor markers in cerebrospinal fluid. Clin. Lab. Med. 5:303–315, 1985.
38. Johnson, T.S., Katz, R.L., and Pershouse, M.: Flow cytometric applications in cytopathology. Anal. Quant. Cytol. Histol. 10:423–458, 1988.
39. Joint Commission Accreditation Manual for Hospitals: The Joint Commission on Accreditation of Healthcare Organizations, Chicago, 1989, p. 158.
40. Kajiwara, K., Nishizaki, T., Orita, T., et al.: Silver colloid staining technique for analysis of glioma malignancy. J. Neurosurg. 73:113–117, 1990.
41. Kawasaki, E.S., Clark, S.S., Coyne, M.Y., et al.: Diagnosis of chronic myeloid and acute lymphocytic leukemia by detection of leukemia-specific mRNA sequences amplified in vitro. Proc. Natl. Acad. Sci. U.S.A. 85:5698–5702, 1988.
42. Keren, D.F. (Ed.): Flow Cytometry in Clinical Diagnosis. American Society of Clinical Pathologists. ASCP Press, Chicago, 1989.
43. Koskiniemi, M.: Malignancy markers in the cerebrospinal fluid. Eur. J. Pediatr. 148:3–8, 1988.
44. Koss, L.G., Czerniak, B., Herz, F., and Wersto, R.P.: Flow cytometric measurements of DNA and other cell components in human tumors: a critical appraisal. Hum. Pathol. 20:528–548, 1989.
45. Kros, J.M., Van Eden, C.G., Stefanko, S.Z., et al.: Prognostic implications of glial fibrillary acidic protein containing cell types in oligodendrogliomas. Cancer 66:1204–1212, 1990.
46. Kunishio, K., Mishima, N., Matsuhisa, T., et al.: Immunohistochemical demonstration of DNA polymerase alpha in human brain tumor cells. J. Neurosurg. 72:268–272, 1990.
47. Lauer, S.J., Kirchner, P.A., and Camitta, B.M.: Identification of leukemic cells in the cerebrospinal fluid from children with acute lymphoblastic leukemia: advances and dilemmas. Am. J. Pediatr. Hematol. Oncol. 11:64–73, 1989.
48. Linder, J.: Overview of digital imaging in pathology: the fifth wave. Am. J. Clin. Pathol. 94(Suppl. 1):S30-S34, 1990.
49. Linder, J.: Editorial. The coming era of cytologic automation. Am. J. Clin. Pathol. 96:293–294, 1991.
49a. Matsumoto, T., Tani, E., Kaba, K., Shindo, H.,

and Miyaji, K.: Expression of P-glycoprotein in human glioma cell lines and surgical glioma specimens. J. Neurosurg. 74:460–466, 1991.

50. Maygarden, S.J., and McLendon, W.W.: Pathology and laboratory medicine. JAMA 265: 3154–3156, 1991.
51. M.D. Computing. Official Journal of the American Medical Informatics Association. Springer-Verlag, New York.
52. Melamed, M.R., Mullaney, P.F., and Mendelsohn, M.L. (Eds.): Flow Cytometry and Sorting, Ed 2. John Wiley and Sons, New York, 1979.
53. Miller, D.C., Koslow, M., Budzilovich, G.N., et al.: Synaptophysin: a sensitive and specific marker for ganglion cells in central nervous system neoplasms. Hum. Pathol. 21:271–276, 1990.
54. Miller, R.T.: Immunohistochemistry in the community practice of pathology: part II. Lab. Med. 22:527–532, 1991.
55. Nadji, M., and Ganjei, P.: Immunocytochemistry in diagnostic cytology: a 12-year perspective. Am. J. Clin. Pathol. 94:470–475, 1990.
56. Nishizaki, T., Orita, T., Furutani, Y., et al.: Flow-cytometric DNA analysis and immunohistochemical measurement of Ki-67 and BUdR labeling in human brain tumors. J. Neurosurg. 70:379–384, 1989.
57. Osterag, C.B., Volk, B., Shibata, T., Burger, P., et al.: The monoclonal antibody Ki-67 as a marker for proliferating cells in stereotactic biopsies of brain tumours. Acta Neurochir. 89:117–121, 1987.
58. Platt, M.S., Igel, H.J., and Novak, R.W.: Getting onto patient floors: a proposed, proactive quality assurance function for pathologists. Lab. Med. 22:540–542, 1991.
59. Redner, A., Andreeff, M., Miller, D.R., Steinherz, P., and Melamed, M.: Recognition of central nervous system leukemia by flow cytometry. Cytometry 5:614–618, 1984.
60. Rhodes, R.H.: Diagnostic immunostaining of the nervous system. Chapter 16 in: Taylor, C.R. (Ed.): Immunomicroscopy: A Diagnostic Tool for the Surgical Pathologist. W.B. Saunders, Philadelphia, 1986, pp. 334–362.
61. Rooney, M.T., and Henry, J.B.: Molecular markers of malignant neoplasms. Chapter 14 in: Henry, J.B. (Ed.): Clinical Diagnosis and Management by Laboratory Methods. 18th Ed. W.B. Saunders, Philadelphia, 1991, pp. 285–307.
62. Ross, D.W.: Molecular markers of cancer. Arch. Pathol. Lab. Med. 115:402, 1991.
63. Russell, D.S., and Rubinstein, L.J.: Pathology of Tumors of the Nervous System. Williams & Wilkins, Baltimore, 1989.
64. Salonen, R., Ilonen, J., Jagerroos, H., et al.: Lymphocyte subsets in the cerebrospinal fluid in active multiple sclerosis. Ann. Neurol. 25:500–502, 1989.
65. Schlom, J.: Innovations in monoclonal antibody tumor targeting. Diagnostic and therapeutic implications. JAMA 261:744–746, 1989.
66. Schultz, E.K., and Brown, R.A.: The pathologist's workstation. Issues and an early prototype. Am. J. Clin. Pathol. 95(Suppl. 1):S50-S57, 1991.
67. Schwartsmann, G., VanDerVijgh, W.J.F., Klein, I., et al.: Pharmacokinetics of brequinar sodium (NSC 368390; DUP 785) in cerebrospinal fluid. Eur. J. Cancer Clin. Oncol. 24:1903–1904, 1988.
68. Shapiro, H.M. (Ed.): Practical Flow Cytometry, 2nd Ed. Alan R. Liss, New York, 1988.
69. Shibata, T., Burger, P.C., and Kleihues, P.: Ki-67 immunoperoxidase stain as a marker for the histological grading of nervous system tumours. Acta Neurochir. Suppl. 43:103–106, 1988.
70. Shibata, D., Martin, W.J., and Arnheim, N.: Analysis of DNA sequences in forty-year-old paraffin-embedded thin-tissue sections: a bridge between molecular biology and classical histology. Cancer Res. 48:4564–4566, 1988.
71. Shibata, D., Nichols, P., Sherrod, A., Rabinowitz, A., Bernstien-Singer, L., and Hu, E.: Detection of occult CNS involvement of follicular small cleaved lymphoma by the polymerase chain reaction. Mod. Pathol. 3:71–75, 1990.
72. Standards for Laboratory Accreditation. Commission on Laboratory Accreditation, College of American Pathologists, Skokie, IL, 1988, p. 87.
73. Stewart, C.E.: Basic Quality Assurance Practices for Clinical Laboratories. J.B. Lippincott, Philadelphia, 1987.
74. Takahashi, H., Wakabayashi, K., Kawai, K., et al.: Neuroendocrine markers in central nervous system neuronal tumor (gangliocytoma and ganglioglioma). Acta Neuropathol. 77:237–243, 1989.
75. Taylor, C.R.: Immunomicroscopy: A Diagnostic Tool for the Surgical Pathologist. Volume 19 in: Bennington, J.L. (Ed.): Major Problems in Pathology. W.B. Saunders, Philadelphia, 1986.
76. Trojanowski, J.Q., Atkinson, B., and Lee, V.M.Y.: An immunocytochemical study of normal and abnormal human cerebrospinal fluid with monoclonal antibodies to glial fibrillary acidic protein. Acta Cytol. 30:235–239, 1986.
77. Ullen, H., Falkner, U.G., Collins, V.P. and Auer, G.U.: Methodologic aspect of nuclear DNA assessment of gliomas with astrocytic and/or oligodendrocytic differentiation. Correlation of image and flow cytometric studies on paraffin-embedded specimens. Anal. Quant. Cytol. Histol. 13:168–176, 1991.
78. Vielh, P.: Flow Cytometry. Guides to Clinical Aspiration Biopsy. Igaku-Shoin, New York, 1991.
79. Vick, W.W., Wikstrand, C.J., Bullard, D.E., Kemshead, J., et al.: The use of a panel of monoclonal antibodies in the evaluation of cytologic

specimens from the central nervous system. Acta Cytol. 31:815–824, 1987.
80. Wakely, P.E., Favara, B.E., and Galliani, C.A.: Diagnostic histopathologic criteria in pediatric tumors: an eclectic review. Crit. Rev. Oncol. Hematol. 6:261–262, 1986.
81. Wallace, R.M., Bigner, S.H., and Johnston, W.W.: Metastatic breast carcinoma in cerebrospinal fluid. A cytomorphometric study. Acta Cytol. 26:787–792, 1982.
82. Weller, R.O. (Ed.): Nervous System; Muscle and Eyes. Vol. 4 in: Symmers, W.C. (Ed.): Systemic Pathology, 3rd Ed. Churchill Livingstone, New York, 1990.
83. Weinstein, R.S., and Coon, J.S.: Editorial. Laboratory Assessment of P-glycoprotein in cancer chemosensitivity testing. Hum. Pathol. 21:785–786, 1990.
84. Weinstein, R.S., Jakate, S.M., Dominquez, J.M., Lebowitz, M.D., Koukoulis, G.K., Kuszak, J.R., Klusens, L.F., Grogan, T.M., Saclarides, T.J., Robinson, I.B., and Coon, J.S.: Relationship of the expression of the multidrug resistance gene product (P-glycoprotein) in human colon carcinoma to local tumor aggressiveness and lymph node metastasis. Cancer Res. 51:2720–2726, 1991.
85. Wied, G.L.: Clinical cytology: past, present and future. Beitr. Onkol. 38:1–58, 1990.
86. Wied, G.L., Bartels, P.H., Bibbo, M., and Dytch, H.E.: Image analysis in quantitative cytopathology and histopathology. Hum. Pathol. 20:549–571, 1989.
87. Williams, N.N., and Daly, J.M.: Flow cytometry and prognostic implications in patients with solid tumors. Surg. Gynecol. Obstet. 171:257–266, 1990.
87a. Wittchow, R., and Landas, S.K.: Glial fibrillary acidic protein expression in pleomorphic adenoma, chordoma, and astrocytoma. A comparison of three antibodies. Arch. Pathol. Lab. Med. 115:1030–1033, 1991.
87b. Wright, P.A., and Wynford-Thomas, D.: The polymerase chain reaction: miracle or mirage? A critical review of its uses and limitations in diagnosis and research. J. Pathol. 162:99–117, 1990.
88. Yam, I.T., English, M.C., Janckila, A.J., Ziesmer, S., and Li, C.Y.: Immunocytochemistry of cerebrospinal fluid. Acta Cytol. 31:825–833, 1987.
89. Yasnoff, W.A.: Weighing pros and cons of CD-ROM publishing. Am. Med. News, May 18, 1990, p. 17.

Appendix

SPECIAL STAINS

A. Preparation of Parlodion Solution
B. Poly-L-Lysine Adhesive Slides
C. Blood Elimination Techniques
D. Cell Block Technique
E. Preparing Membrane Filters for Staining
F. Rapid Papanicolaou Stain (Gill 2)
G. Modified Papanicolaou Stain for Manual Staining of Cytocentrifugation and Direct Smear Preparations (Gill 1)
H. Modified Papanicolaou Stain for Manual Staining of Filters (Gill 1)
I. Destaining Technique for Cytological Preparations
J. Destaining Procedure—Direct Smear and Cytocentrifugation Preparations
K. Destaining Procedure—Membrane Filters
L. Diff-Quik (Wright's) Stain
M. Hematoxylin and Eosin Method for Frozen Sections and Smear Preparations
N. Removal of Mercury Precipitated Pigment
O. Cytochemical (Special) Stains
  1. Acid-Fast Stain
  2. Fontana-Masson Stain
  3. Gomori's Methenamine-Silver (GMS) Nitrate Technique
  4. Gram Stain
  5. Iron Stain
  6. Mucicarmine Stain
  7. Oil Red O Fat Stain
  8. Oil Red O Stain (Alternate Method)
  9. PAS Stain
  10. PAS/Diastase Digestion Method
  11. Toluidine Blue O Stain
  12. Toluidine Blue Stain
P. Coverslipping

A. Preparation of Parlodion Solution

Purpose:

For coating cellular sediment on slides to prevent cell loss.

Materials:

1. 200 ml 95% ETOH
2. 200 ml Ether technical brand - anhydrous
3. 1 gram of parlodion[a]

Procedure:

1. Mix ingredients and allow to stand overnight. By the morning the parlodion will have dissolved.
2. The slides to be fixed may be covered with the parlodion solution by using a pipette and applying it dropwise to the slide. Cytocentrifuge specimens should be held horizontally during this procedure.
3. The slide is then immediately put into the fixative of choice to allow for fixation of the cells and hardening of the parlodion.
4. The parlodion coat need not be removed, as it does not stain and floaters do not become attached to it. However, if you wish to dissolve the coating, a dish of acetone may be placed between the 100% alcohol and xylene for a brief bath.
5. Do not allow the parlodion mixture to evaporate, as ether crystals could form and are explosive.

B. Poly-L-Lysine Adhesive Slides

PLL technique used at the University of Rochester Medical Center, Rochester, NY, U.S.A. (Courtesy of S.F. Patten and F.W. Patten)

Poly-L-Lysine (PLL) can be used to coat glass slides in the preparation of frozen and/or paraffin tissue sections for immunohistochemical staining and for cytology preparations (i.e., CSF, fine needle aspirates, effusions). When applied as a monolayer, high-molecular-weight PLL (350 K mw) changes the negative charge of the glass surface to a positive one, which will then bind negatively charged tissues strongly.

Materials:

1. Poly-L-Lysine (PLL) (Sigma P 1524). One gram of PLL will coat approximately 28,000 microscopic glass slides.
2. Deionized water, phosphate buffered saline (PBS), or TRIS-HCL. (We keep 10 liters of PBS on stock. The use of PBS leaves a film or precipitate on the glass slide that dissolves in 95% ETOH and does not alter the cytomorphology or staining reaction. The use of TRIS-HCL leaves less of a precipitate.
3. Clean microscopic glass slides and staining racks.
4. 50-ml plastic centrifuge tubes with screw caps.

Method:

Stock Solution

1. Make up a 10x stock solution of PLL by dissolving 250 mg of PLL in 500 ml of PBS or TRIS-HCL - pH 7.
2. Place 40 ml of the solution in 50-ml plastic centrifuge tubes and freeze.

Slides (total 600–700 coated)

1. Thaw one tube of 40 ml of PLL (10x stock).
2. Add 360 ml of PBS; mix.
3. Place solution in staining dish.
4. Carefully rack clean glass slides, being careful not to fingerprint slides. Rubber gloves may be used to facilitate this.
5. Dip racked slides in the solution and let sit for a minimum of 10 minutes.
6. Remove slides and allow to air dry overnight, or place in an oven at 50°C until dried. Keep away from dust while drying.
7. Use PLL within 48 hours after thawing.

[a] Parlodion (strips). A purified pyroxylin (Mallinckrodt) comes in 1-lb (453.6-gm) containers of individual strips, each of which weighs approximately 1 gram. (Consider each strip to be 1 gram, as they are extremely difficult to cut or break.)

C. Blood Elimination Techniques

1. Glacial Acetic Acid Preparation of Bloody Specimens

Purpose:

To eliminate erythrocytes from cytologic specimens prior to cell concentration and preparation.

Indications for Use:

Glacial acetic acid preparation should be used on all grossly bloody body fluids.

Materials:

2% Glacial acetic acid
In a clean glass storage container, place 2 ml of glacial acetic acid, add 98 ml of distilled water.

Procedure:

1. In a small centrifuge tube (15 ml), place a small amount of representative sample and dilute with saline to a total volume of approximately 4 to 5 ml.
2. Add approximately 3 times the diluted specimen volume of 2% glacial acetic acid.
3. Place on aliquot mixer for 5 minutes.
4. Centrifuge at 1500 rpm for 5 minutes.
5. Decant supernate and resuspend button. Since most RBCs have been lysed, the suspension can be more concentrated than normal without obscuring diagnostic cells.
6. Make cytocentrifuge preparations of the material.

2. Saponization Procedure

Purpose:

To eliminate erythrocytes from cytologic specimens prior to cell concentration and preparation.

Indications for Use:

Saponization should be used on all grossly bloody specimens that are greater than 10 cc in volume.

Materials:

1% (w/v) saponin in distilled water.
1. In a clean beaker, mix 50 ml distilled water and 0.5 g powdered saponin.
2. Filter through Grade 1 Whatman paper into another clean beaker.

Procedure:

1. Prepare fresh saponin solution.
2. Agitate specimen container to distribute cellular material.
3. Divide specimen equally between two centrifuge tubes.
4. Mix the specimen in one tube with an equal volume of saponin. Agitate.
5. Discard unused saponin solution.
6. Centrifuge both specimens at 1500 rpm for 10 minutes.
7. Remove supernate.
8. Prepare six cytospins:
   Three from the saponized specimen
   Three from the unsaponized specimen.

NOTE: To preserve cellular morphology, slides made from saponized specimens should be prepared immediately.

Reference:

Gary W. Gill, CT (ASCP) CMIAC: *The Shandon Cytospin 2 in Diagnostic Cytology: Technique, Tips and Troubleshooting*. Johns Hopkins University School of Medicine, Baltimore, Maryland 21205.

D. Cell Block Technique

1. Pour specimen into centrifuge tubes labeled with the specimen accession number.
2. Centrifuge at 1500 rpm for 10 minutes.
3. Decant supernatant. Add 95% ETOH to cell button and agitate thoroughly.
4. Centrifuge again with fixative.
5. Remove tube from the centrifuge and allow sediment to harden for at least 20 minutes.
6. If a specimen fails to harden adequately, decant the 95% ETOH fixative and add acetone. Agitate thoroughly and centrifuge again.

7. Carefully remove sediment button from tube with a clean metal spatula and place on a small piece of premoistened lens paper.
8. Fold lens paper over specimen, place in a labeled cassette, and close. Immerse in 10% buffered formalin and deliver to Surgical Pathology.

E. Preparing Membrane Filters for Staining

Procedure:

1. With a clean Millipore forceps, carefully lift filter, keeping cell side up.
2. Place filter in filter holder, keeping cell side up; or attach filter to glass slide (cell side up) with alligator clip.
3. Place filter holder in staining tray.
4. Stain manually or on an automated Papanicolaou stainer.

F. Rapid Papanicolaou Stain (Gill 2)

Purpose:

1. Rapid preliminary assessment of fine needle aspiration material.
2. "Stat" assessment of intraoperative procedures, i.e., brain aspirations, scrapes, and smears.
3. Rapid assessment of any specimen for which a physician has requested a "stat" report.

Procedure:

Step	Solution	Time (Interval)
1.	Distilled H_2O	1 minute
2.	Gill 2 hematoxylin	10 seconds
3.	Distilled H_2O	1 minute
4.	Distilled H_2O	Until clear
5.	Distilled H_2O	Until clear
6.	95% ETOH	1 minute
7.	OG-6	1 minute
8.	95% ETOH	½ minute
9.	95% ETOH	½ minute
10.	EA-50	1½ minutes
11.	95% ETOH	½ minute
12.	95% ETOH	½ minute
13.	100% ETOH	1 minute
14.	Xylene	1 minute
15.	Xylene	5 minutes

G. Modified Papanicolaou Stain for Manual Staining of Cytocentrifugation and Direct Smear Preparations (Gill 1)

Purpose:

Recommended for the highest quality manual staining of cytocentrifugation and direct smear preparations. This procedure is used primarily for CSF, fine needle aspirations, and smears.

Procedure:

Step	Solution	Time (Interval)
1.	Distilled H_2O	1 minute
2.	Gill 1 hematoxylin	1 minute
3.	Distilled H_2O	10 (1-second) dips
4.	Distilled H_2O	10 (1-second) dips
5.	Scott's tap H_2O	10 (1-second) dips
6.	Distilled H_2O	10 (1-second) dips
7.	95% ETOH	10 (1-second) dips
8.	95% ETOH	10 (1-second) dips
9.	OG-6	1½ minutes
10.	95% ETOH	10 (1-second) dips
11.	95% ETOH	10 (1-second) dips
12.	EA-50	1½ minutes
13.	95% ETOH	10 (1-second) dips
14.	95% ETOH	10 (1-second) dips
15.	100% ETOH	10 (1-second) dips
16.	100% ETOH	2 minutes
17.	Xylene	1 minute (until clear)
18.	Xylene	1 minute
19.	Xylene	5 minutes

H. Modified Papanicolaou Stain for Manual Staining of Filters (Gill 1)

Purpose:

Staining of all membrane filter preparations, including spinal fluids, aspirates, and other cytologic procedures where membrane filters have been prepared.

Procedure:

Step	Solution	Time (Interval)
1.	Distilled H_2O	1 minute
2.	Gill 1 hematoxylin	30 seconds/agitate gently
3.	Distilled H_2O	10 (1-second) dips
4.	Distilled H_2O	10 (1-second) dips
5.	Acid-H_2O (0.25%)	10 (1-second) dips
6.	Distilled H_2O	5 (1-second) dips
7.	Scott's Tap H_2O	5 (1-second) dips
8.	Distilled H_2O	10 (1-second) dips
9.	95% ETOH	10 (1-second) dips
10.	95% ETOH	10 (1-second) dips
11.	OG-6	1½ minutes
12.	95% ETOH	10 (1-second) dips
13.	95% ETOH	10 (1-second) dips
14.	EA-50	1½ minutes
15.	95% ETOH	10 (1-second) dips
16.	95% ETOH	10 (1-second) dips
17.	1-propanol	10 (1-second) dips
18.	1-propanol	2 minutes
19.	Xylene 1	1 minute (until clear)
20.	Xylene 2	1 minute
21.	Xylene 3	5 minutes

I. Destaining Technique for Cytological Preparations

Purpose:

The purpose of destaining cytological smears is to rejuvenate tinctorial qualities in poorly stained smears and/or old, badly oxidized smears.

Procedure:

Removing the Coverslip

1. Very old slides may be placed on a metal tray and put in the freezer compartment for several hours. The coverslips can then be carefully removed using the edge of a razor blade. These slides then need to be soaked in xylene to soften and remove excess mounting medium, as in 2 below.
2. Recent cases need to be soaked in xylene for several days in order to dislodge coverslips. Place slides "tag end down" in the staining rack. This helps to keep the adhesive material from the tags off the slide. It is important to change this xylene after 1 or 2 days so that artifacts and debris are not introduced onto the preparation.

Destaining the Smear

1. Once the coverslips have been removed, place the slides in the following solutions for the times indicated:

a.	1:1 solution of absolute alcohol and xylene	1–5 minutes
b.	Absolute ethanol	1–5 minutes
c.	Absolute ethanol	1–5 minutes
d.	95% ethanol	1–5 minutes
e.	95% ethanol	1–5 minutes
f.	50% ethanol	1–5 minutes
g.	Running water bath	5 minutes
h.	Dilute hydrochloric acid (carefully add 5 or 6 drops of concentrated HCl to the existing staining dish, to ensure complete removal of nuclear and cytoplasmic stain)	Up to 45 minutes: until nuclear stain is gone
i.	Running water bath	5 minutes

Restaining the Smear

To restain the slides, follow the standard staining protocol for gyn or non-gyn cases.

J. Destaining Procedure—Direct Smear and Cytocentrifugation Preparations

Purpose:

To prepare less optimally stained slides for restaining, prior to:

1. Review of original diagnosis.
2. Photography.
3. Utilization as teaching material.

Procedure:

Step	Solution	Time (Interval)
1.	Xylene	Until coverslip comes off
2.	100% ETOH	1 minute
3.	100% ETOH	1 minute
4.	95% ETOH	1 minute
5.	95% ETOH	1 minute
6.	Distilled H_2O	1 minute
7.	Distilled H_2O	1 minute
8.	0.5% HCl	5 minutes–1 hour
9.	Running tap H_2O	10–15 minutes
10.	Scott's tap H_2O	5 minutes
11.	Running tap H_2O	5 minutes
12.	Restain using approved procedure	

Reference:

Koss LG: *Diagnostic Cytology and Its Histopathologic Bases,* 3rd Ed. J.B. Lippincott, Philadelphia, 1979, p. 1221.

K. Destaining Procedure—Membrane Filters

Purpose:

To prepare less optimally stained membrane filter preparations for restaining, prior to:
1. Reviews of original diagnosis.
2. Photography.
3. Utilization as teaching material.

Procedure:

Step	Solution	Time (Interval)
1.	Xylene	Until coverslip comes off
2.	Xylene	30 minutes (minimum)
3.	1-Propanol	1 minute
4.	1-Propanol	1 minute
5.	95% ETOH	20 dips
6.	95% ETOH	20 dips
7.	Distilled H_2O	1 minute
8.	Distilled H_2O	1 minute
9.	0.5% HCl	5 minutes–1 hour
10.	Running distilled H_2O	2–5 minutes
11.	Restain using approved procedure	

Reference:

Adapted from Gelman Application Bulletin 100 "Diagnostic Cytology by Membrane Filter," 1978.

L. Diff-Quik (Wright's) Stain

Purpose:

1. Characterization of hematopoietic cells (especially eosinophils in body fluids).
2. Rapid quantitation of cellular material in determination of whether or not to filter a specimen.
3. Identification of stromal matrix.

Principle:

Metachromatic staining of hematopoietic cells.

Reagents:

Diff-Quik kit commercially available from Baxter Scientific, Order #B4132-1.
Diff-Quik Fixative Solution: 1.8 mg/L triarylmethane dye in methyl alcohol. **WARNING: Methyl alcohol is poisonous. Do not breathe vapor or allow contact with skin, eyes, or clothing. Do not drink.** For further information see package insert or MSDS.
Diff-Quik Solution I: 1.0 gm/L xanthene dye and 0.01% sodium azide in buffer. **WARNING: In combination with lead and copper plumbing, sodium azide may form explosive**

metal azides. If discarded into sink, flush with a large volume of water to prevent azide buildup.
Diff-Quik Solution II: 0.625 gm/L azure A and 0.625 gm/L methylene blue in buffer.

Procedure:

1. Prepare slide and allow to air dry.
2. Dip slide in Diff-Quik fixative for 10 seconds (10 1-second dips). Allow excess to drain.
3. Dip slide in Diff-Quik Solution I for 10 seconds (10 1-second dips). Allow excess to drain.
4. Dip slide in Diff-Quik Solution II for 12 seconds (12 1-second dips). Allow excess to drain.
5. Rinse slide with distilled or deionized water. Allow to dry.
6. Dip in xylene and coverslip using permanent mounting medium.

Results:

Erythrocytes:	Pink or yellowish-red
Platelets:	Violet to purple granules
Leukocytes:	
Neutrophils:	
Nucleus	Dark blue
Cytoplasm	Pale pink
Granules	Reddish lilac
Eosinophils:	
Nucleus	Blue
Cytoplasm	Blue
Granules	Red to red-orange
Basophils:	
Nucleus	Purple or dark blue
Granules	Dark purple (almost black)
Monocytes:	
Nucleus (lobate)	Violet
Cytoplasm	Sky blue
Lymphocytes:	
Nucleus	Violet
Cytoplasm	Dark blue
Epithelial (lining) cells:	
Nucleus	Violet
Cytoplasm	Sky blue
Macrophages:	
Nucleus	Violet
Cytoplasm	Blue to dark blue
Bacteria:	Blue
Stromal matrix:	Purple to blue

Controls:

Routine material makes an adequate control.

Reference:

Package insert supplied with the American Scientific Products Diff-Quik Stain Set (Product number: B4132-1).
Comment: Staining times may vary, especially as solutions age. In Solution I, 10 to 20 seconds may be necessary, and in solution II 12 to 30 seconds in order to obtain the desired degree of color, particularly in CNS smear preparations.

M. Hematoxylin and Eosin Method for Frozen Sections and Smear Preparations

Reagents:

Lerner III Hematoxylin[b]
Eosin-Y (alcoholic)[b]
Bluing reagent[b]

Procedure:

1.	Fix in 95% alcohol	30 seconds
2.	70% alcohol	10 dips
3.	Tap H_2O	10 dips (or until clear)
4.	Hematoxylin	30 seconds
5.	Bluing reagent	5 dips
6.	70% alcohol	10 dips
7.	Eosin-Y (alcoholic)	10 dips
8.	95% alcohol	10 dips
9.	100% alcohol	10 dips
10.	100% alcohol	10 dips
11.	Xylene	10 dips (or until clear)
12.	Xylene	10 dips
13.	Mount with Permount	

[b] Lerner Laboratories, 171 Industry Drive, Pittsburgh, PA 15275, U.S.A.

N. Removal of Mercury Precipitated Pigment

When a fixative containing mercuric chloride is employed one can expect a random distribution of brown to black artifactual deposits throughout the tissue section. This may be removed by the following method:

1. Deparaffinize and hydrate to water.
2. Place in Gram's or Lugol's iodine solution for 15 minutes.

Gram's Iodine:	
Iodine	1.0 gm
Potassium iodide	2.0 gm
Distilled water	300 ml
Lugol's Iodine:	
Iodine	1.0 gm
Potassium iodide	2.0 gm
Distilled water	100 ml

3. Rinse in tap water.
4. Place in 5% aqueous sodium thiosulfate (hypo) for 3 minutes.
5. Wash in tap water for 10 minutes or longer.
6. Stain as desired.

Reference:

Histopathology Laboratories, Armed Forces Institute of Pathology, Washington, D.C., 20305.

O. Cytochemical (Special) Stains

1. Acid-Fast Stain

Purpose:

The cell walls of certain bacteria contain long-chain fatty acids (mycolic acids), lending them the property of resistance to destaining of basic dyes by acid alcohol.

Principle:

Bacteria of the genus *Mycobacterium* are the microorganisms for which the acid-fast stain is most often used.

Reagents:

T.B. Kinyoun Stain Kit, commercially available from CMS, Order # L12318

1. Basic fuchsin with 5% phenol.
2. 3% hydrochloric acid in ethanol.
3. 0.3% aqueous solution of methylene blue.

Procedure:

Kinyoun's Cold Acid-fast Stain

1. Fix slides in 95% ETOH for 10 minutes.
2. Place in distilled water for 1 minute.
3. Flood slides with Kinyoun's Basic Fuchsin and allow to stain for 3 minutes at room temperature.
4. Rinse with distilled water to prevent tap water contaminants from being introduced.
5. Decolorize with acid-alcohol until no more red color runs from the smear.
6. Rinse with distilled water and drain standing water from slide surface by tipping slide.
7. Flood slide with methylene blue counterstain and allow to stain for 30 seconds.
8. Rinse with distilled water and allow to air dry.
9. Coverslip with Permount.
10. Examine under high dry magnification and confirm acid-fast structures under oil immersion.

Results:

The acid-fast organisms should be stained a bright red; other organisms and the background material should be stained blue.

Controls:

A control must be run with each procedure. Controls are made up with broth solutions of autoclaved *Mycobacterium tuberculosis* placed in any body fluid and prepared by cytocentrifugation.

Reference:

Finegold and Baron: *Bailey and Scott's Diagnostic Microbiology*, 7th ed. C.V. Mosby, St. Louis, 1986, p. 603.

2. Fontana-Masson Stain

Purpose:

Demonstration of melanin pigment.

Principle:

Melanin has an affinity for silver nitrate.

Reagents:

Silver Nitrate Solution (Fontana):
Dissolve 10 gm of silver nitrate in 100 ml of distilled water. To 95 ml of this solution, add ammonium hydroxide until a clear solution with no precipitate is obtained. Add, drop by drop, enough of the remaining 5 ml of silver nitrate solution to cause the clear solution above to become slightly cloudy. Let stand overnight before using. When ready to use, dilute each 25 ml of silver solution with 75 ml of distilled water and filter.

Gold Chloride Solution:

Gold chloride, 1% aqueous	10.0 ml
Distilled water	40.0 ml

5% Sodium Thiosulfate (Hypo) Solution:

Sodium thiosulfate	5.0 gm
Distilled water	100 ml

Nuclear Fast Red (Kernechtrot) Solution:
Dissolve 0.1 gm nuclear fast red in 100 ml of 5% solution of aluminum sulfate with aid of heat. Cool, filter, add grain of thymol as a preservative.

Procedure:

1. Hydrate to distilled water.
2. Silver nitrate solution at 56°C for 1 hour. Sections should be light brown.
3. Rinse sections in distilled water.
4. Gold chloride solution for 10 minutes.
5. Rinse in distilled water, three changes.
6. Sodium thiosulfate solution for 5 minutes.
7. Rinse in distilled water.
8. Nuclear fast red solution for 5 minutes.
9. Rinse in distilled water, two changes.
10. Dehydrate in 95% alcohol, absolute alcohol, and clear in xylene, two changes each.
11. Mount with Permount.

Results:

Silver reducing substances:	Black
Nuclei:	Pink

Controls:

Cytospins of previously positive melanoma aspirate.

Reference:

Masson P: Am. J. Pathol. 4:181-212, 1928.

3. Gomori's Methenamine-Silver (GMS) Nitrate Technique (Grocott's Application to Fungi)

Purpose:

Demonstration of fungi and *Pneumocystis carinii*.

Principle:

Fungi and *Pneumocystis carinii* are demonstrated by impregnation with silver nitrate.

Reagents:

1.	*10% Chromic Acid*	
	Chromic acid	10.0 gm
	Distilled water	100.0 ml
2.	*5% Silver Nitrate Solution*	
	Silver nitrate	5.0 gm
	Distilled water	100.0 ml
3.	*35% Methenamine Solution*	
	Hexamethylenetetramine, SUP	3.0 gm
	Distilled water	100.0 ml
4.	*5% Borax Solution*	
	Borax (sodium borate)	5.0 gm
	Distilled water	100.0 ml
5.	*Stock Methenamine-Silver Solution*	
	5% silver nitrate	5.0 ml
	3% methenamine	100.0 ml
6.	*Working Methenamine-Silver Nitrate Solution*	
	Borax, 5% solution	2.0 ml
	Distilled water	25.0 ml
	Mix and add:	
	Methenamine-silver nitrate, stock	25.0 ml
7.	*1% Sodium Bisulfite Solution*	
	Sodium bisulfite	1.0 gm
	Distilled water	100.0 ml
8.	*0.1% Gold Chloride*	
	Gold chloride, 1%	10.0 ml
	Distilled water	90.0 ml
9.	*2% Sodium Thiosulfate Solution (Hypo)*	
	Sodium thiosulfate	2.0 gm
	Distilled water	100.0 ml

10. *Stock Light Green Solution*

Light green, S.F. (yellow)	0.2 gm
Distilled water	100.0 ml
Glacial acetic acid	0.2 ml

11. *Working Light Green Solution*

Light green, stock solution	10.0 ml
Distilled water	30.0 ml

Procedure:

1. Hydrate in distilled water for 5 minutes.
2. Oxidize in chromic acid solution (10% chromic—10 minutes). Solution may be kept until dark brown in color.
3. Wash in running tap water for a few seconds.
4. Rinse in 1% sodium bisulfite for 1 minute to remove any residual chromic acid.
5. Wash in tap water for 5–10 minutes.
6. Wash with 3 or 4 changes of distilled water.
7. Place in working methenamine-silver nitrate solution at 60° for 60–90 minutes until section turns yellowish brown. Check for adequate silver impregnation under microscope. Fungi should be dark brown at this stage. Solution may be preheated.
8. Rinse in 6 changes of distilled water.
9. Tone in 0.1% gold chloride solution for 2–5 minutes. Solution may be reused.
10. Rinse in distilled water.
11. Remove unreduced silver with 2% sodium thiosulfate solution for 2–5 minutes. Solution may be reused.
12. Wash thoroughly in tap water.
13. Counterstain with working light green solution for 1–2 minutes. Solution may be reused.
14. Dehydrate, clear, and mount.

Results:

Fungi and *Pneumocystis carinii*:	Sharply delineated in black
Mucin:	Taupe to dark gray
Inner parts of mycelia and hyphae:	Old rose
Background:	Pale green

Controls:

A control must be run with each procedure. Previously positive *Pneumocystis* material is recommended; however, a positive fungus control may be used and the time increased in working silver by 15 minutes to properly demonstrate *Pneumocystis*.

Reference:

Grocott RG: Am. J. Clin. Pathol. 25:975–979, 1955 (AFIP modification).

4. Gram Stain

Purpose:

The Gram stain is used to stain microorganisms from cultures and specimens by the differential Gram method.

Principle:

The Gram stain divides all bacterial species into two large groups: those that take up the basic dye, crystal violet (Gram-positive), and those that allow the crystal violet dye to wash out easily with decolorizer (alcohol) and then are stained by the counterstain, safranin (Gram-negative).

Reagents:

Difco Gram Stain Kit, commercially available from CMS, order #3328-32-1.

1. 1% aqueous solution crystal violet.
2. Gram iodine.
3. Mixture of acetone and alcohol.
4. Safranin.

Procedure:

1. Fix slides in ETOH for 10 minutes.
2. Place slides in distilled water for 1 minute.
3. Flood slide with crystal violet and stain for 1 minute.
4. Remove crystal violet by gently washing with cold tap water.
5. Flood slides with Gram iodine and retain on slide for 1 minute.
6. Remove iodine by gently washing with tap water.
7. Decolorize with Gram decolorizer until solvent running from slide is colorless (15–30 seconds).
8. Wash slides gently in cold tap water.
9. Flood slides with safranin and stain for 1 minute.

10. Wash slides with cold tap water and allow to dry.
11. Coverslip with Permount.
12. Examine under high dry magnification and confirm bacteria under oil immersion.

Results:

Gram-positive microorganisms should be stained a blue-black; Gram-negative microorganisms should be stained red.

Controls:

A control must be run with each procedure. Controls are made up with broth suspensions of *Staphylococcus aureus* (Gram-positive) and *Escherichia coli* (Gram-negative) placed in any body fluid and prepared by cytocentrifugation.

Reference:

Finegold and Baron: *Bailey and Scott's Diagnostic Microbiology*. 7th ed. C. V. Mosby, St. Louis, 1986, pp. 76–77.

5. Iron Stain

Purpose:

Demonstration of iron pigment.

Principle:

Iron pigment reacts with potassium ferrocyanide to form a reaction known as Prussian blue.

Reagents:

2% Potassium Ferrocyanide:	
Potassium ferrocyanide	2.0 gm
Distilled water	100.0 ml
2% Hydrochloric Acid Solution:	
Hydrochloric acid, concentrated	2.0 ml
Distilled water	98.0 ml

Procedure:

1. Deparaffinize and hydrate to distilled water.
2. Place slides in a freshly prepared mixture of equal parts 2% potassium ferrocyanide and 2% hydrochloric acid at 56°C for 20 minutes.
3. Wash thoroughly in several changes of distilled water.
4. Counterstain with eosin for required time using routine stain setup.
5. Dehydrate, clear, and mount.

Results:

Hemosiderin (iron):	Blue
Background:	Pink

Controls:

A control must be run with each procedure (e.g., preparations of specimens with hemosiderin-laden macrophages present).

Reference:

Lillie RD: *Histopathologic Technic and Practical Histochemistry*. 3rd ed. McGraw-Hill, New York, 1965, p. 406.

6. Mucicarmine Stain

Purpose:

Demonstration of mucin and capsule of *Cryptococcus neoformans*.

Principle:

Mucin and capsule of *C. neoformans* are stained positive with mucicarmine solution.

Reagents:

Weigert's Iron Hematoxylin Solution:	
Solution A	
Hematoxylin crystals	1.0 gm
Alcohol, 95%	100.0 ml
Solution B	
Ferric chloride, 29% aqueous	1.0 ml
Distilled water	23.7 ml
Hydrochloric acid, concentrated	0.25 ml

Working Solution:
Equal parts of Solution A and Solution B for use.

Mucicarmine Solution:	
Carmine	1.0 gm
Aluminum chloride, anhydrous	0.5 gm
Distilled water	2.0 ml

Mix stain in small evaporating dish. Heat on electric hot plate for 2 minutes. Liquid becomes black and syrupy. Dilute with 100 ml of 50% alcohol and let stand for 24 hours. Filter.

Dilute 1 part mucicarmine solution with 4 parts tap water for use.

0.25% Metanil Yellow Solution:

Metanil yellow	0.25 gm
Distilled water	100.0 ml
Glacial acetic acid	0.25 ml

Procedure:

1. Deparaffinize and hydrate to distilled water.
2. Working solution of Weigert's hematoxylin for 7 minutes.
3. Wash in running water for 10 minutes.
4. Diluted mucicarmine solution for 60 minutes.
5. Rinse quickly in distilled water.
6. Metanil yellow solution for 1 minute.
7. Rinse quickly in distilled water.
8. Dehydrate, clear, and mount.

Results:

Mucin:	Deep rose to red
Capsule of *C. neoformans*:	Deep rose to red
Nuclei:	Black
Other tissue elements:	Yellow

Controls:

A control must be run with each procedure (e.g., cytospin preparations of previously positive mucin-producing cells).

Reference:

Mallory FB: *Pathological Technique*. Hafner Publishing Co., New York, 1961, p. 130.

7. Oil Red O Fat Stain

Purpose:

Stains for fat.

Principle:

Unfixed and undissolved fat stains positively with oil red O.

Reagents:

0.5% Oil Red O Solution:

Oil red O	0.5 gm
Propylene glycol, 100%	100.0 ml

Add a small amount of propylene glycol to the oil red O and mix well; crush larger pieces. Gradually add the remainder of the propylene glycol, stirring periodically. Heat gently until the solution reaches 95°C. Do not allow to go over 100°C. Stir while heating. Filter through coarse filter paper while still warm. Allow to stand overnight at room temperature.

85% Propylene Glycol Solution:

Propylene glycol, 100%	85.0 ml
Distilled water	15.0 ml

Gills Hematoxylin Solution: Commercially available from Surgipath, Order #HX-100.

Procedure:

1. Prepare slides and allow to air dry.
2. Place in absolute propylene glycol for 2 minutes.
3. Place in oil red O for 1 hour.
4. Differentiate in 85% propylene glycol solution for 1 minute.
5. Rinse in distilled water for 2 changes.
6. Stain in Gills hematoxylin for 2 minutes.
7. Rinse in distilled water for 2 changes.
8. Mount with Aqua Mount.

Results:

Fat:	Red to orange
Nuclei:	Blue

Control:

Cytospin preparations of previously positive cases.

Reference:

Histopathology Laboratories, Armed Forces Institute of Pathology, Washington, D.C., 20305.

8. Oil Red O Fat Stain (Alternate Method)

Reagents:

Oil red O (Harleco)
10% neutral buffered formalin
Propylene glycol, 100%

Lerner-III Hematoxylin (Lerner Laboratories[c])

Purpose:

Rapid fat stain for frozen section.

Procedure:

1. Cut and mount frozen sections on clear slide.
2. Fix sections in 10% buffered neutral formalin for 10 minutes.
3. Remove excess formalin by rinsing slides in several changes of distilled H_2O for 2–5 minutes.
4. Dehydrate in two changes of propylene glycol for 3–5 minutes, moving slides occasionally.
5. Stain in oil red O solution for 5–7 minutes at 60°C, moving slide occasionally.
6. Differentiate and hydrate in 85% propylene glycol, moving slides back and forth for 3 minutes.
7. Rinse slides thoroughly in several changes of distilled H_2O.
8. Counterstain in hematoxylin for 2 minutes.
9. Blue sections in running tap H_2O for 2 minutes.
10. Distilled H_2O rinse.
11. Coverslip with aqueous mounting media and seal edges of coverslip (e.g., Geltol permanent aqueous mounting medium).

Results:

Fat:	Red
Nuclei:	Blue

Reference:

Package insert

9. PAS Stain

Purpose:

Demonstration of fungi and glycogen.

Principle:

Carbohydrates stain PAS positive by immersion in basic fuchsin solution and developed by running tap water.

[c] Lerner Laboratories, 171 Industry Drive, Pittsburgh, PA 15275, U.S.A.

Reagents:

Schiff Reagent Solution:
Dissolve 1.10 gm basic fuchsin in 200.0 ml hot distilled water. Bring to boiling point. Cool to 50°C. Filter and add 20.0 ml normal hydrochloric acid. Cool further and add 1.0 gm anhydrous sodium bisulfite or sodium metabisulfite. Keep in the dark for 48 hours until solution becomes straw colored. Store in refrigerator.

Normal Hydrochloric Acid Solution:

Hydrochloric acid, sp. gr. 1.19	83.5 ml
Distilled water	916.5 ml

Test for Schiff Reagent Solution:
Pour a few drops of Schiff reagent solution into 10 ml of 37–40% formaldehyde in a watch glass. If the solution turns reddish purple rapidly, it is good. If the reaction is delayed and the resulting color deep blue-purple, the solution is breaking down.

0.5% Periodic Acid Solution:

Periodic acid	0.5 gm
Distilled water	100.0 ml

0.2% Light Green Solution (Stock):

Light green, SF yellowish	0.2 gm
Distilled water	100.0 ml
Glacial acetic acid	0.2 ml

Light Green Solution (Working):

Light green (stock)	10.0 ml
Distilled water	50.0 ml

Harris Hematoxylin:
Available on routine stain setup.

Procedure:

1. Fix slides in 95% ETOH for 10 minutes. Hydrate to distilled water. Several changes.
2. Oxidize in periodic acid solution for 5 minutes (made fresh each time).
3. Rinse in distilled water.
4. Schiff reagent solution for 15 minutes.
5. Wash in running water for 10 minutes for pink color to develop.
6. Gill's hematoxylin for required time, or light green counterstain for a few seconds. Light green is recommended for counterstaining section in which fungi are to be demonstrated (1 minute). Omit steps 7 and 8 if light green is used.
7. Wash in running water.
8. Dehydrate, clear, and mount.

Results:

Glycogen, mucin, reticulin, fibrin or thrombi, hyalin, hyalin deposits in basement membranes, and amyloid infiltration may show a positive reaction.

Positive reaction:	Rose to purplish red
Nuclei:	Blue
Fungi:	Red
Background:	Pale green (with light green counterstain).

Controls:

A control must be run with each procedure (e.g., cytospin preparations of specimens containing fungi; small intestine mucosa).

Reference:

McManus JFA: Stain Technology 23: 99–108, 1948 (AFIP modification). Copyright by Williams & Wilkins Co., Baltimore, MD.

10. PAS/Diastase Digestion Method

Purpose:

Elimination of glycogen within the cytoplasm of cells.

Principle:

Diastase enzymatically breaks down glycogen.

Reagents:

Phosphate Buffer Solution pH 6.0:

Sodium chloride	8.0 gm
Sodium phosphate, dibasic	0.282 gm
Sodium phosphate, monobasic	1.97 gm
Distilled water	100.0 ml

Diastase Digestion Solution:

Diastase of malt	0.1 gm
Phosphate buffer solution, pH 6.0	100.0 ml

Mix just before use.

Procedure:

1. Fix slides in 95% ETOH.
2. Place slides in preheated diastase solution at 37°C for 1 hour. (If human saliva is substituted for diastase, solution slides kept at room temperature for 20 minutes.)
3. Wash in running water for 5 minutes.
4. Stain with periodic acid-Schiff or other appropriate procedure.

Results:

Staining attributable to glycogen is selectively eliminated.

Reference:

McManus JFA: Stain Technology 23: 99–108, 1948 (AFIP modification). Copyright by Williams & Wilkins Co., Baltimore, MD.

11. Toluidine Blue O Stain

Purpose:

Rapid demonstration of *Pneumocystis carinii.*

Principle:

Toluidine blue O stain is taken up by the cysts after treatment with sulfation reagent.

Reagents:

Toluidine Blue O Working Solution (0.15%):

Toluidine blue O	0.17 g
Distilled water	60.0 ml
Concentrated HS	2.0 ml
Absolute ETOH	140.0 ml

Dissolve dye in water, add HS, then alcohol. Solution is stable for 1 year. Filter before use.

Sulfation Reagent:

Glacial acetic acid (chilled to 10°C)	45.0 ml
Concentrated sulfuric acid	15.0 ml

Slowly add concentrated sulfuric acid to a coplin jar containing chilled glacial acetic acid and mix. Discard reagent after 1 week of use.

Procedure:

1. Fix slide in 95% ETOH.
2. Place slides in sulfation reagent for 5 minutes.
3. Place in running tap water for 1 minute.
4. Place in toluidine blue O (working) for 5 minutes.
5. Dehydrate, clear, and mount.

Results:

P. carinii cysts:	Purple or violet
Background:	Green to pale blue

Reference:

Hummer DA: Cytodiagnosis of *Pneumocystis carinii* infection using toluidine blue O. Lab. Med. 19:821–823, 1988.

12. Toluidine Blue Stain

Purpose:

Toluidine blue is a rapid stain for wet sediment examination. It may be used as a control for setting up new cytopreparatory procedures, as a check on the cellular preservation of a sample, as a method of estimating the cellularity of a sample, to help achieve a monolayer of cells, and to prevent overloading filter preparations.

Principle:

Toluidine blue dye is taken up by all cells in the sample.

Reagents:

Toluidine blue, C.I. No. 52040	0.5 gm
95% ETOH	20.0 ml
Distilled water	80.0 ml

Dissolve dye in alcohol and add water. Filter and store in a dark bottle in the refrigerator.

Procedure:

1. Centrifuge specimen and remove most of the supernatant.
2. Place a drop of centrifuged specimen on single-end frosted slide.
3. Place a small drop of dye on the slide near the specimen and mix them together with applicator stick.
4. Coverslip (do not use mounting medium) and let stand for 2–5 minutes.

Results:

Cytoplasm stains light blue-purple. Nucleus stains dark blue-purple.

Reference:

Koss LG: *Diagnostic Cytology and Its Histopathologic Bases*. 3rd ed. JB Lippincott, Philadelphia, 1979, pp. 1242–1243.

P. Coverslipping

Procedure:

1. Smears

Smears should be taken *one at a time* from xylol, drained, and examined as to thickness or thinness of material. If smear is thin only one or two drops of mounting medium is necessary.[d] Drop medium on smear, being careful not to contaminate the specimen with the carrier of the medium. Touch edge of coverslip along edge of slide and slowly lower coverslip over smear. Drain on both sides and push out any bubbles that remain with the forceps. If too many bubbles persist, remove the coverslip, rinse smear in xylol, drain, and recover. If smear is too thick, take a clean coverslip and, using corner, scrape off thickest pieces of smear. Rinse slide in xylol, drain, and coverslip. Thicker smears require from 3 to 4 drops of mounting medium, depending on the consistency of the smear. Drain slide on both sides and push out any bubbles that persist. Rescrape and recover if necessary. Make sure edges are well drained and no mounting media is on top of coverslip or on bottom of glass slide.

2. Filters (Millipore and Gelman)

The filters are removed from the staining rack *one at a time*. Carefully remove from holder or remove the paper clips holding the filter to the slide. Using clean Millipore forceps, lift the filter out, trim the edges with a clean pair of scissors, and lay the filter on clean paper toweling. Using a lint-free tissue or clean gauze square, dry an all-frosted slide. Place 3–4 drops of Permount on the slide. Pick up the filter with the forceps and place it carefully, cell side up, on the slide, taking care not to allow air bubbles between

[d] Cytospin—1 drop of mounting medium.

filter and slide. Place an additional 3–4 drops of Permount on the filter, taking care not to contaminate the dispenser by touching the filter. Touch edge of coverslip on edge of slide and slowly lower on the filter. If air bubbles persist after a *minimum* effort to press them out with forceps, remove the coverslip and repeat the procedure. Clean excess Permount from top of coverslip gently with corner of gauze or with brush.

Color Plates

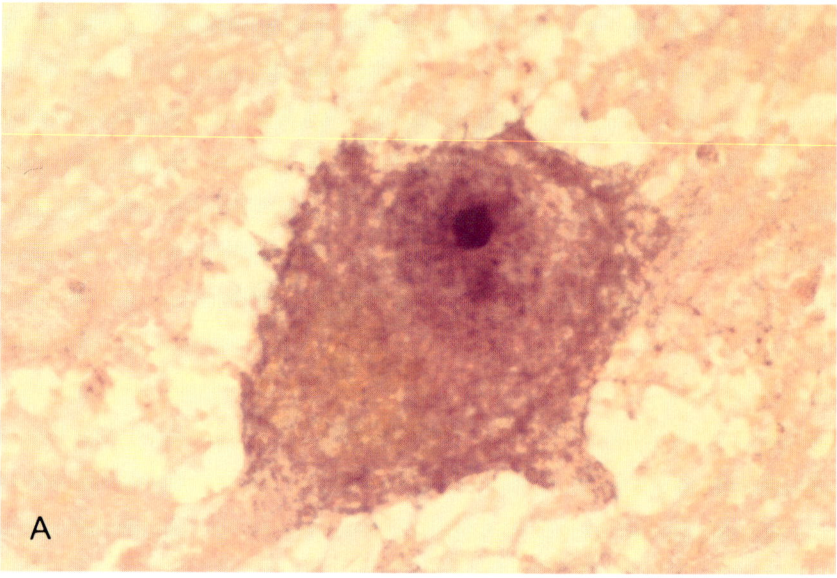

Figure 2.1. Neurons. **A,** Neuron demonstrating classical nuclear and cytoplasmic appearance. The cytoplasmic membrane appears shaggy due to adherent synaptic boutons and possibly glial fibrils. Some golden brown lipofuscin pigment is visible in the cytoplasm. The nucleolus is prominent. (Thalamus, smear preparation, H&E, ×400.)

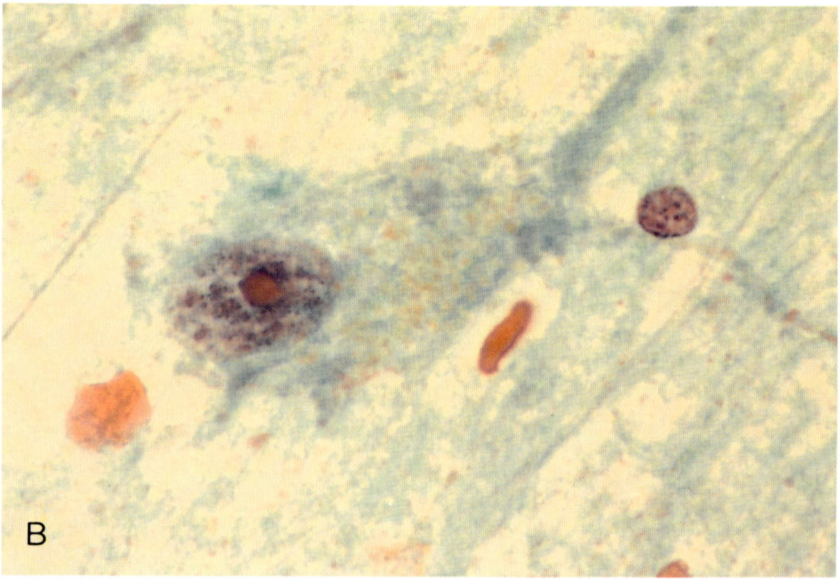

Figure 2.1. Neurons. **B,** Large neuron, with lipofuscin. (Thalamus, smear preparation, Pap stain, ×400.)

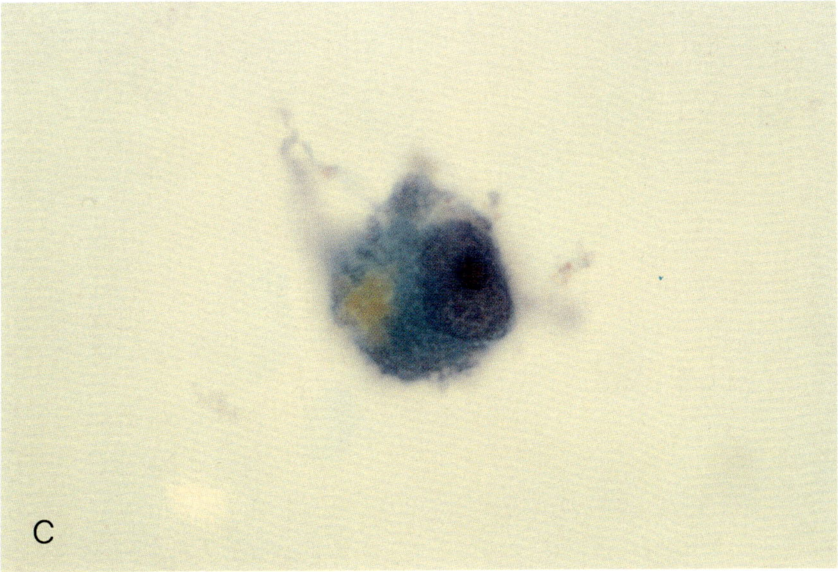

Figure 2.1. Neurons. **C,** Neuron appearance in cytospin preparation. Lipofuscin is more obvious due to the clear background. (Thalamus, cytospin, Pap stain, ×400.)

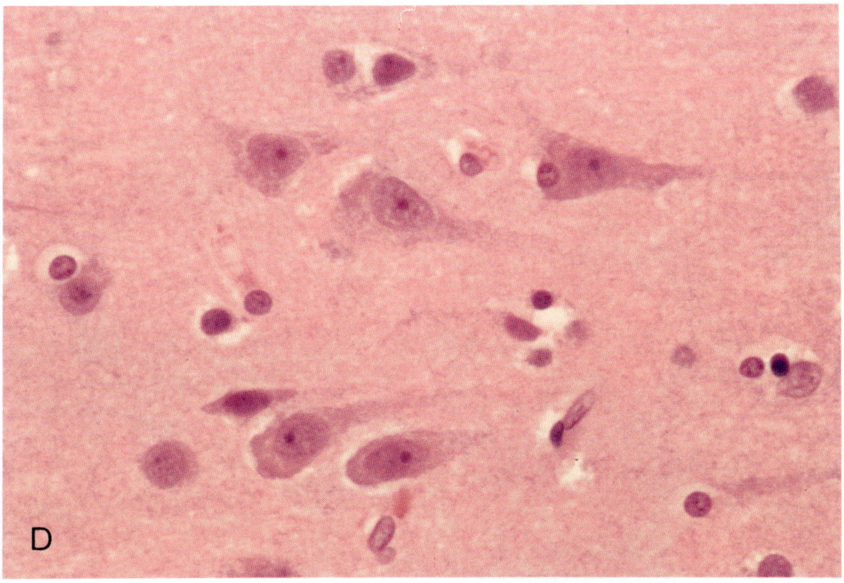

Figure 2.1. Neurons. **D,** Comparison of neuronal and glial nuclei. Large neurons with conspicuous cytoplasm contrast with the ''bare'' nuclei of glia. Oligodendrocyte nuclei resemble lymphocytes. Astrocyte nuclei are slightly larger and less chromatin rich. (Cerebral cortex, frontal lobe, paraffin section, H&E, ×160.)

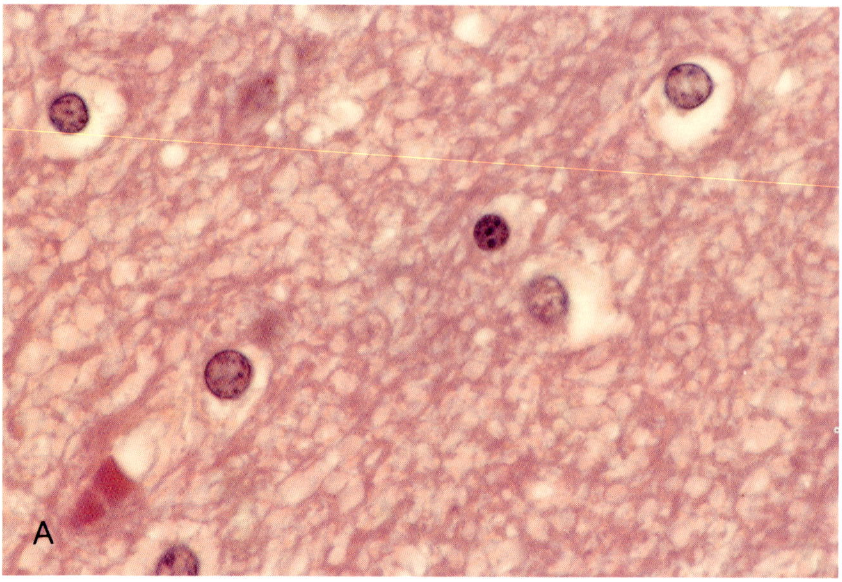

Figure 2.2. White matter. **A,** Appearance of normal white matter. The fibrillar background consists primarily of neuronal and neuroglial processes, with nuclei of astrocytes (larger, more vesicular nuclei) and oligodendrocytes (small, lymphocyte-like nuclei) present. Note the low cellularity and the perinuclear clear areas resulting from fixation artifact. (Cerebellum, paraffin section, H&E, ×400.)

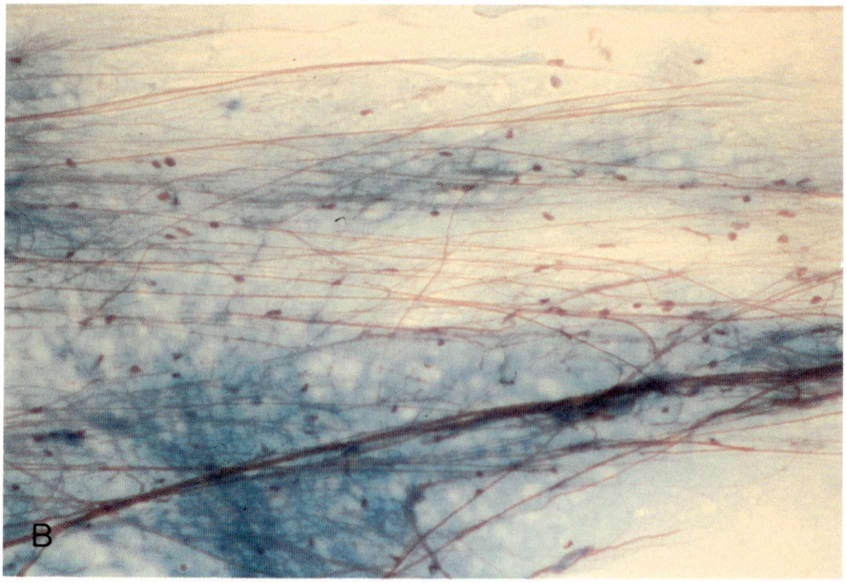

Figure 2.2. White matter. **B,** Normal white matter from spinal cord, demonstrating large red axons on a background of smaller (blue-green) axons and glial fibrils and nuclei. (Smear preparation, Pap stain, ×64.)

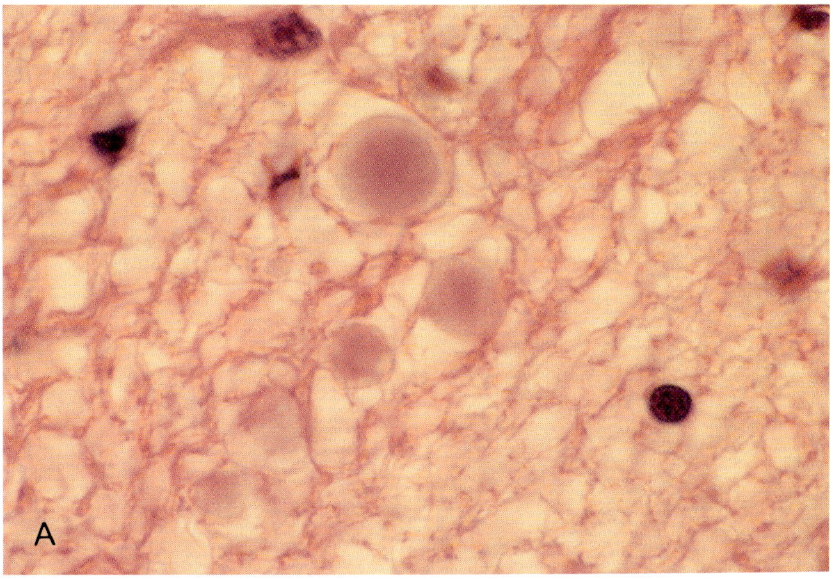

Figure 2.3. Corpora amylacea. **A,** Ovoid pink bodies in subpial neuropil. (Uncus, paraffin section, H&E, ×400.)

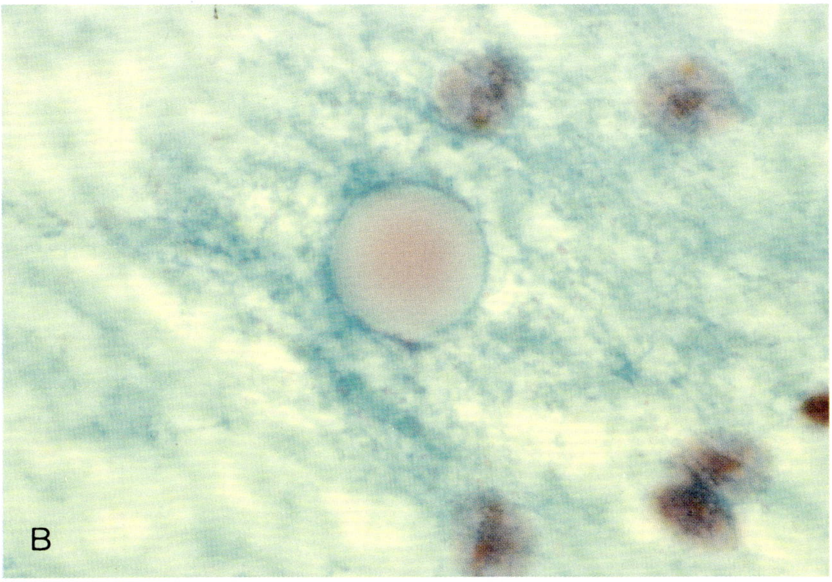

Figure 2.3. Corpora amylacea. **B,** Varying shades of pink to violet are typical of Papanicolaou-stained corpora amylacea. (Uncus, smear preparation, Pap stain, ×400.)

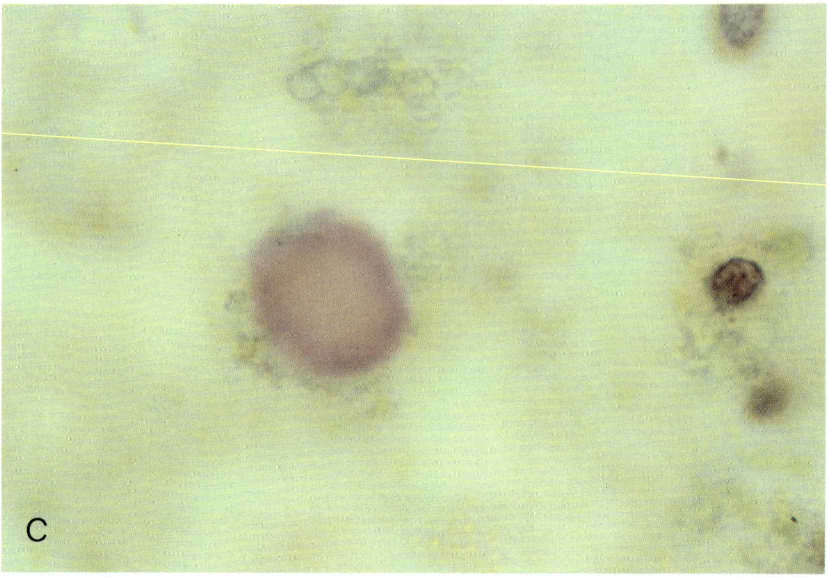

Figure 2.3. Corpora amylacea. **C.** (Uncus, membrane filtration, Pap stain, ×400.)

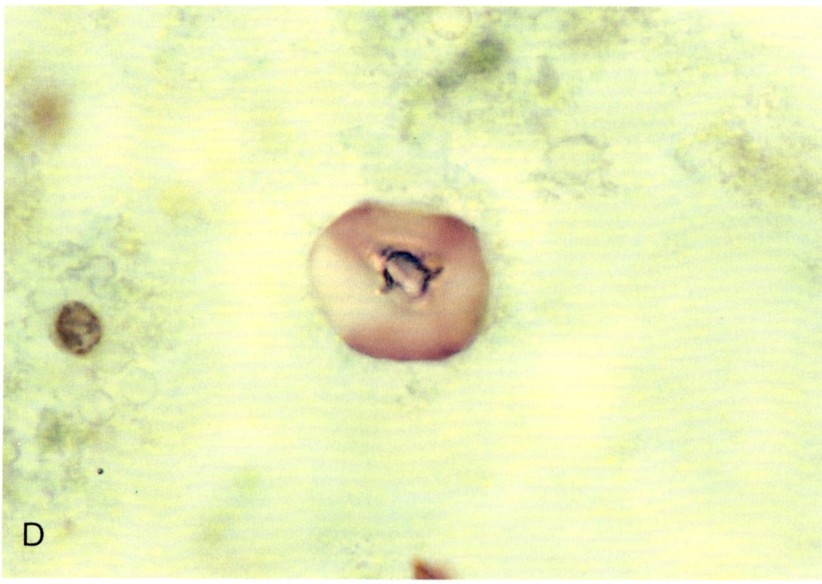

Figure 2.3. Corpora amylacea. **D,** Talc crystal. Note lamination and central birefringence in contrast to corpora amylacea. (Uncus, membrane filtration, Pap stain, ×400.)

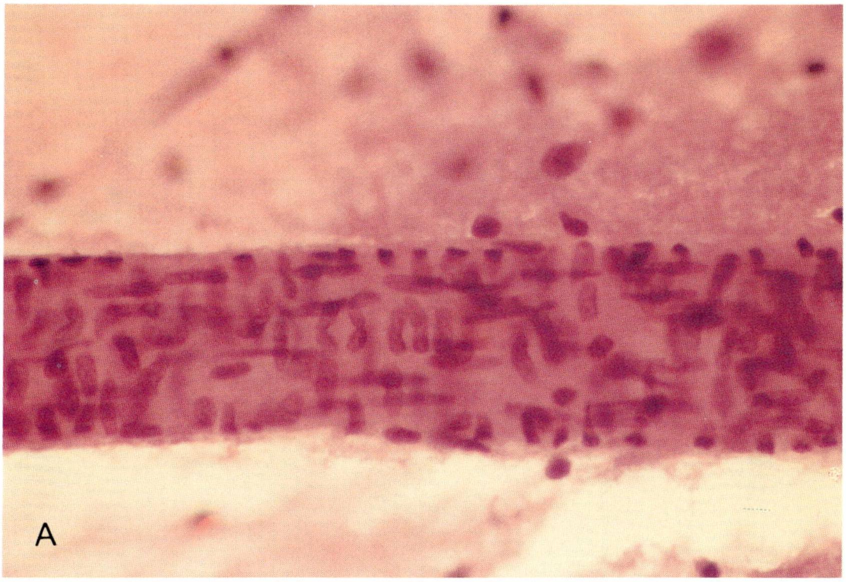

Figure 2.4. Vasculature. **A,** Arteriole, demonstrating bidirectional nuclear orientation. Longitudinal nuclei are endothelial cells, and nuclei perpendicular to the long axis of the vessel are predominantly smooth muscle nuclei. (Frontal lobe, smear preparation, H&E, ×160.)

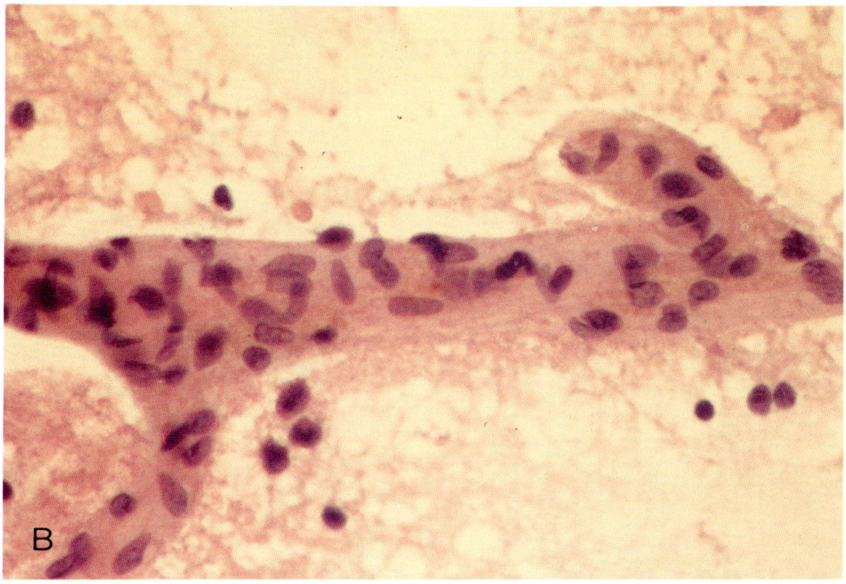

Figure 2.4. Vasculature. **B,** Venule. (Frontal lobe, smear preparation, H&E, ×160.)

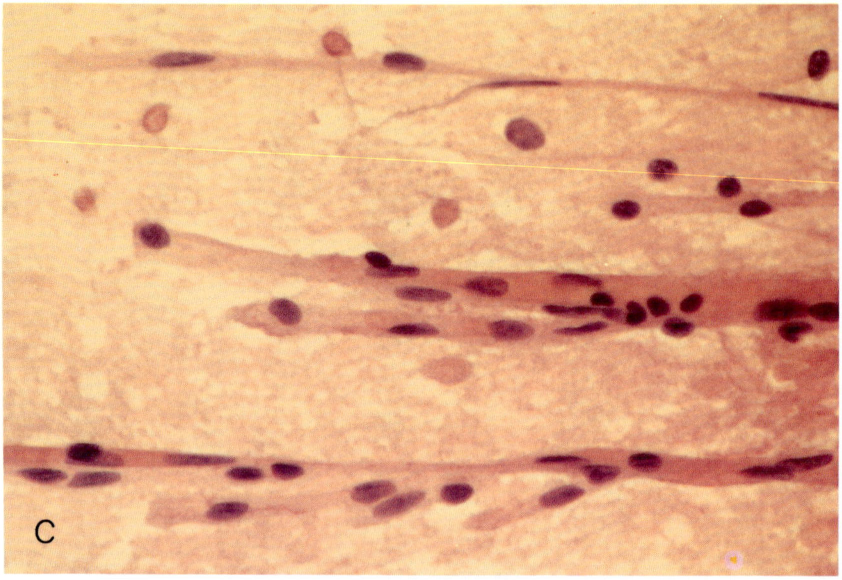

Figure 2.4. Vasculature. **C,** Transition of capillaries to small venules. (Frontal lobe, smear preparation, H&E, ×160.)

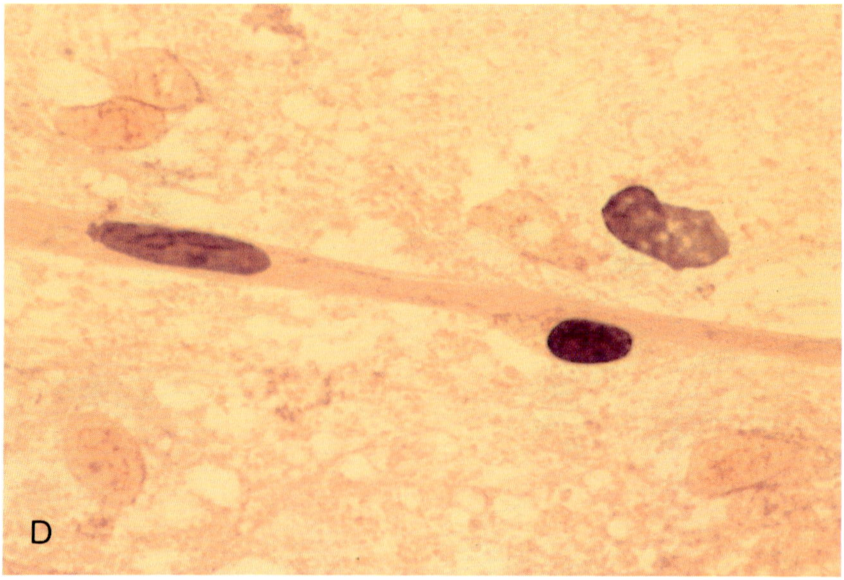

Figure 2.4. Vasculature. **D,** Detail of capillary demonstrating elongate endothelial cell nucleus and more ovoid hyperchromatic pericyte nucleus. (Frontal lobe, smear preparation, H&E, ×400.)

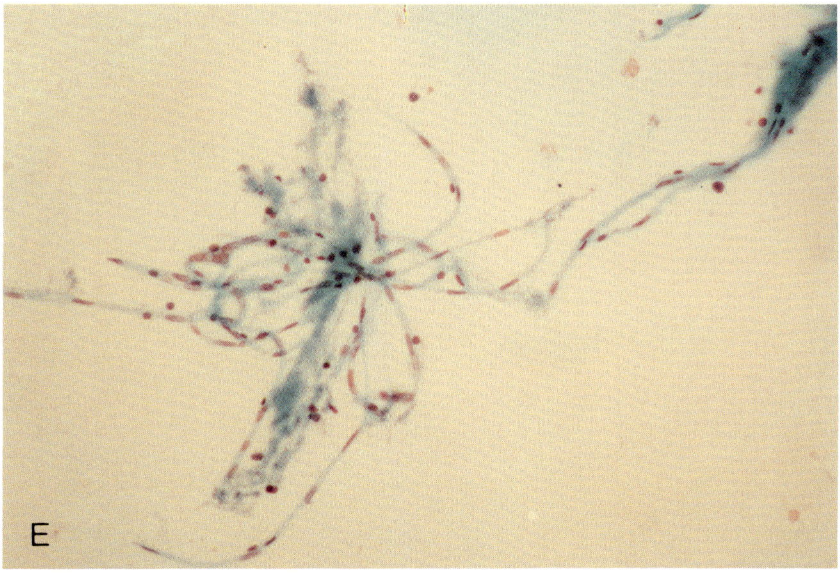

Figure 2.4. Vasculature. **E,** Capillaries and other small vessels are often a prominent component of cerebral cortex cytopreparations. (Lateral temporal lobe, cytospin, Pap stain, ×64.)

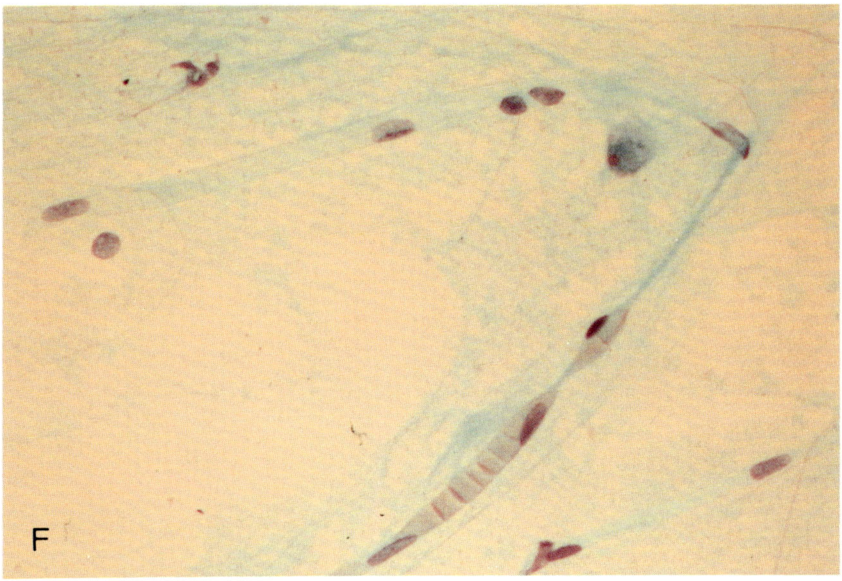

Figure 2.4. Vasculature. **F,** Tightly packed intraluminal RBCs within capillaries may produce an unusual cross-striped pattern with the Pap stain. (Basis pontis, smear preparation, Pap stain, ×160.)

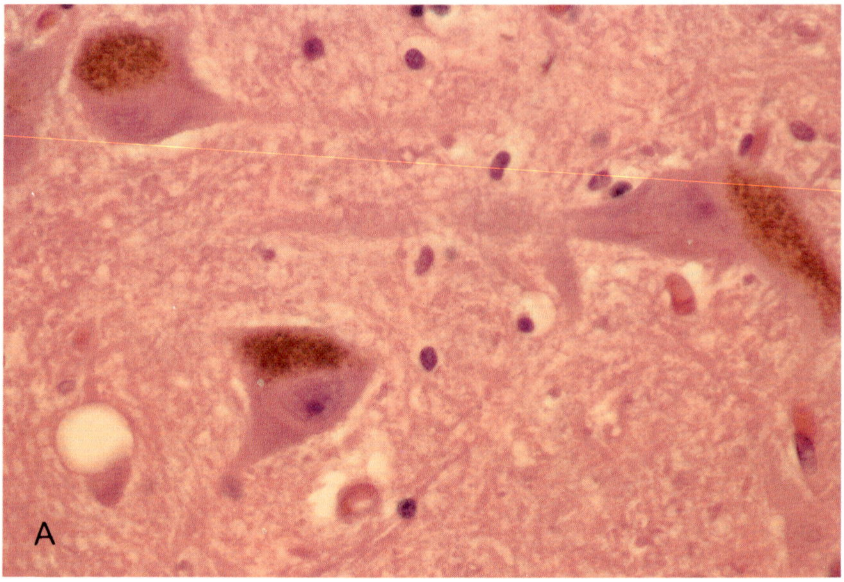

Figure 2.5. Melanin-containing neurons. **A,** Melanin-containing neurons within substantia nigra. (Paraffin section, H&E, ×160.)

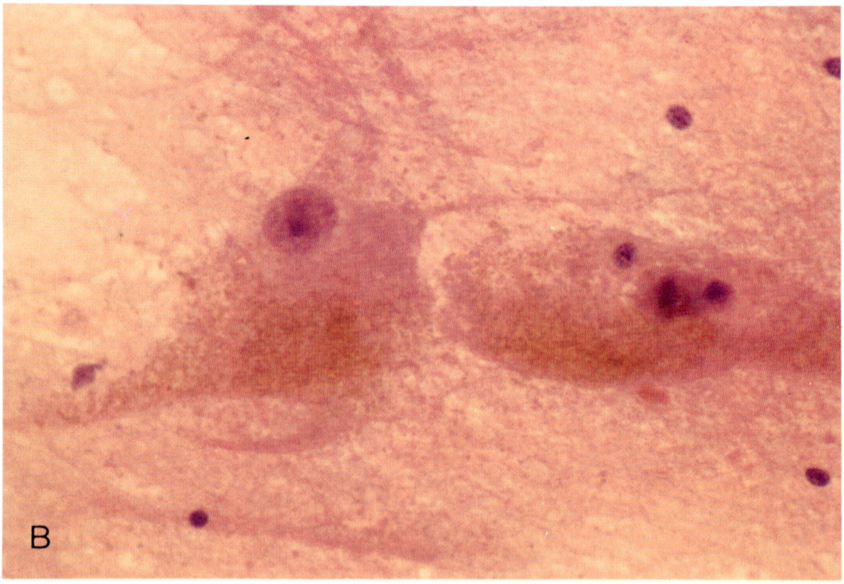

Figure 2.5. Melanin-containing neurons. **B,** Melanin-containing neurons in smears often demonstrate rather delicate cytoplasm, easily disrupted. These pigmented neurons are more intact than many that are encountered in such areas. Note that cells appear larger in smears than in paraffin sections (see **A**). (Substantia nigra, smear preparation, H&E, ×160.)

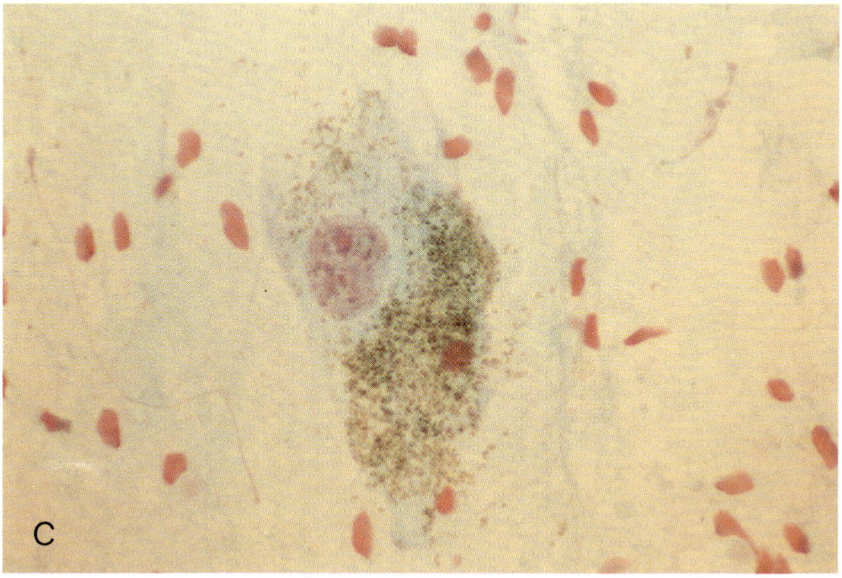

Figure 2.5. Melanin-containing neurons. **C,** The melanin stains olive green with the Pap stain. (Substantia nigra, smear preparation, Pap stain, ×160.)

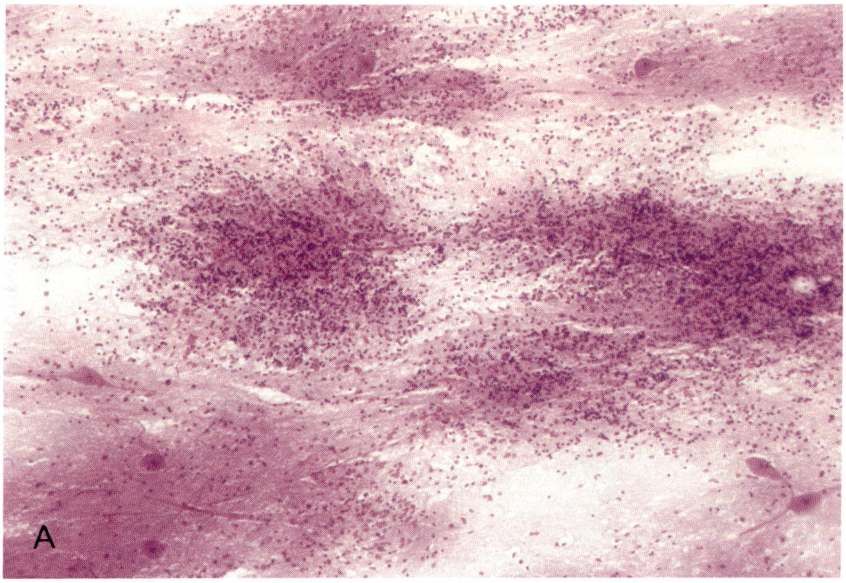

Figure 2.6. Cerebellar cortex. **A,** The cerebellar cortex is the most hypercellular zone in the normal gray matter of the neuraxis. (Smear preparation, H&E, ×40.)

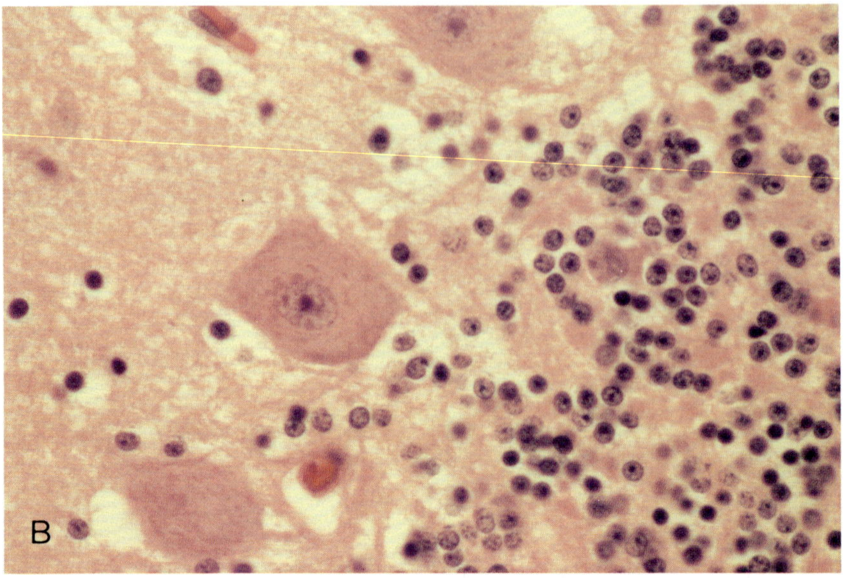

Figure 2.6. Cerebellar cortex. **B,** The major cell components of the cerebellar cortex are demonstrated in this section. The hypocellular zone on the left is the molecular layer, the row of large cells diagonally crossing the field constitutes the Purkinje cell layer, and the hypercellular zone on the right is the granular cell layer. A slightly larger neuron present within the granular layer is a Golgi type 2 cell. Bergmann glia are inconspicuous in the normal cerebellar cortex. (Paraffin section, H&E, ×160.)

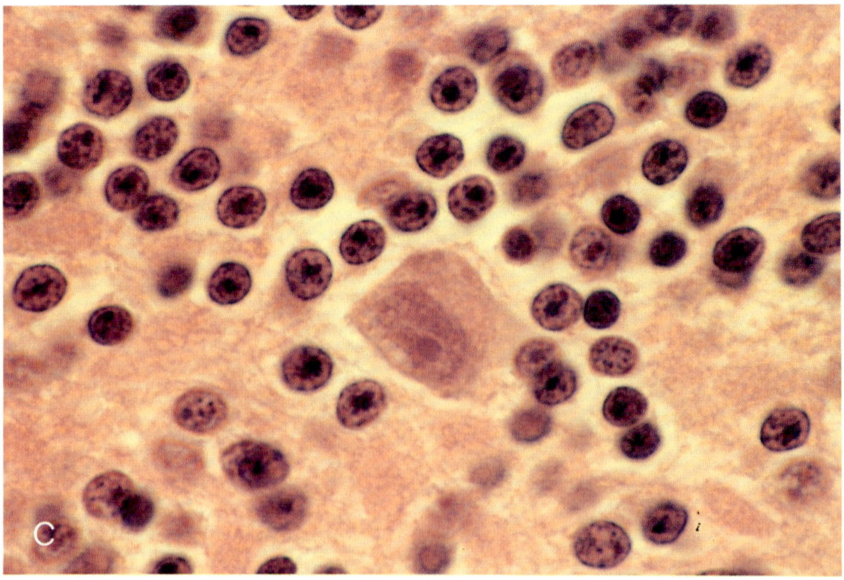

Figure 2.6. Cerebellar cortex. **C,** Detail of cerebellar cortex granular layer demonstrates a Golgi type 2 neuron in the center of the field surrounded by granule cells. Many of the latter have a central condensation of chromatin, giving a targetoid appearance. (Paraffin section, H&E, ×400.)

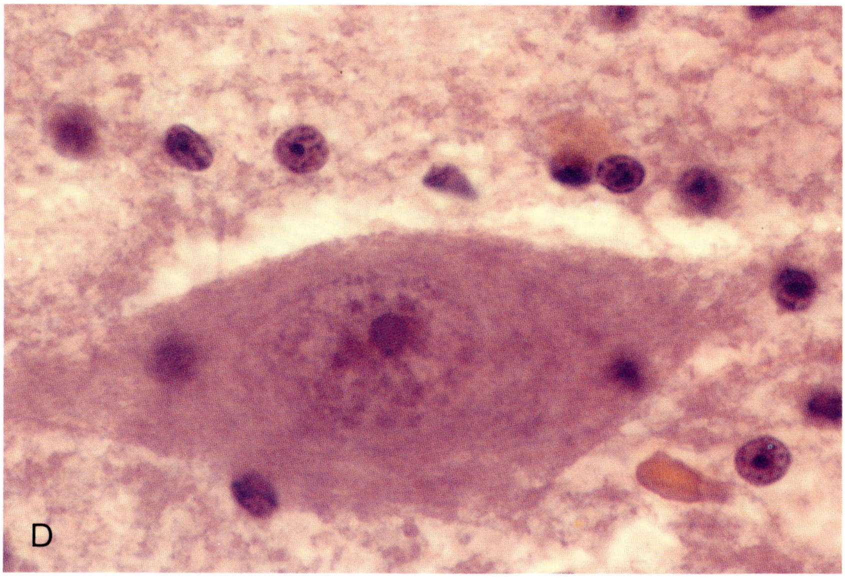

Figure 2.6. Cerebellar cortex. **D,** Purkinje cell with some surrounding granule cells and probably glia. Note the persistence of the targetoid appearance of the granular cell nuclei in Fig. 2.6**D**, **E**, and **F**. (Smear preparation, H&E, ×400.)

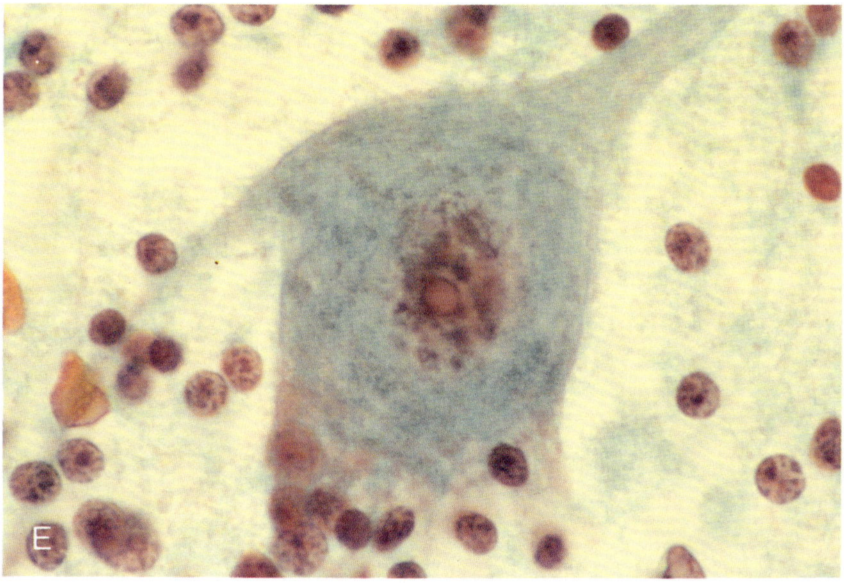

Figure 2.6. Cerebellar cortex. **E,** Appearance of cerebellar cortex using Pap stain. (Smear preparation, Pap stain, ×400.)

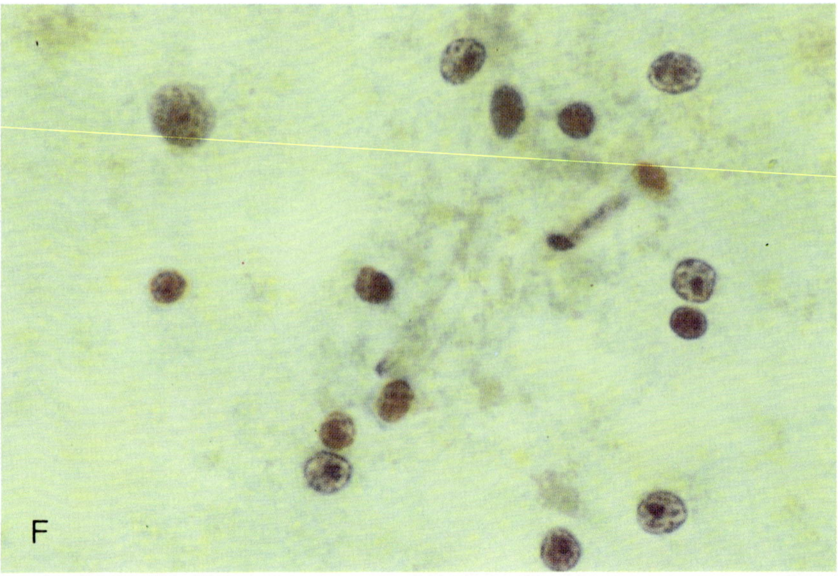

Figure 2.6. Cerebellar cortex. **F,** The characteristic nuclear appearance of granule cells persists with a variety of cytopreparatory techniques, including cytospins and membrane filter preparations. (Membrane filtration, Pap stain, ×400.)

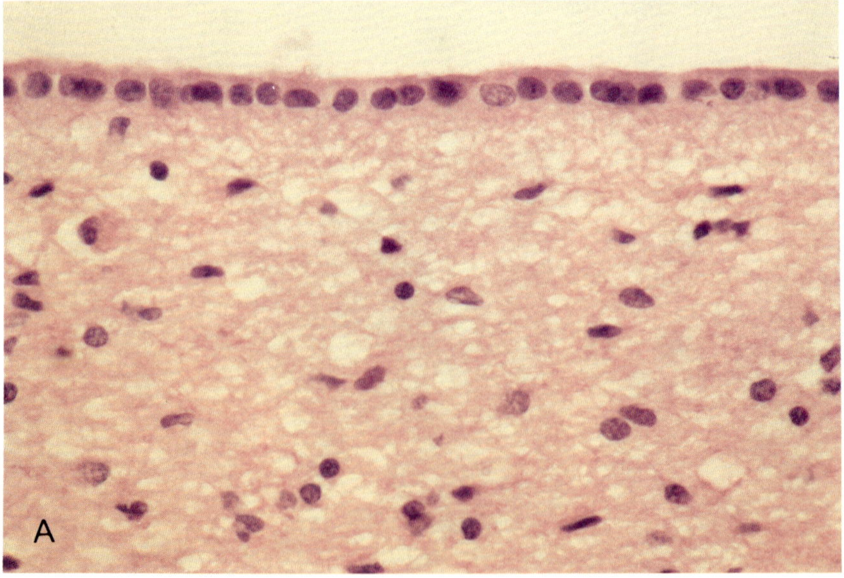

Figure 2.7. Ependyma. **A,** The ependyma consists of a single layer of cuboidal cells lining the ventricular surfaces and aqueduct. Cilia may be present. (Lateral ventricular surface, paraffin section, H&E, ×160.)

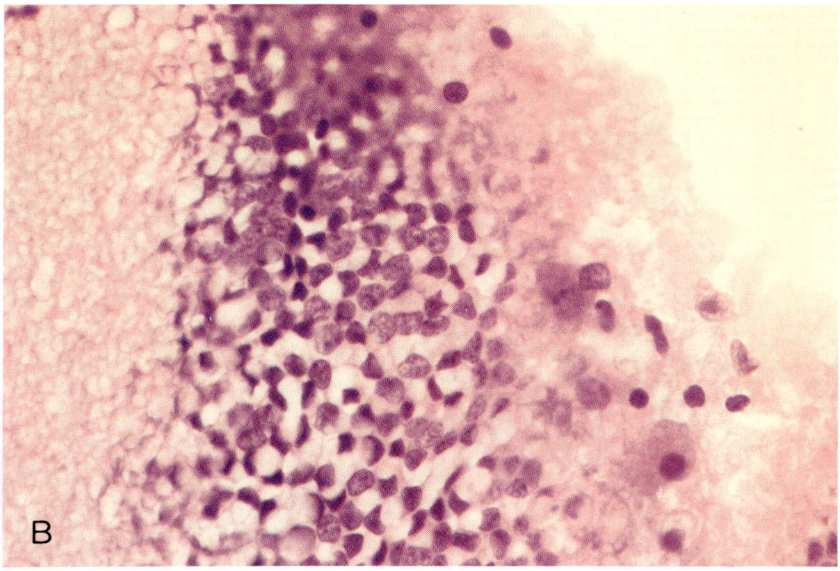

Figure 2.7. Ependyma. **B,** Tangential sections of paraffin-embedded tissue give some impression of the organization of the ependymal cell layer but often demonstrate artifacts, including shrunken nuclei and vacuoles. (Temporal horn, lateral ventricle, paraffin section, H&E, ×160.)

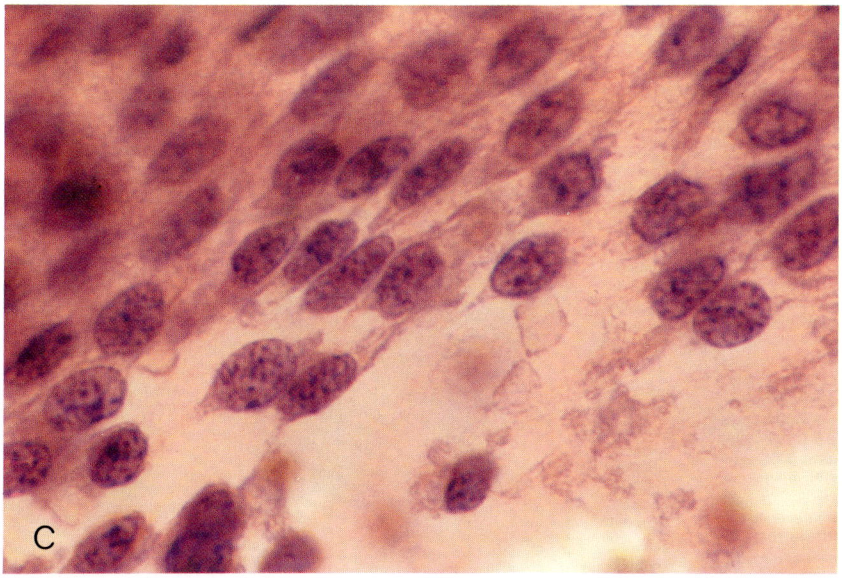

Figure 2.7. Ependyma. **C,** The ependymal nuclei contain finely distributed chromatin and inconspicuous nucleoli. They tend to have delicate processes that extend in bipolar fashion from the long axis of the nucleus (probably related to mechanical distortion during the smear technique) and are rather regularly placed on the lining surface. Nuclei at the edge of the smear tend to be separated from their rather delicate cytoplasm, without clear intact individual cell membranes surviving smear techniques. (Lateral ventricle lining, smear preparation, H&E, ×400.)

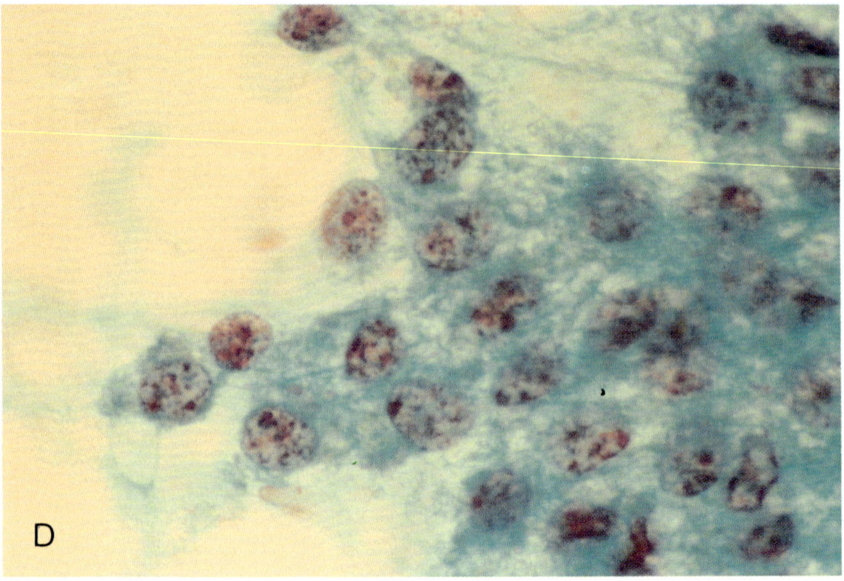

Figure 2.7. Ependyma. **D,** Ependymal surfaces stained with the Pap technique demonstrate the small nucleoli, delicate fibrillar cytoplasm, and lack of clear cell membranes, as noted in the H&E smear. Cells separated from the edge of the ependymal sheet appear as bare nuclei, with little or no residual cytoplasm. (Lateral ventricle, smear preparation, Pap stain, ×400.)

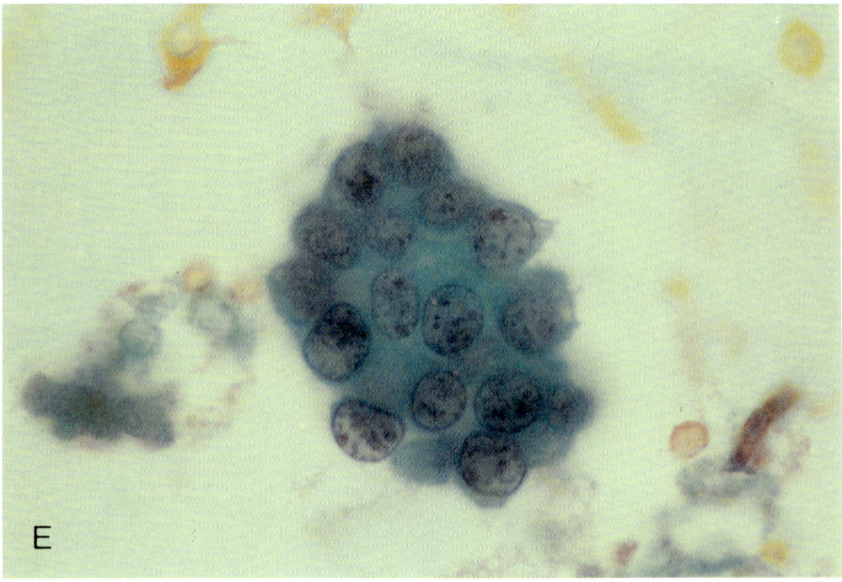

Figure 2.7. Ependyma. **E,** Cytospin preparations, as well as membrane filter techniques, may show ependymal cells in clumps or as single cells, with cells at the edge of the clumps or the single cells having little residual cytoplasm. (Lateral ventricle ependyma, cytospin, Pap stain, ×400.)

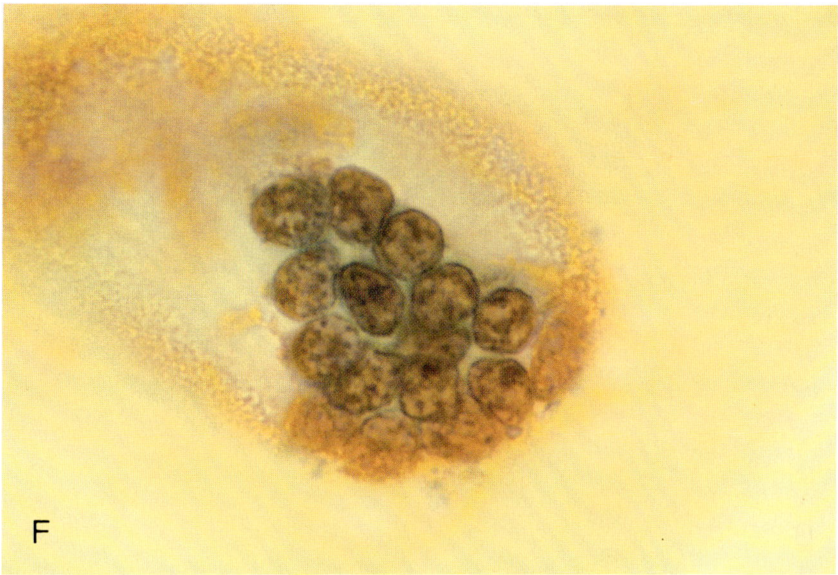

Figure 2.7. Ependyma. **F,** Occasionally, normal ependymal cell clumps may demonstrate rather tightly cohesive cells with some tendency toward nuclear molding, reminiscent of the medulloblastoma and morphologically similar tumors. (Lateral ventricle ependyma, cytospin, Pap stain, ×400.)

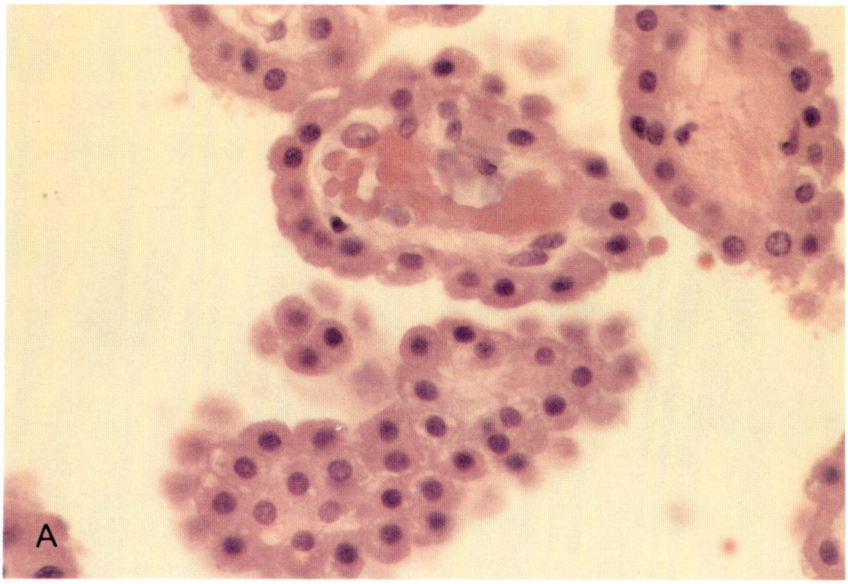

Figure 2.8. Choroid plexus. **A,** Normal choroid plexus consists of papillary fronds composed of a central blood vessel surrounded by connective tissue and other elements, and surfaced by a cuboidal to low columnar simple epithelium. (Paraffin section, H&E, ×160.)

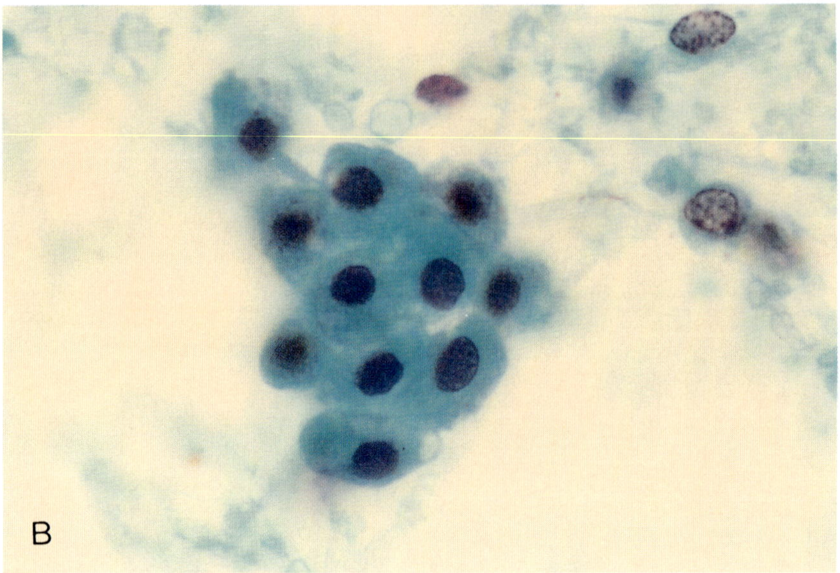

Figure 2.8. Choroid plexus. **B,** The choroid plexus epithelium has a typical mosaic or "ductal" type appearance with distinct cell membranes, polyhedral cells, and nuclei centrally situated in well-preserved cytoplasm. Varying degrees of shrinkage artifact may occur (compared with Fig. 2.8**C** and **D**). (Smear preparation, Pap stain, ×400.)

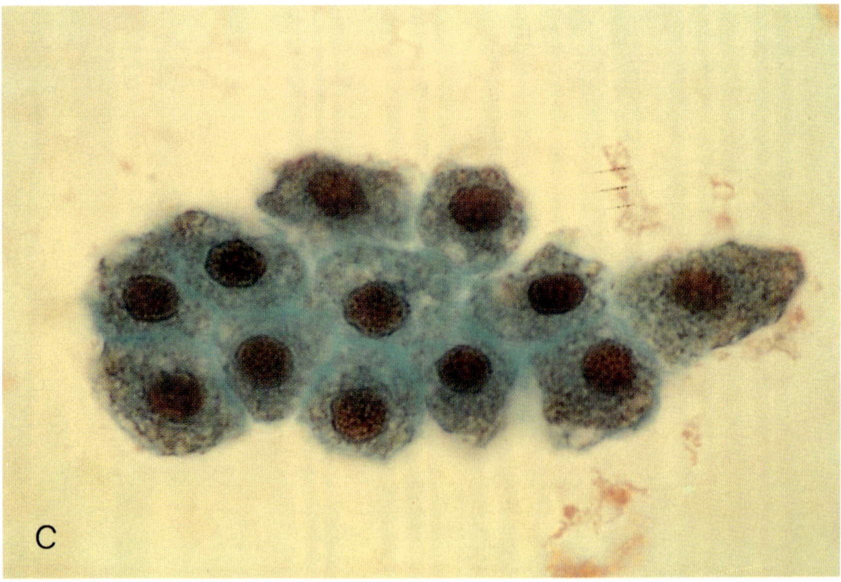

Figure 2.8. Choroid plexus. **C,** At times, choroid plexus cytoplasm may appear vacuolated, probably as a result of a preparation artifact. (Cytospin, Pap stain, ×400.)

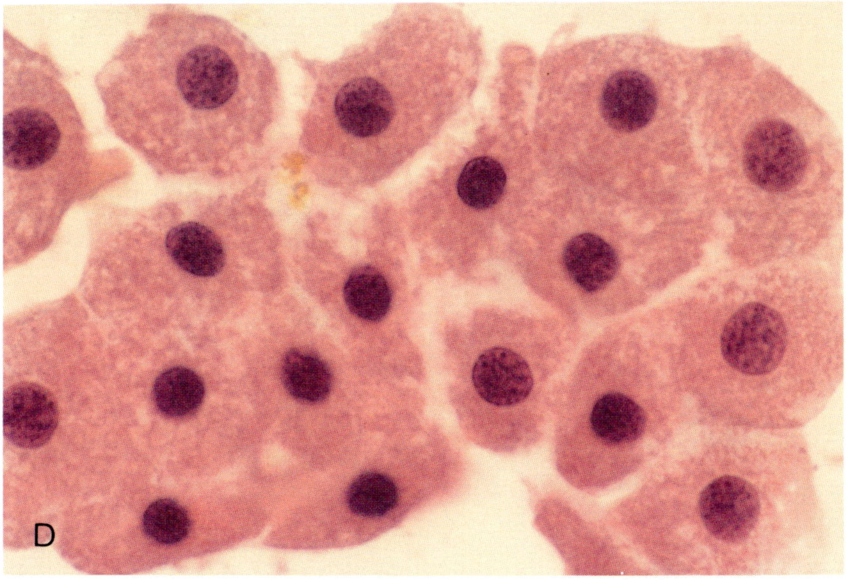

Figure 2.8. Choroid plexus. **D,** At higher magnification, well-preserved choroid plexus epithelium is often somewhat granular. The nuclei tend to be moderately dense but with evenly distributed chromatin. Cell-to-cell junctions are moderately adherent, but single cells are not uncommonly seen in smears as well as in other cytopreparation techniques. (Paraffin section, H&E, ×400.)

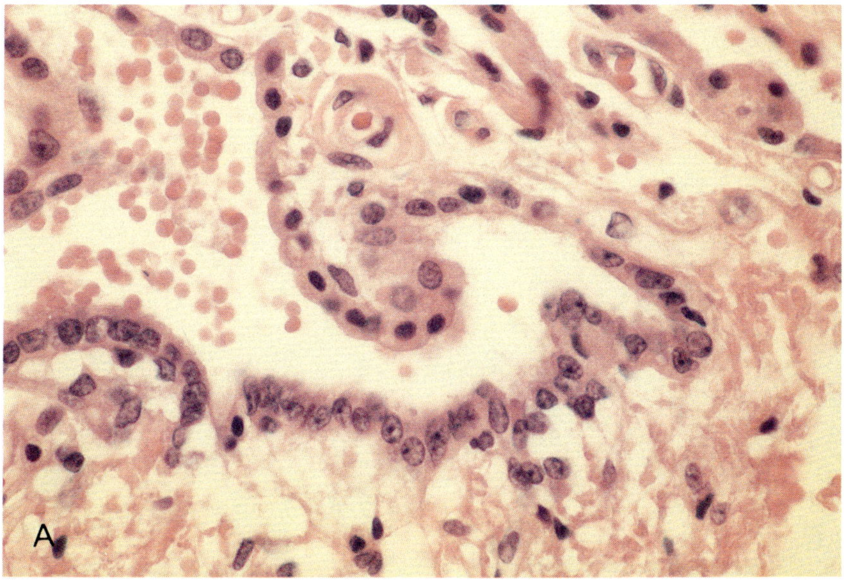

Figure 2.9. Ependyma/choroid plexus. **A,** The transition zone between ependyma and choroid plexus epithelium is rather abrupt, generally only three to four cells wide. (Transition zone, paraffin section, H&E, ×160.)

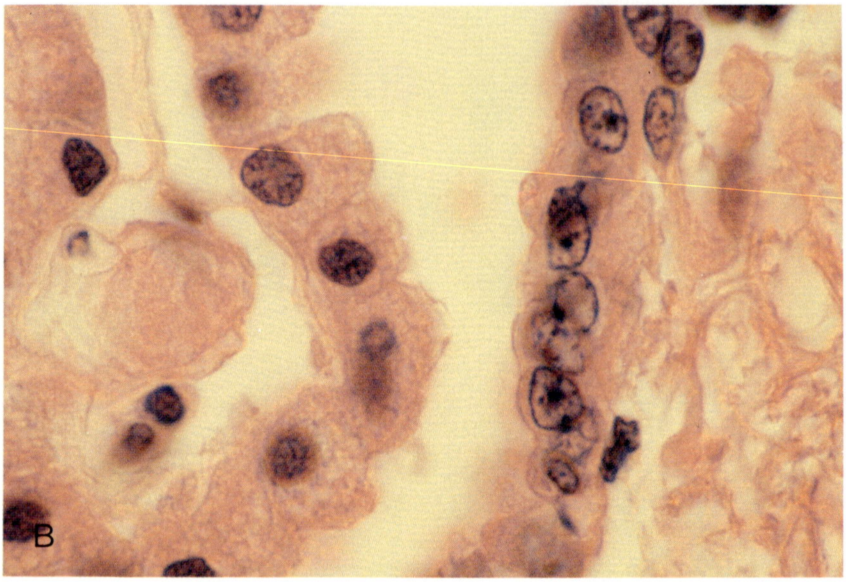

Figure 2.9. Ependyma/choroid plexus. **B,** A comparison of choroid plexus epithelium (left side) and ependyma (right side) discloses clear nuclear differences, within a short distance of the transition zone. This detail is taken from a region very close to that illustrated in Fig. 2.9**A**. (Transition zone, paraffin section, H&E, ×400.)

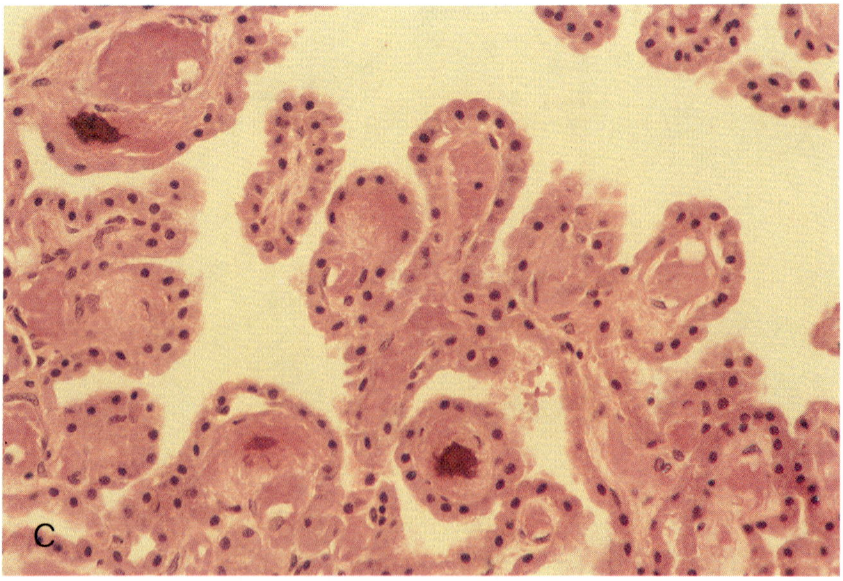

Figure 2.9. Ependyma/choroid plexus. **C,** With aging, fibrous aggregates, sometimes with central calcium deposition, are seen with increasing frequency. These appear as the more densely eosinophilic to basophilic zones within choroid plexus fronds. (Choroid plexus, paraffin section, H&E, ×40.)

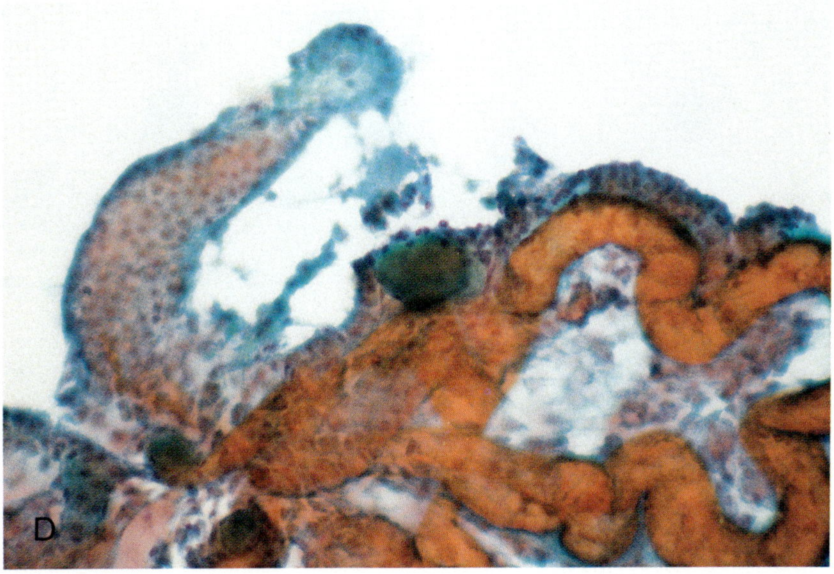

Figure 2.9. Ependyma/choroid plexus. **D,** With Pap stains, choroid plexus vasculature is more prominent, with the three-dimensional appearance of the fronds more easily appreciated in thick portions of smears. Fibrillar aggregates within choroid plexus papillae appear bright green (center and lower left of figure). (Choroid plexus, smear preparation, Pap stain, ×32.)

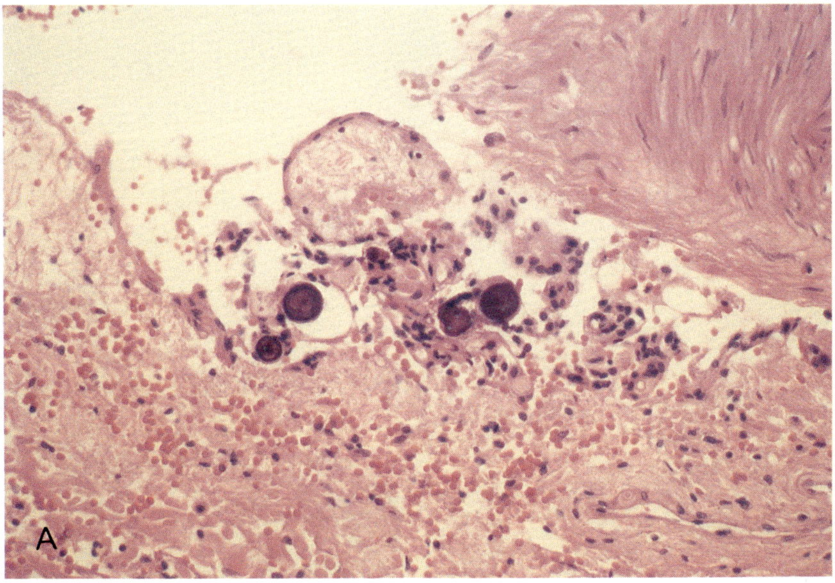

Figure 2.10. Pia-arachnoid. **A,** The pia-arachnoid of normal adults often contains psammoma bodies (dense basophilic laminated ovoids, center) and aggregates of pia-arachnoid cells. (Pia-arachnoid, cerebral hemisphere region, paraffin section, H&E, ×40.)

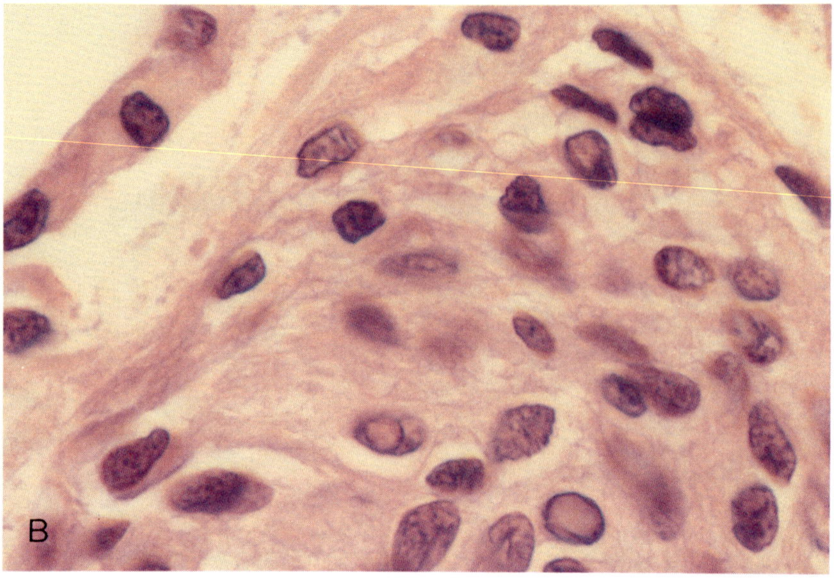

Figure 2.10. Pia-arachnoid. **B,** Detail of pia-arachnoid cells in leptomeningeal cellular aggregate. Occasional nuclei demonstrate folds and cytoplasmic pseudo-inclusions. (Pia-arachnoid, cerebral hemisphere, paraffin section, H&E, ×400.)

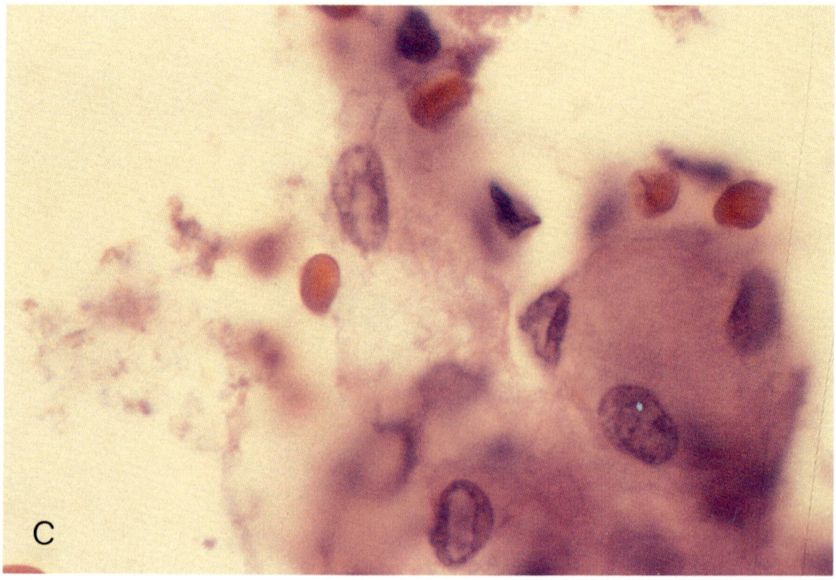

Figure 2.10. Pia-arachnoid. **C,** Pia-arachnoid cell characteristics are well-preserved in smears, and often seen to better advantage. (Pia-arachnoid, cerebral hemisphere, smear preparation, H&E, ×400.)

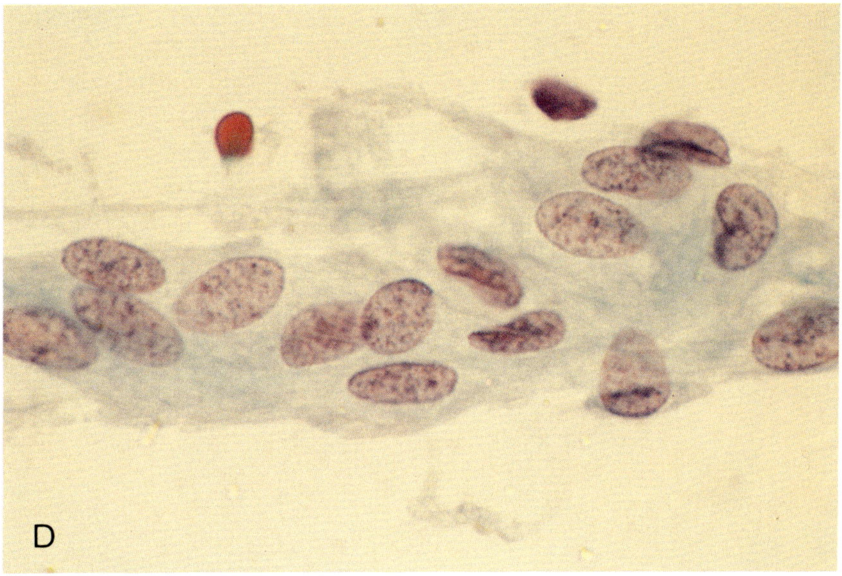

Figure 2.10. Pia-arachnoid. **D,** Pap stain enhances the nuclear detail of pia-arachnoid cells and demonstrates the same features emphasized in Figure 2.10**B** and **C**. (Pia-arachnoid, cerebral hemisphere region, smear preparation, Pap stain, ×400.)

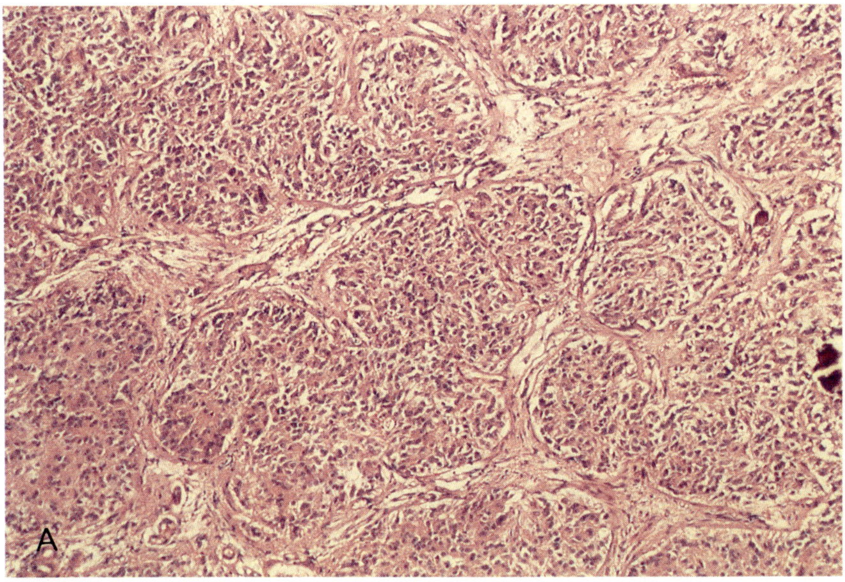

Figure 2.11. Pineal body. **A,** Normal pineal gland typically demonstrates nests of pinealocytes surrounded by delicate blood vessels and fibrous tissue septi. A psammoma body (calcification) is just visible at the right edge of the figure. (Paraffin section, H&E, ×25.)

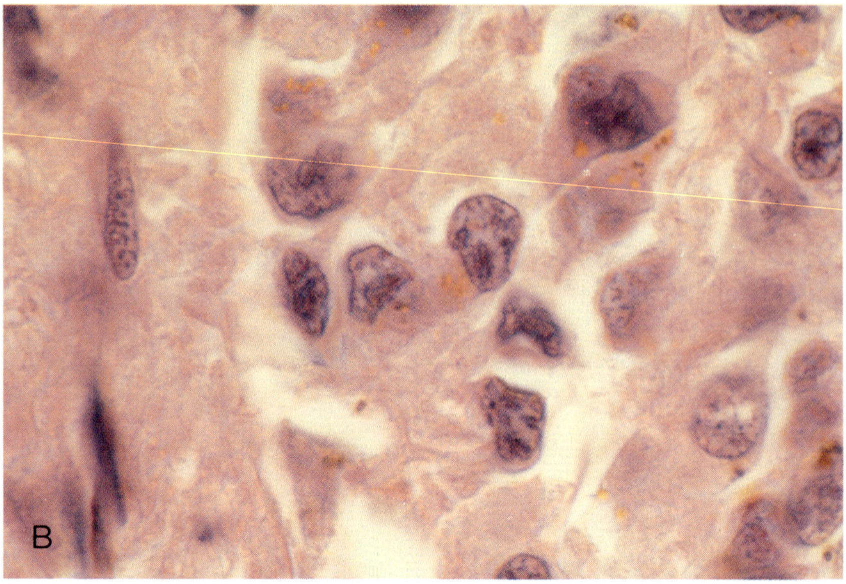

Figure 2.11. Pineal body. **B,** Pinealocytes are present adjacent to a blood vessel wall (vessel on left). The irregularity of the nuclear outline is appreciated even in paraffin sections. (Paraffin section, H&E, ×400.)

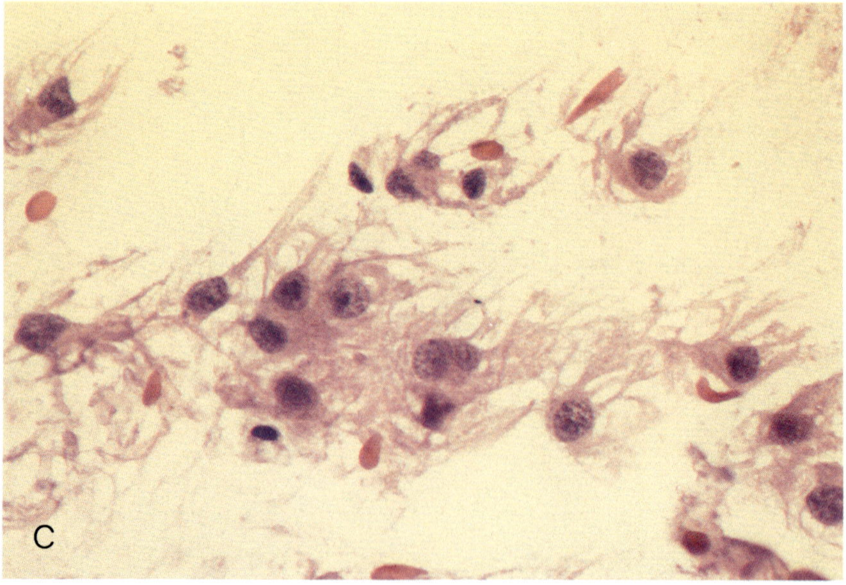

Figure 2.11. Pineal body. **C,** In smear preparations, nuclear characteristics are well demonstrated, and occasionally the terminal expansion of cytoplasmic processes can be appreciated. (Smear preparation, H&E, ×160.)

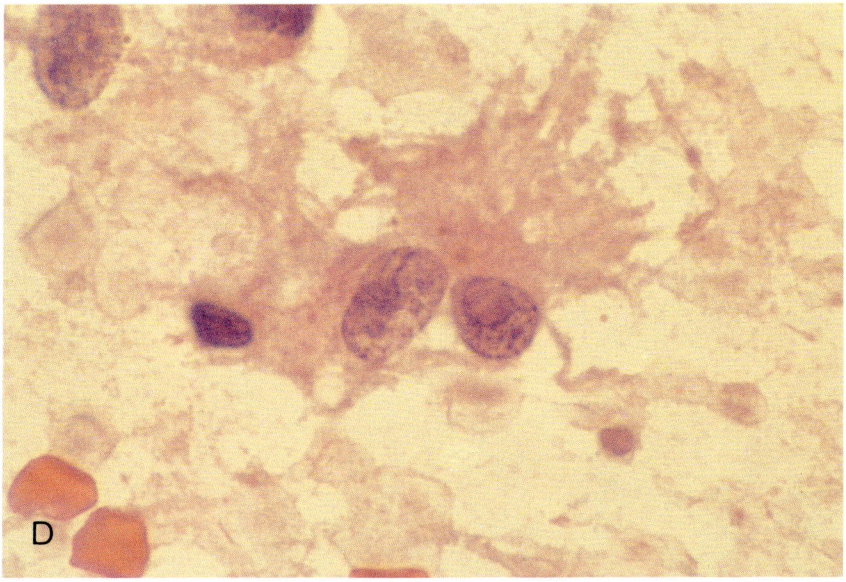

Figure 2.11. Pineal body. **D,** Detail of pinealocyte nuclei. (Smear preparation, H&E, ×400.)

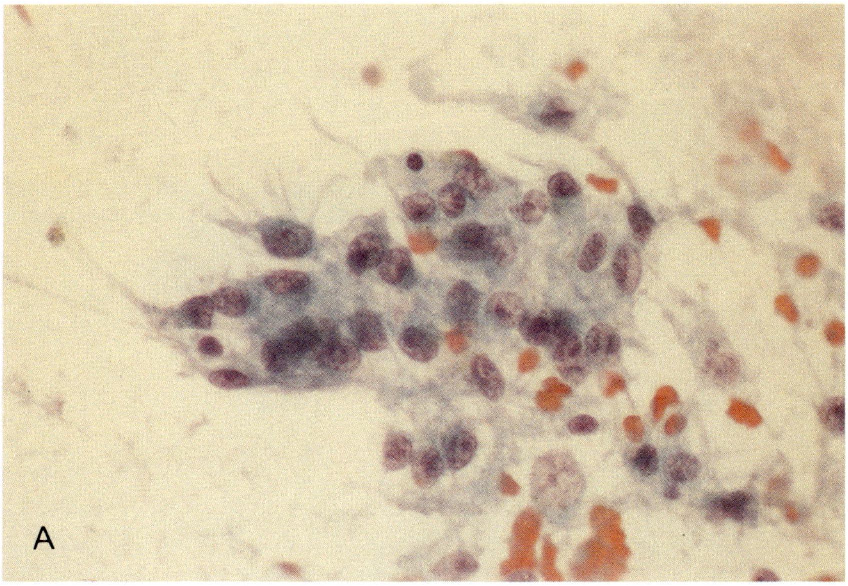

Figure 2.12. Pineal body. **A,** Note the terminal cytoplasmic expansions of occasional pinealocytes. (Smear preparation, Pap stain, ×160.)

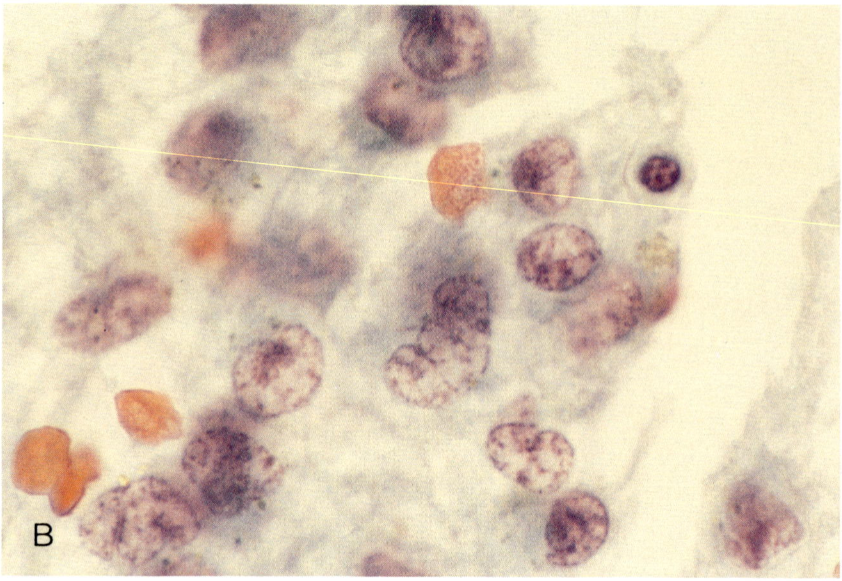

Figure 2.12. Pineal body. **B,** Detail of pinealocytes. Note "salt and pepper" chromatin distribution and nuclear membrane irregularities. (Smear preparation, Pap stain, ×400.)

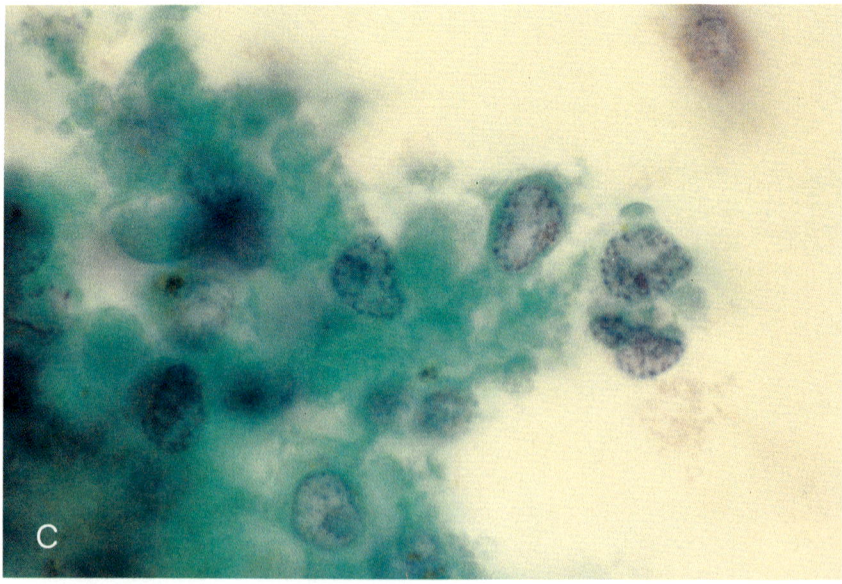

Figure 2.12. Pineal body. **C,** In cytospin preparations, the punctate character of the chromatin appears enhanced. Nuclear irregularities persist. (Cytospin, Pap stain, ×400.)

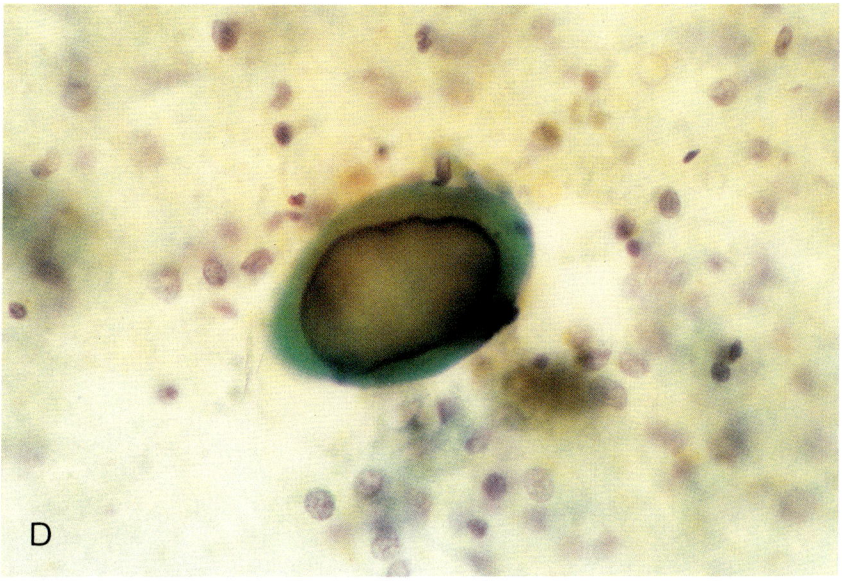

Figure 2.12. Pineal body. **D,** Psammoma bodies may be present in pineal body cytopreparations. (Membrane filtration, Pap stain, ×160.)

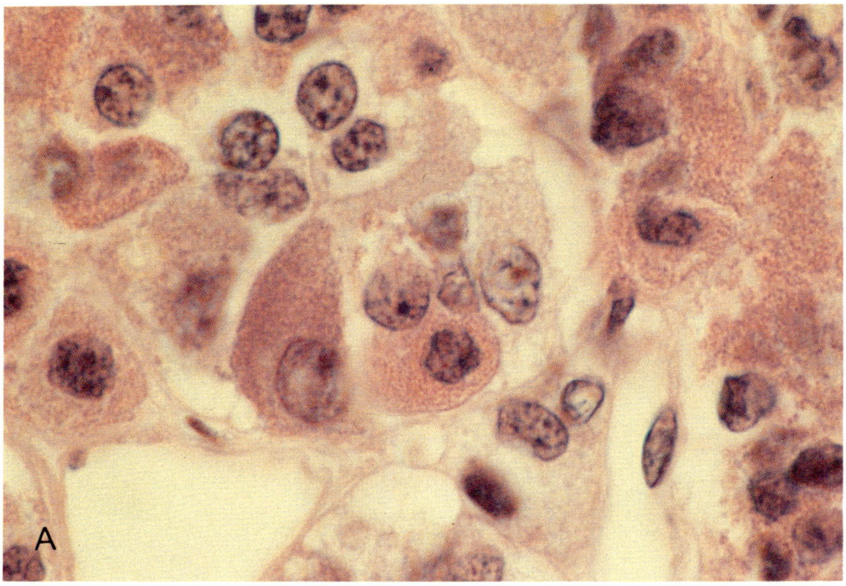

Figure 2.13. Anterior pituitary. **A,** Routine stains may demonstrate three varieties of anterior pituitary cells. In the central nest of cells a basophil (brownish purple) may be seen on the left, an eosinophil (bright red) in the middle, and a chromophobe on the right side. (Paraffin section, H&E, ×400.)

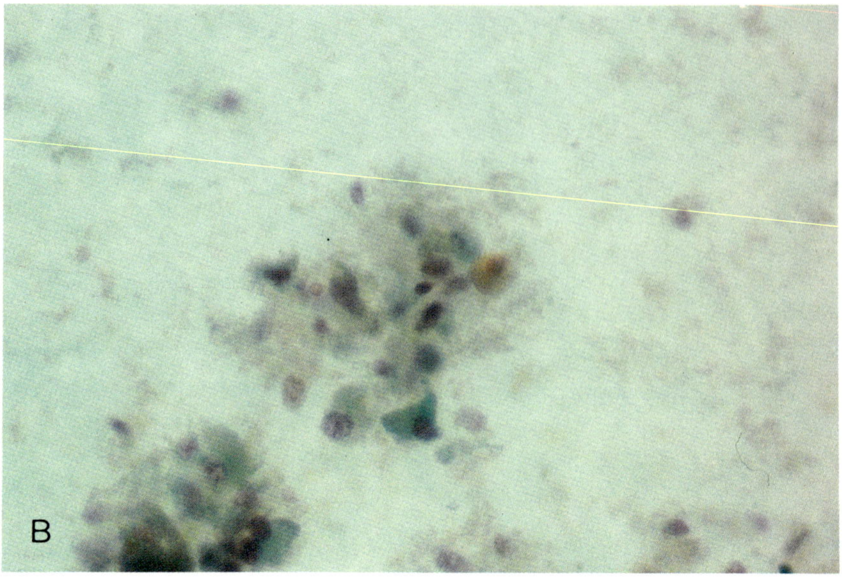

Figure 2.13. Anterior pituitary. **B,** Cytopreparations of anterior pituitary gland are often characterized by a "dirty" background due to the fragile cytoplasm of the cells, contributing to a large amount of cellular amorphous debris. Three cell types, based on cytoplasmic staining characteristics, can be appreciated (i.e., eosinophils are green, basophils brown, and chromophobes pale gray). (Smear preparation, Pap stain, ×160.)

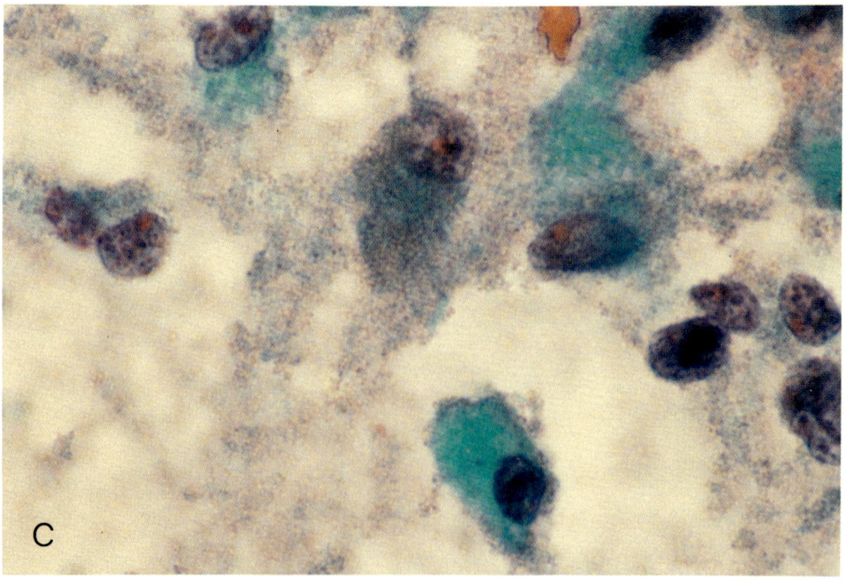

Figure 2.13. Anterior pituitary. **C,** Detail of three cell types on Pap stain. Basophils appear a slightly brownish-green color, eosinophils bright green, and chromophobes demonstrate poorly defined, wispy gray cytoplasm. (Smear preparation, Pap stain, ×400.)

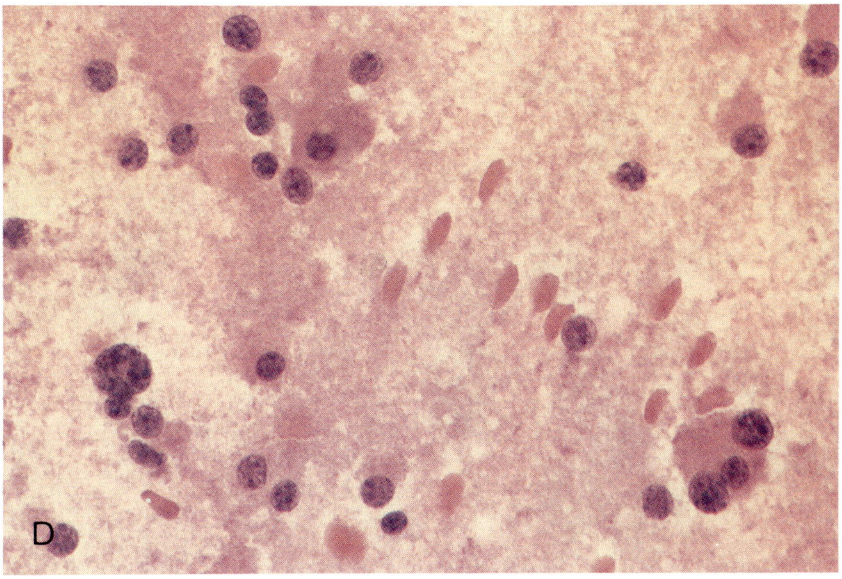

Figure 2.13. Anterior pituitary. **D,** The degree of cellular pleomorphism in the normal gland is better appreciated on smears than on paraffin sections. This field demonstrates moderately pleomorphic cells, including multinucleated cells. (Smear preparation, H&E, ×160.)

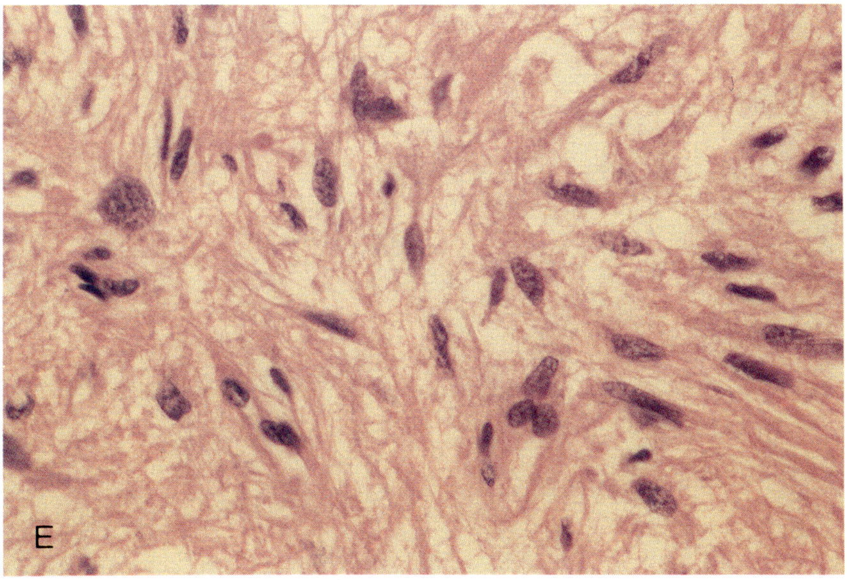

Figure 2.13. Posterior pituitary. **E,** The normal posterior pituitary contains pituicytes that show moderate pleomorphism and a dense, fibrillar background. This may readily mimic a low-grade astrocytoma in certain areas. (Paraffin section, H&E, ×160.)

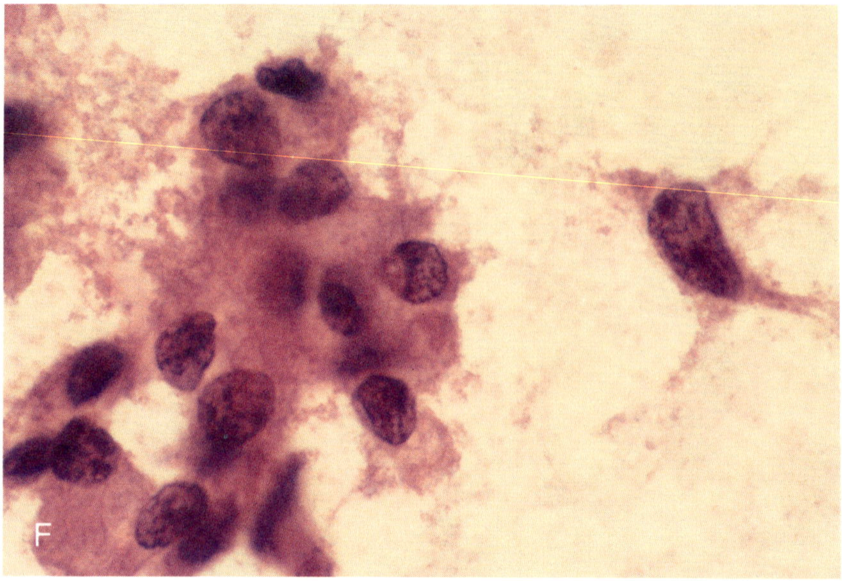

Figure 2.13. Posterior pituitary. **F,** The posterior pituitary tissue does not smear well due to its dense fibrillar nature. Pituicytes demonstrate mild to moderate pleomorphism. (Smear preparation, H&E, ×400.)

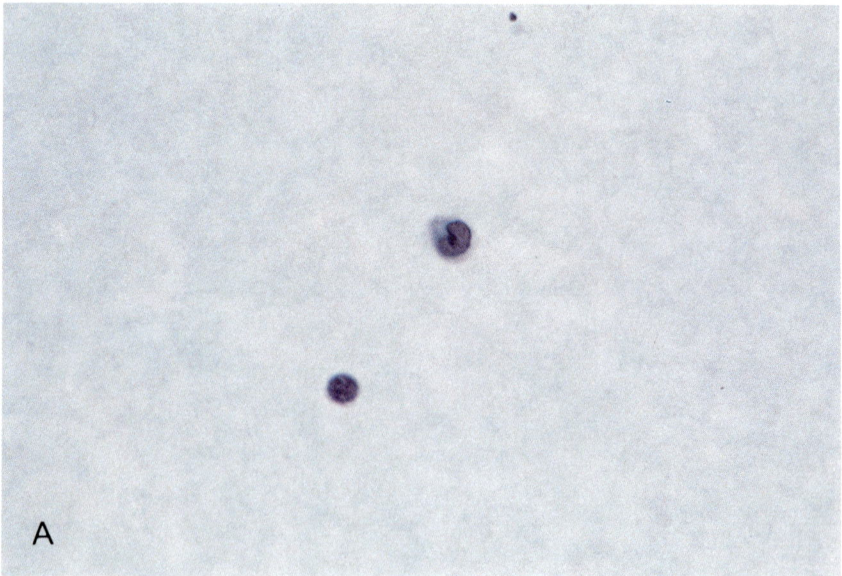

Figure 4.10. **A,** Lymphocyte and larger monocyte; note difference in nuclear staining intensity. (Pap stain, ×160.)

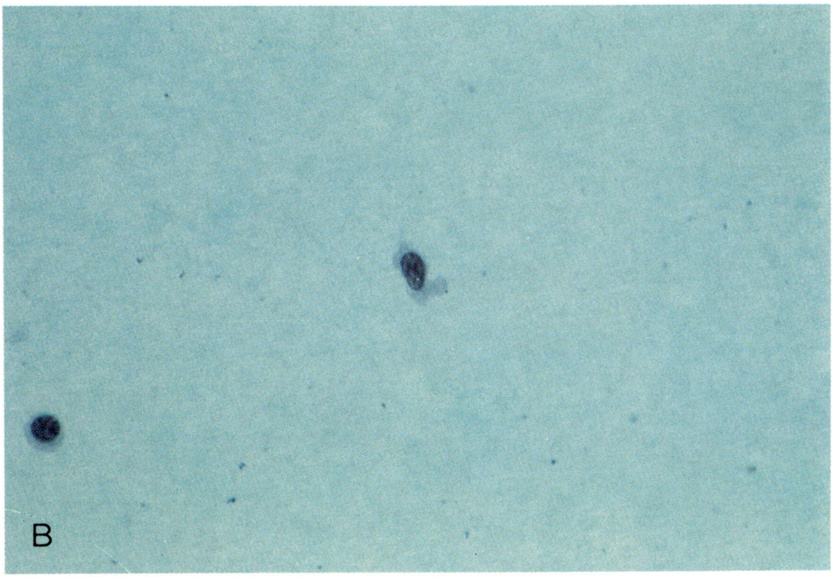

Figure 4.10. B, Lining cell. (Pap stain, ×160.)

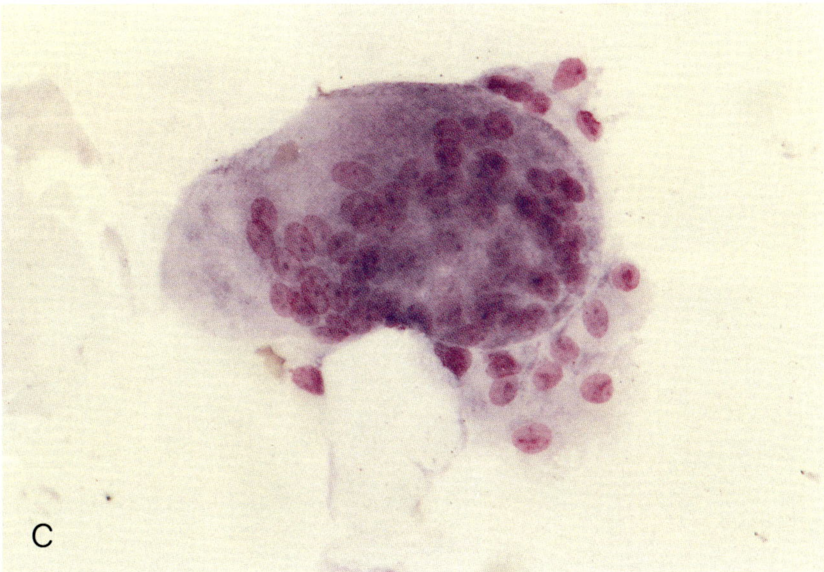

Figure 4.10. C, Multinucleated foreign body-type giant cell in CSF of patient with ventricular shunt (see Chapter 3). (Wright's stain, ×160.)

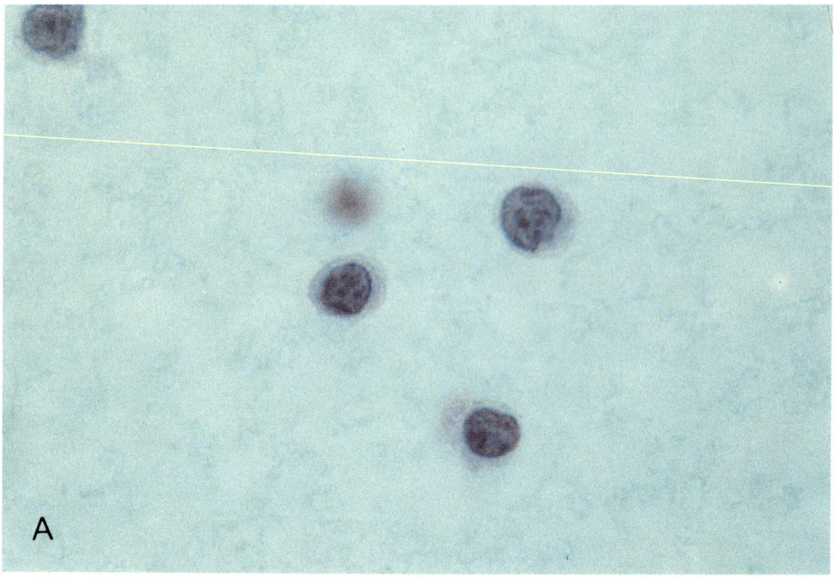

Figure 4.11. A, Reactive monocyte. (Pap stain, ×400.)

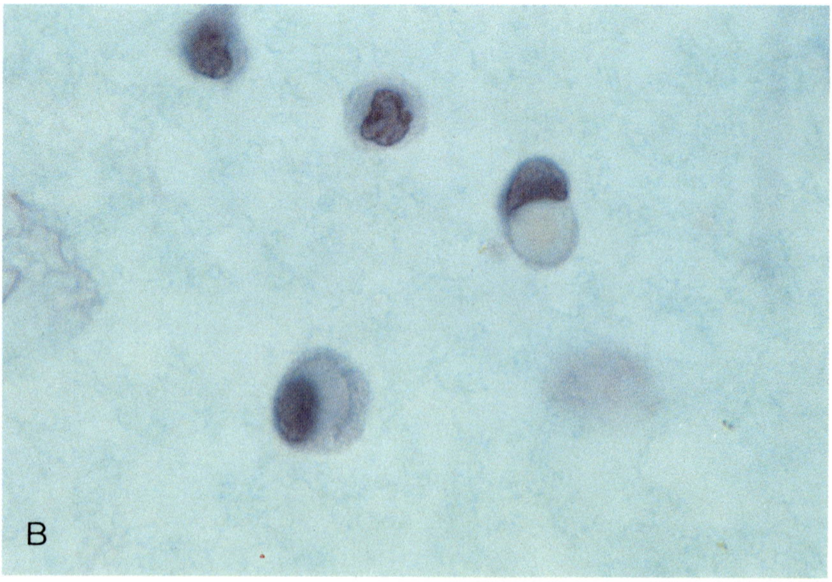

Figure 4.11. B, Macrophages. (Pap stain, ×400.)

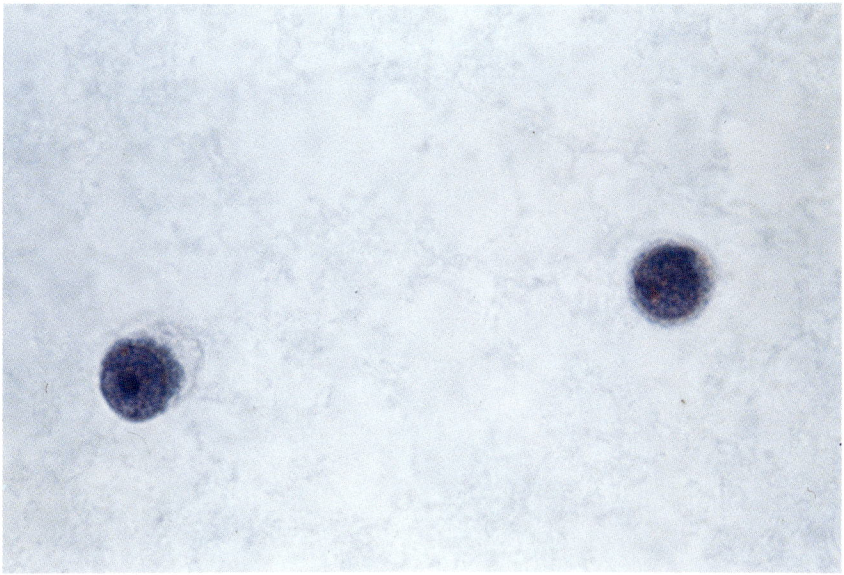

Figure 4.12. Enlarged blastic cells in acute myelogenous leukemia (AML). (Pap stain, ×400.)

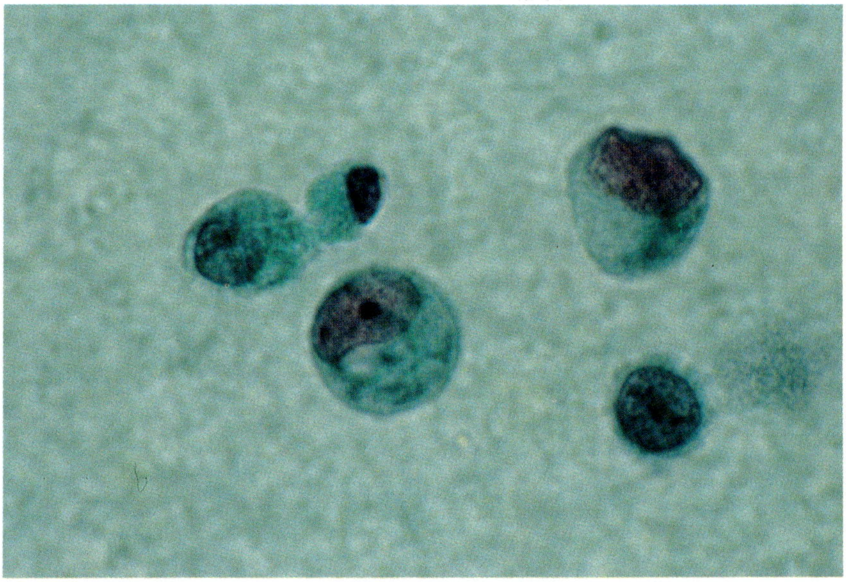

Figure 4.13. Adenocarcinoma; breast primary presenting as large mononuclear cells. (Pap stain, ×400.)

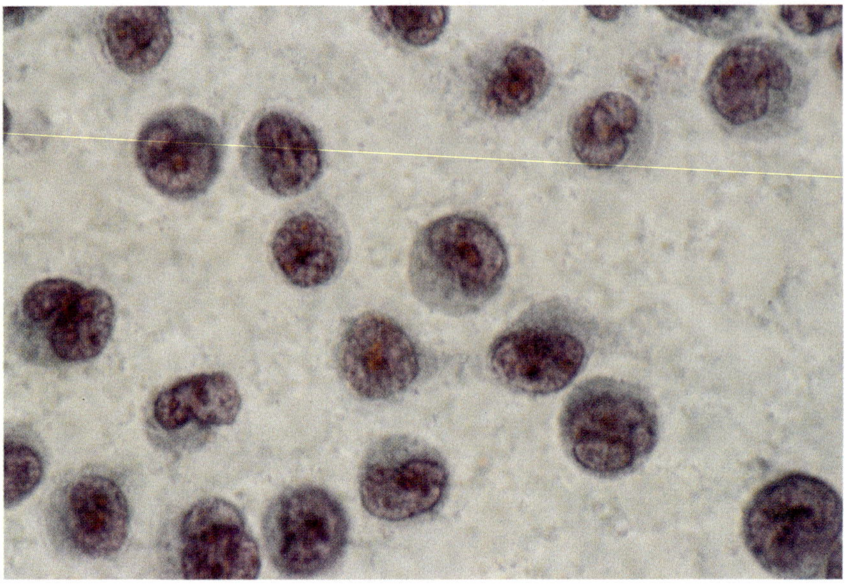

Figure 4.14. Embryonal rhabdomyosarcoma. (Pap stain, ×400.)

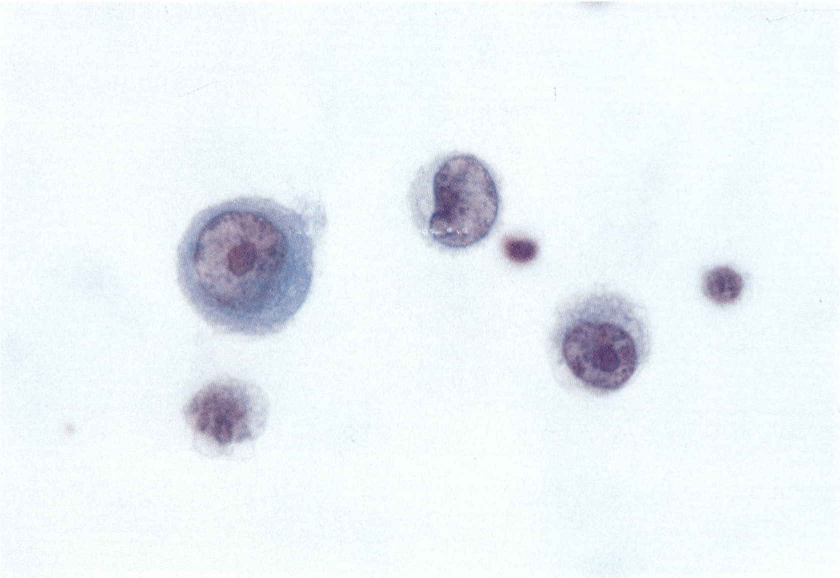

Figure 4.15. Melanoma. (Pap stain, ×400.)

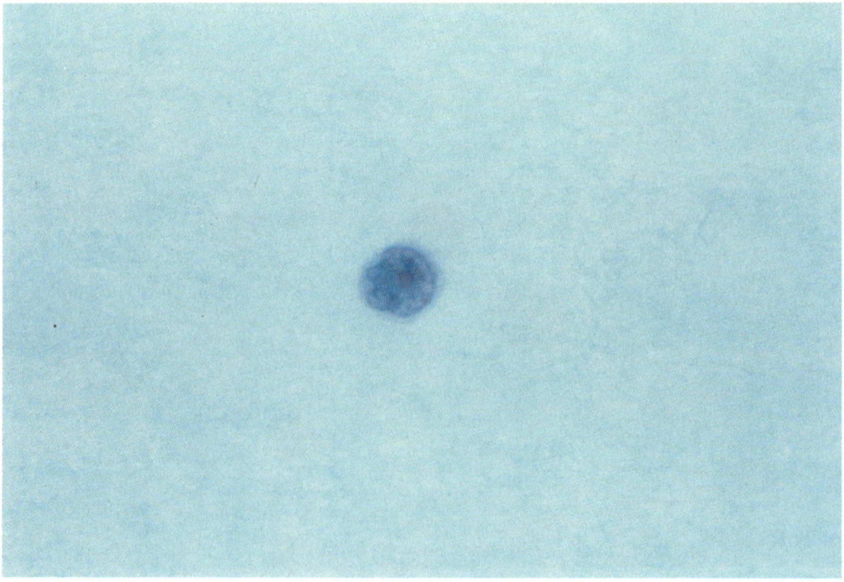

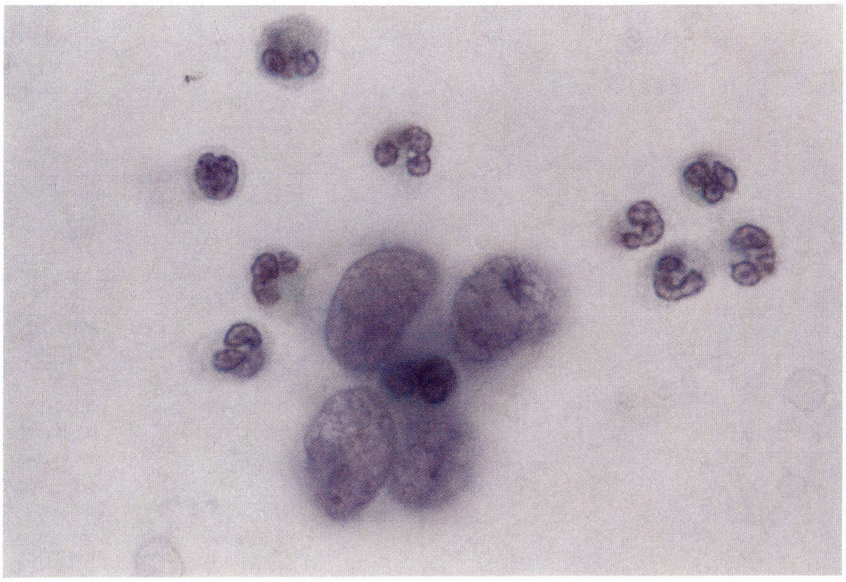

Figure 4.16. Large malignant cells from Ewing's sarcoma and surrounding neutrophils. (Pap stain, ×400.)

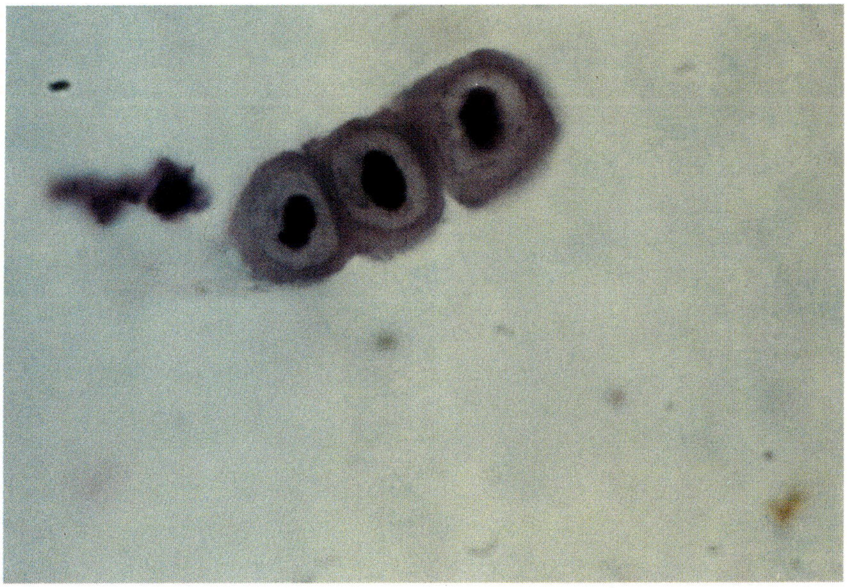

Figure 4.17. Chondrocytes, a CSF contaminant (see Chapter 3). (Pap stain, ×400.)

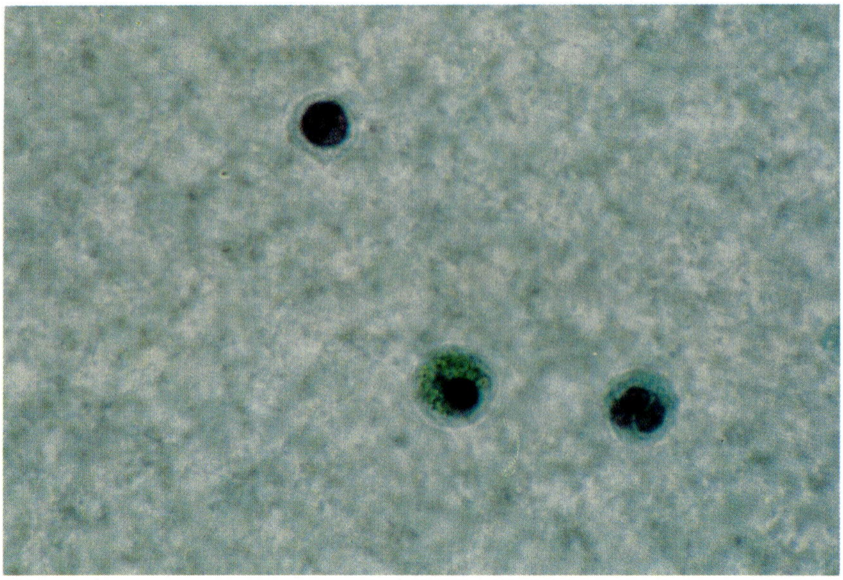

Figure 4.18. Small lymphocyte, neutrophil, and eosinophil. (Pap stain, ×400.)

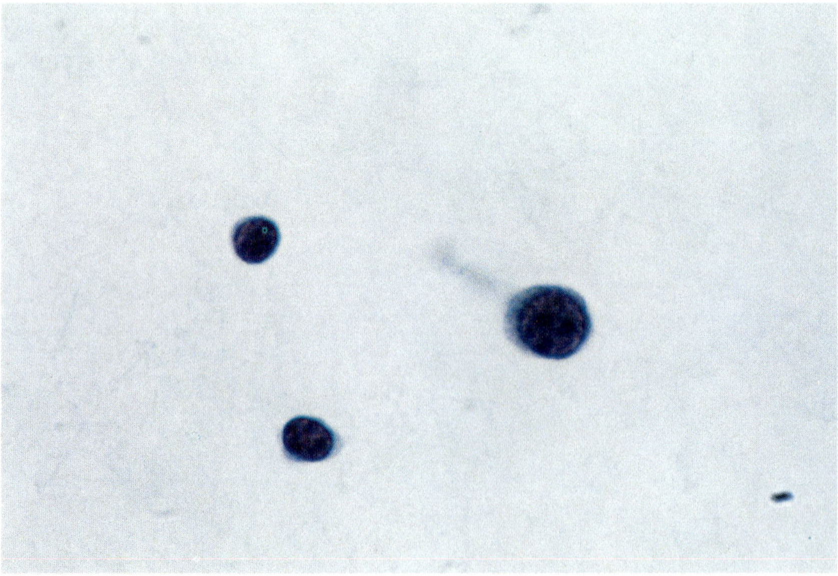

Figure 4.19. Two small lymphocytes and a reactive lymphocyte. (Pap stain, ×400.)

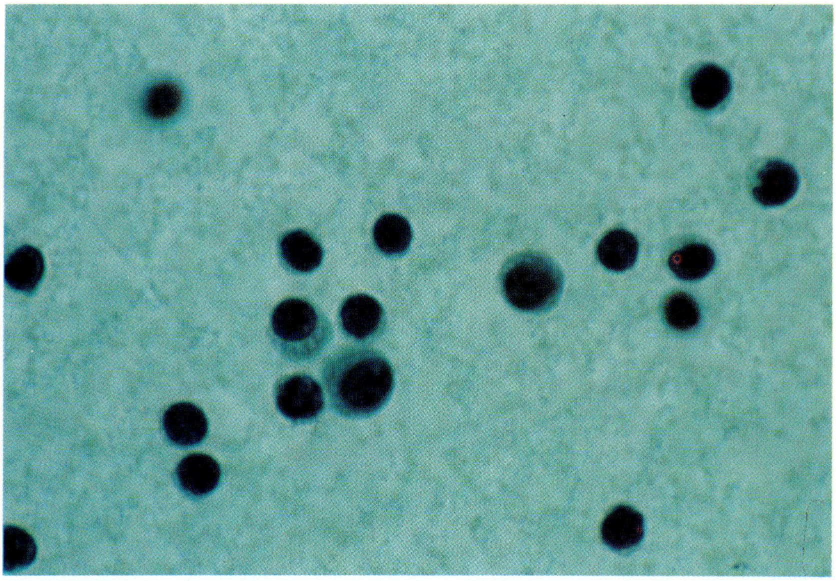

Figure 4.20. Hypercellular specimen with pleomorphism; a heterogeneous population of small, reactive, and atypical lymphocytes and plasmacytoid cells. (Pap stain, ×400.)

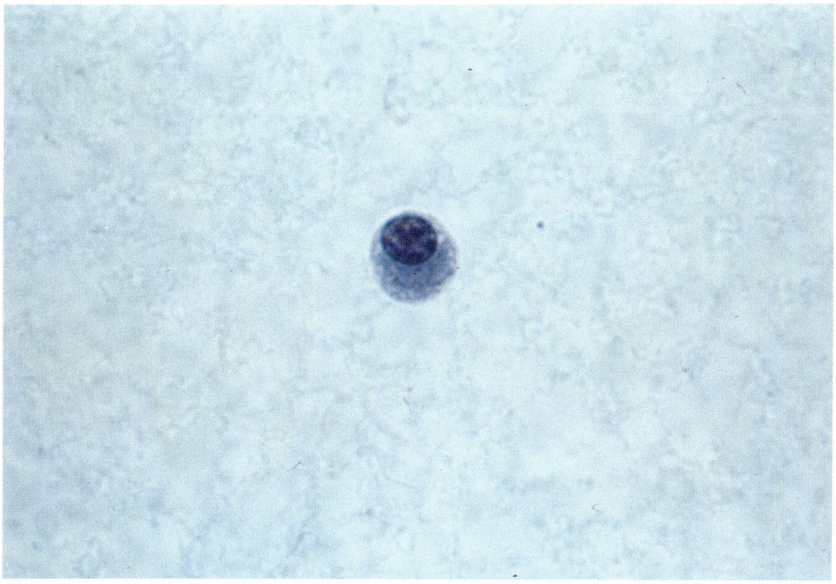

Figure 4.21. Plasma cell. (Pap stain, ×400.)

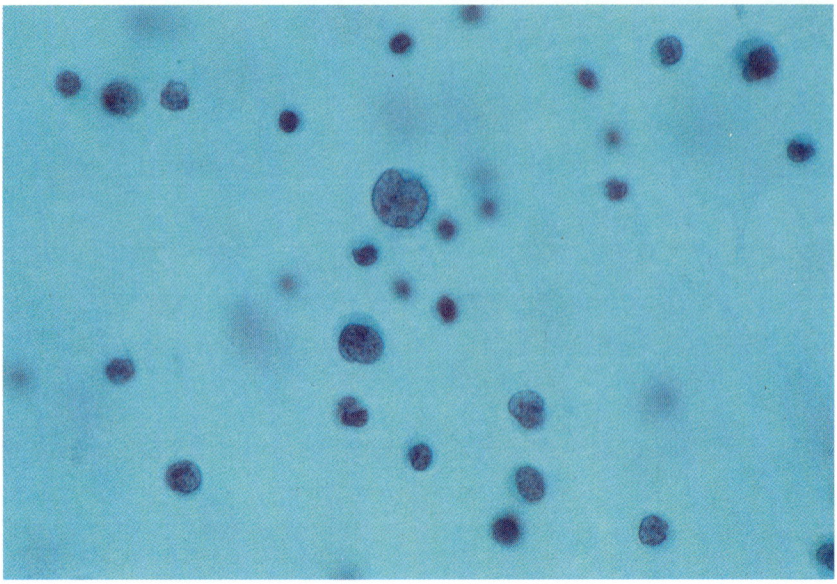

Figure 4.22. Non-Hodgkin's lymphoma with pleocytocytosis. (Pap stain, ×400.)

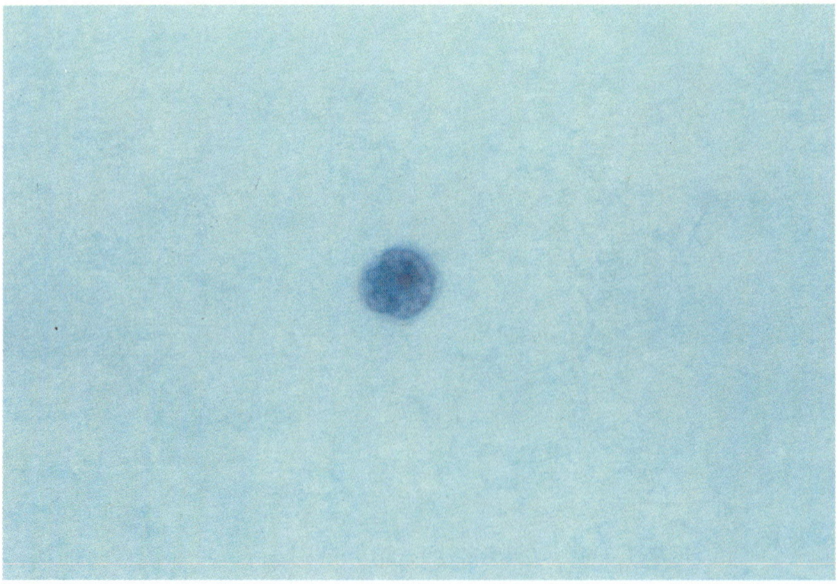

Figure 4.23. Nuclear cleaving in non-Hodgkin's lymphoma. (Pap stain, ×400.)

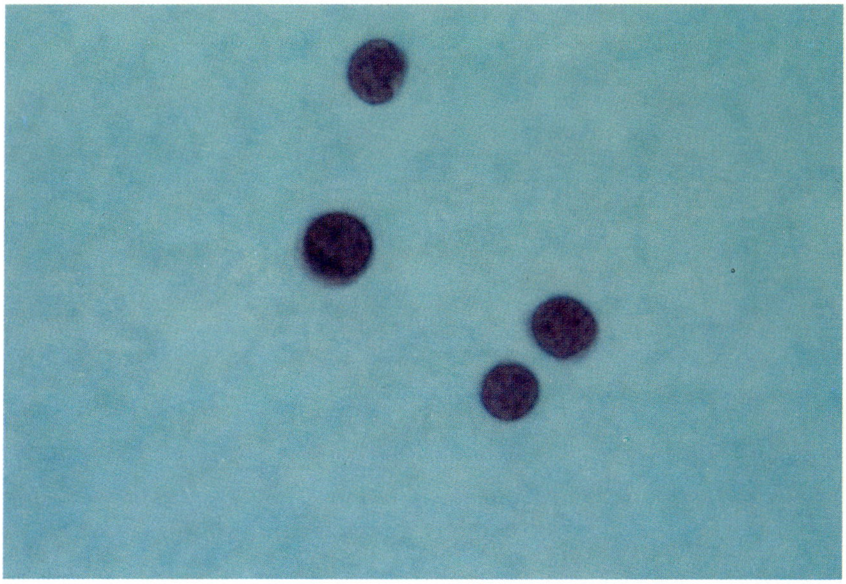

Figure 4.24. Blastic cells from acute lymphocytic leukemia (ALL). (Pap stain, ×400.)

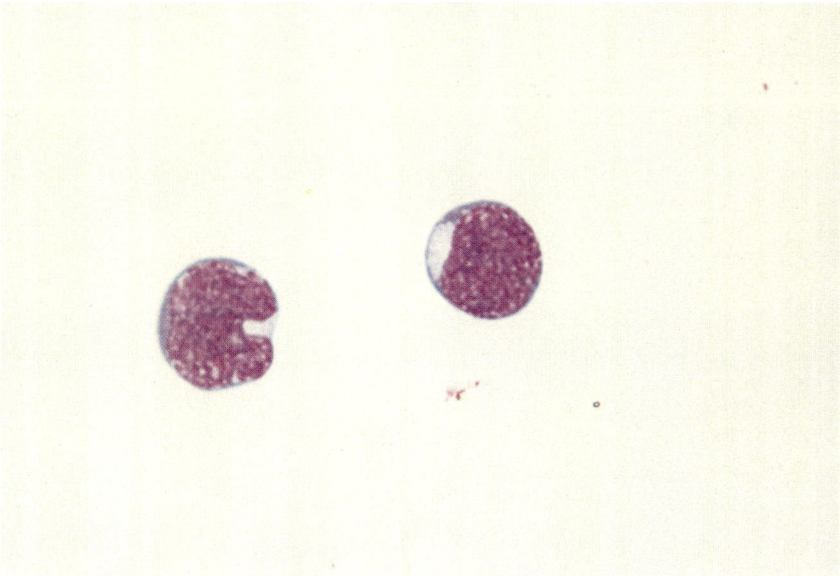

Figure 4.25. Blastic cells from ALL. Note the larger cell size in air-dried preparations (Fig. 4.25) compared to membrane filter preparations (Fig. 4.24). (Wright's stain, ×400.)

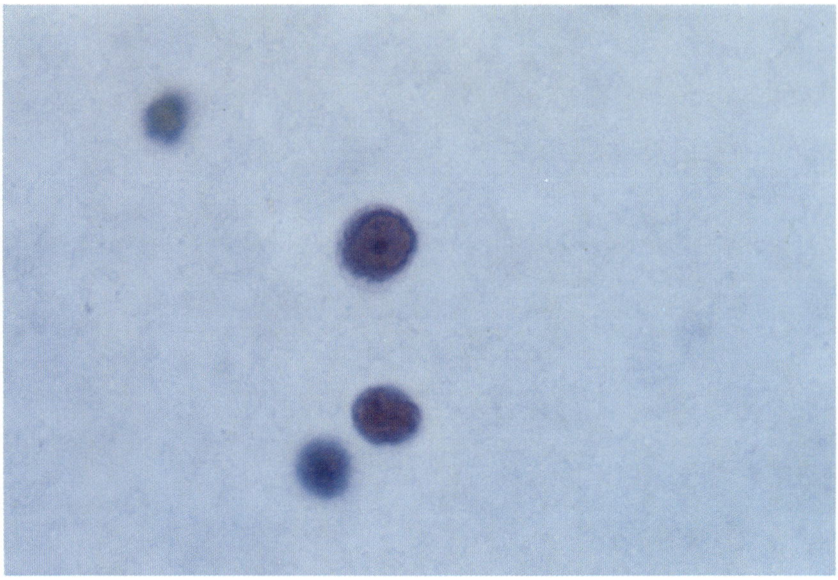

Figure 5.2. Lymphoblasts in CSF in ALL. (Pap stain, ×400.)

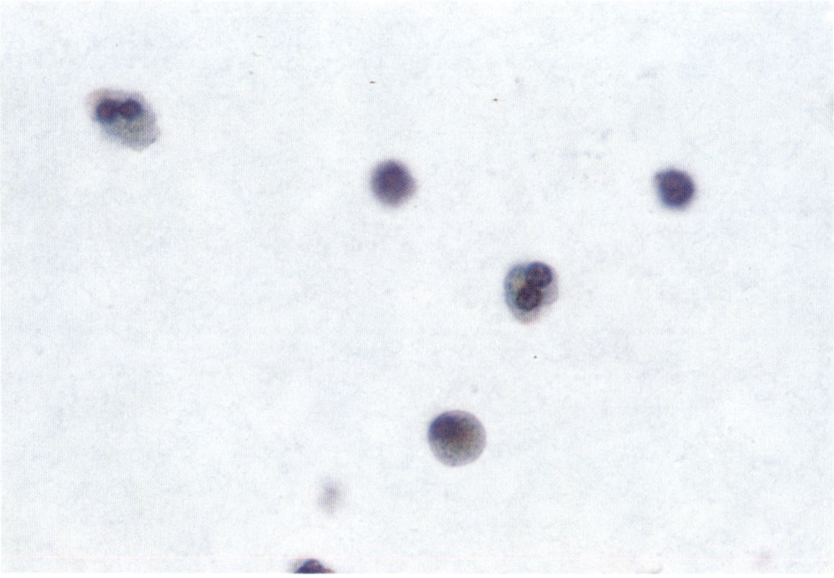

Figure 5.3. Eosinophils in CSF. (Pap stain, ×400.)

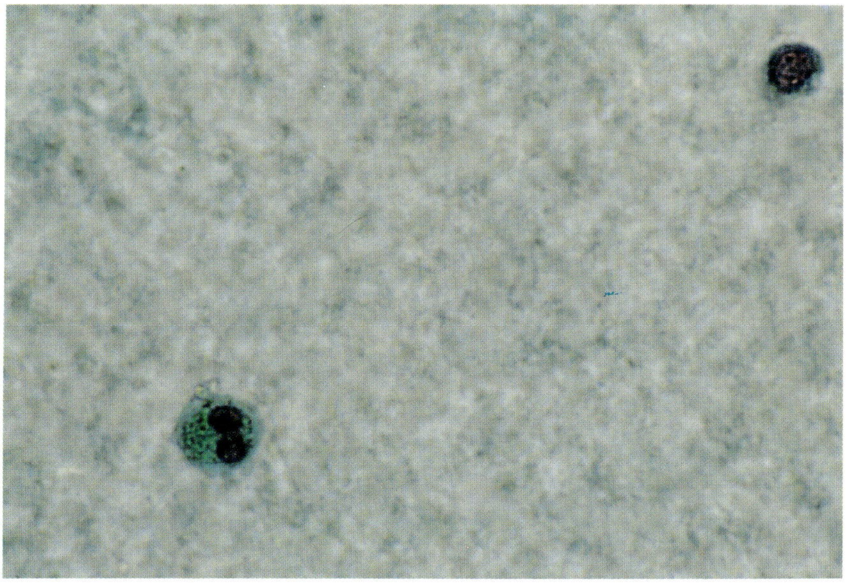

Figure 5.4. Eosinophil and lymphoid cell in CSF. (Pap stain, ×400.)

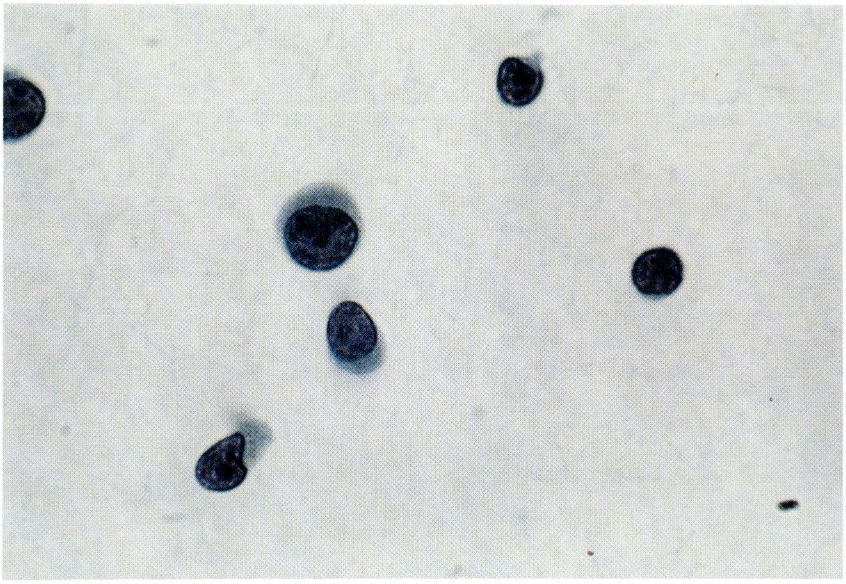

Figure 5.5. Atypical and reactive lymphocytes and plasmacytoid cells. (Pap stain, ×400.)

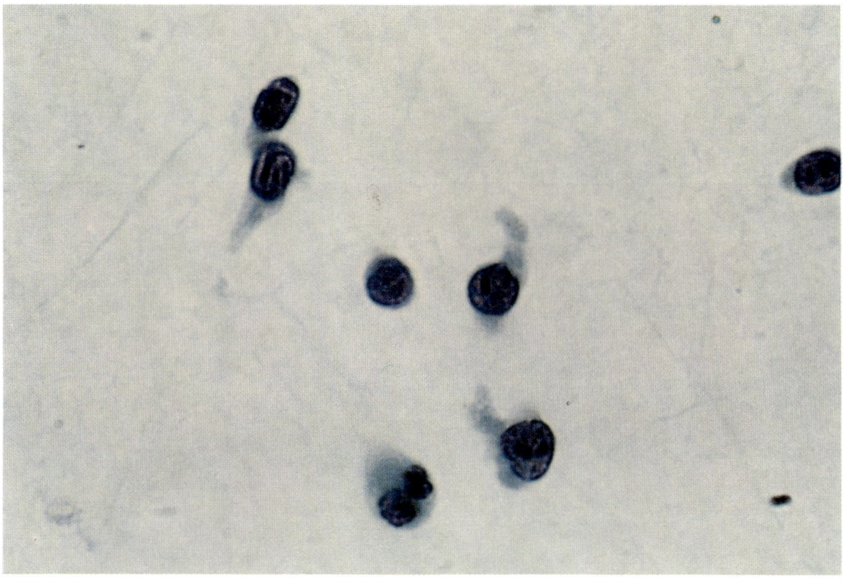

Figure 5.6. Lymphocytes, bilobed leukocyte, and a few elongated "lining cells" in CSF. Nuclear characteristics of the latter are suspicious for origin from atypical lymphoid elements. (Pap stain, ×400.)

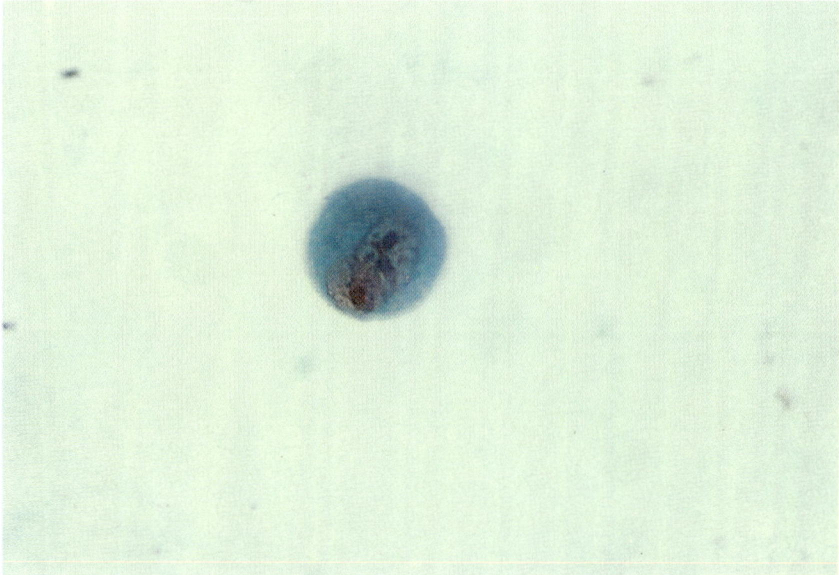

Figure 5.7. Reed-Sternberg cell in CSF. (Pap stain, ×400.)

Figure 6.3. Normal brain tissue sections and smears. **A,** Frontal cerebral cortex, paraffin section. **B,** Smear from frontal cerebral cortex. Normal cerebrum smears easily with only mild pressure, providing a wide distribution of tissue on the slide. **C,** Cerebellar cortex and white matter, paraffin section. **D,** Smear from cerebellum. The tissue smears easily and appears much more cellular than cerebral smears due to granular layer neurons.

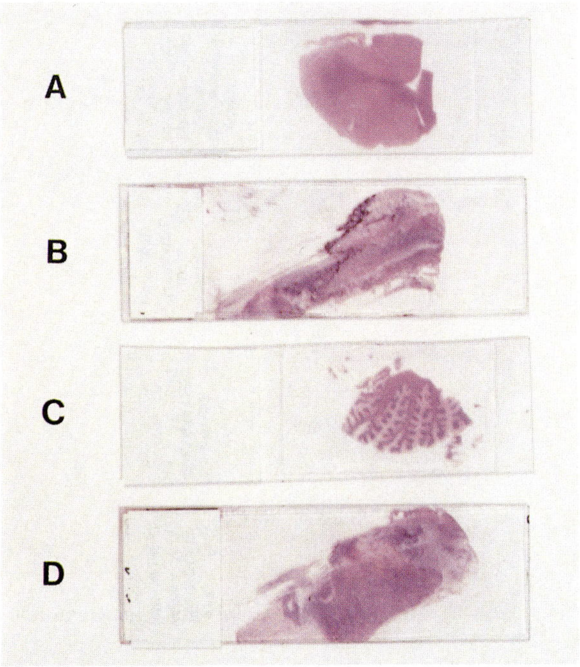

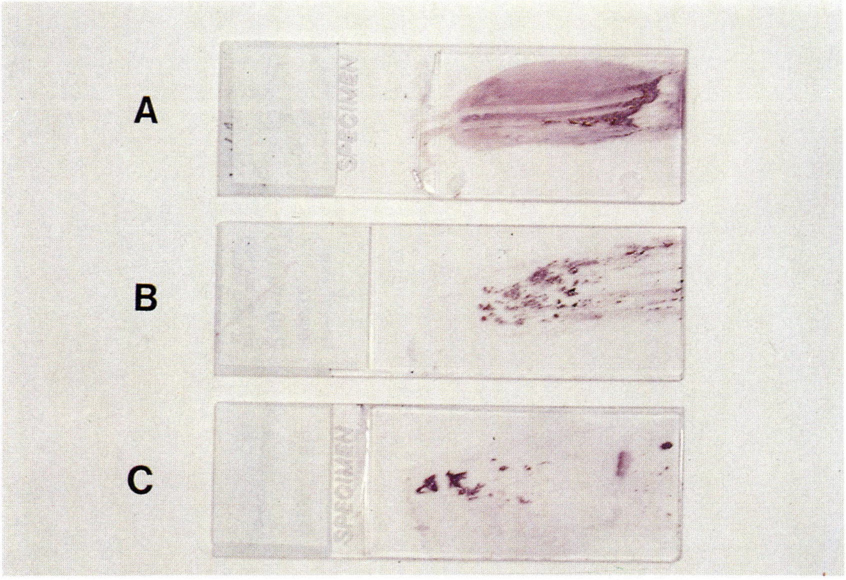

Figure 6.4. Various smear patterns. **A,** Cerebellar capillary hemangioblastoma. This case had a minor intratumoral astrocytic component and smeared easily. **B,** Meningotheliomatous meningioma. Meningotheliomatous and transitional meningiomas often smear more readily than might be expected from their histologic appearance. **C,** Schwannoma. Smears often consist of isolated thick aggregates of cohesive cells; attempts to smear with greater pressure on the slide will produce excessive crush artifacts in such cases (see text).

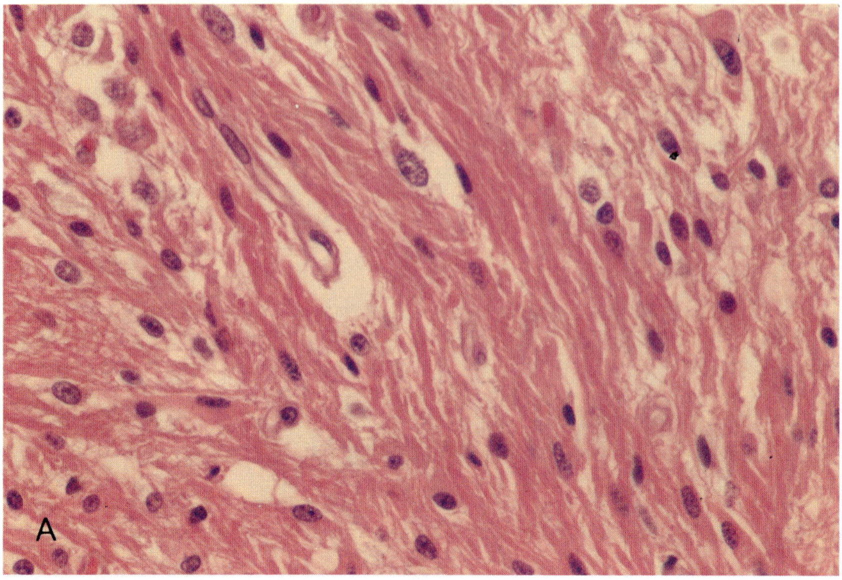

Figure 7.1. **A,** Fibrillary astrocytoma. (Paraffin section, H&E, ×64.)

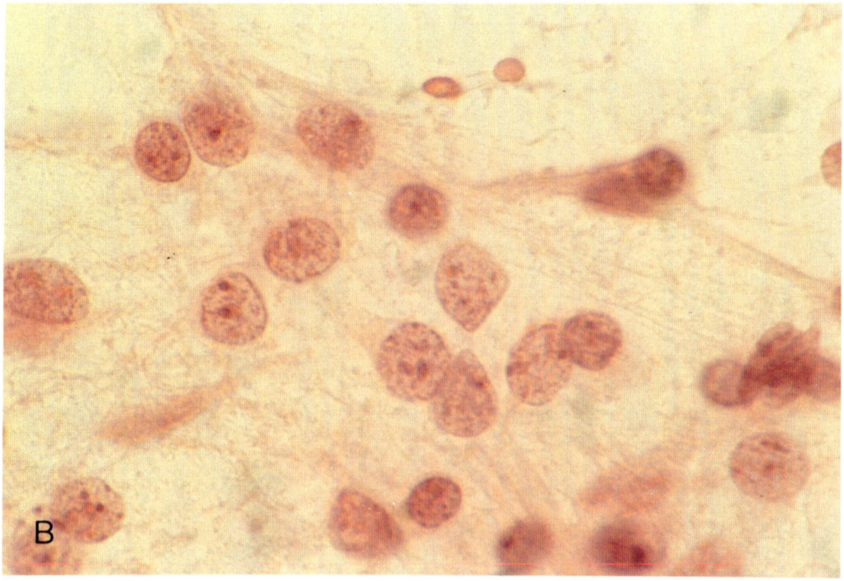

Figure 7.1. **B,** Fibrillary astrocytoma. Bland nuclei with mildly angular outline lie on fine fibrillary background. (Smear preparation, H&E, ×320.)

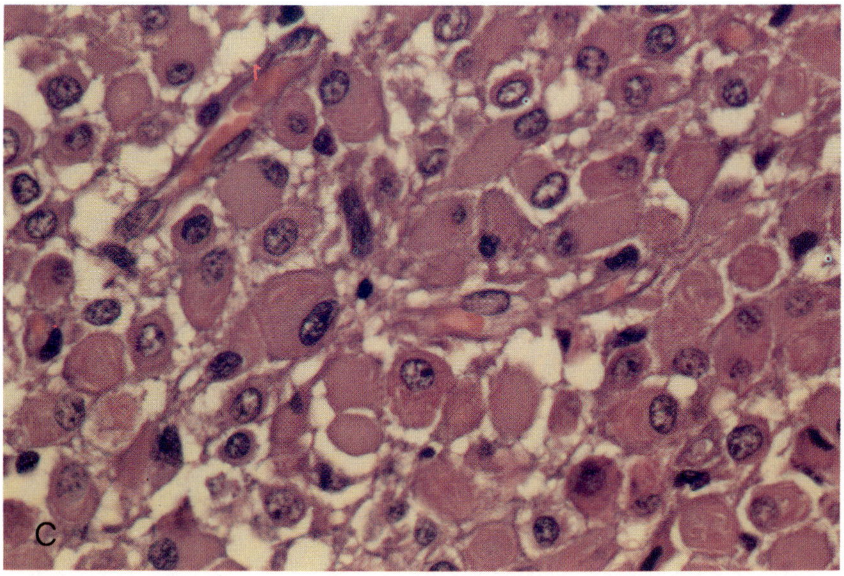

Figure 7.1. C, Gemistocytic astrocytoma. (Paraffin section, H&E, ×128.)

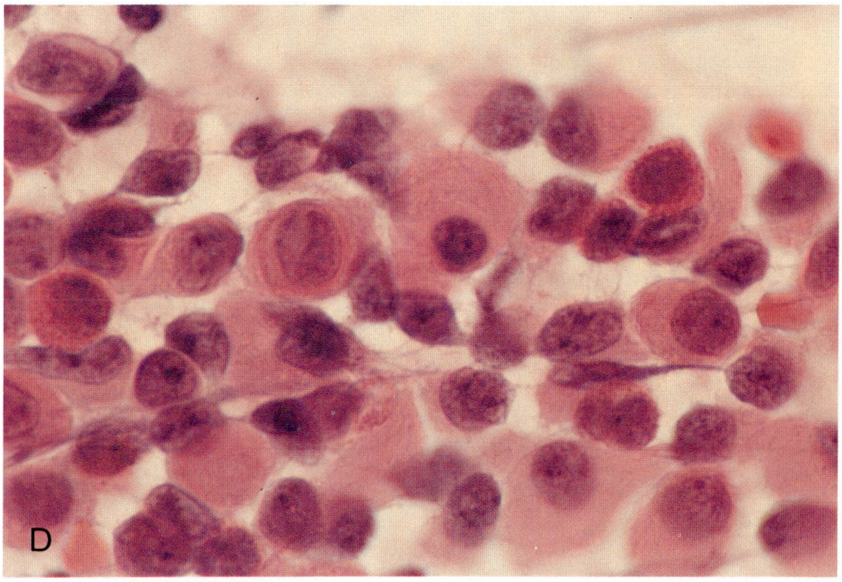

Figure 7.1. D, Gemistocytic astrocytoma. Glial fibrils aggregate at the periphery of the cell cytoplasm in some of the cells. Mild to moderate nuclear pleomorphism and hyperchromicity are evident, and cytoplasm is conspicuous. (Smear preparation, H&E, ×320.)

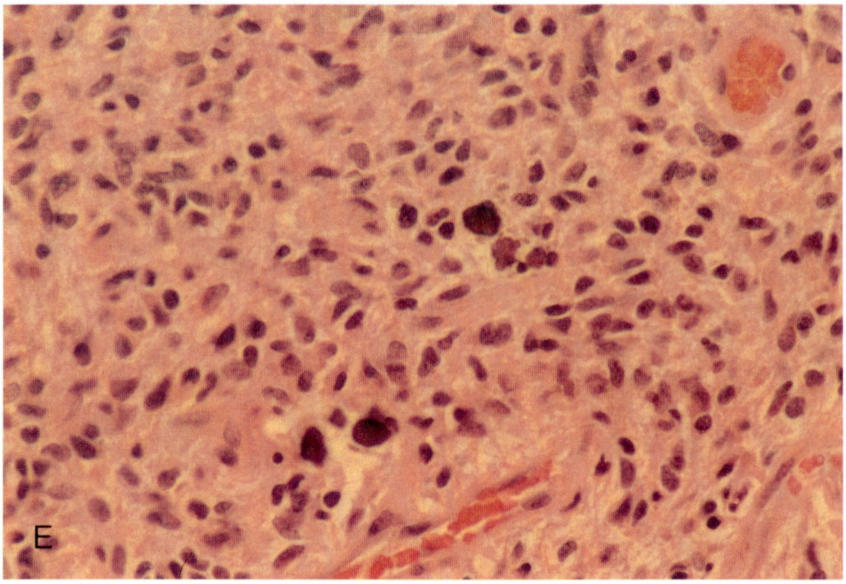

Figure 7.1. E, Anaplastic astrocytoma. Increased cellularity, mild to moderate nuclear pleomorphism, and hyperchromicity. Focal calcification present. (Paraffin section, H&E, ×128.)

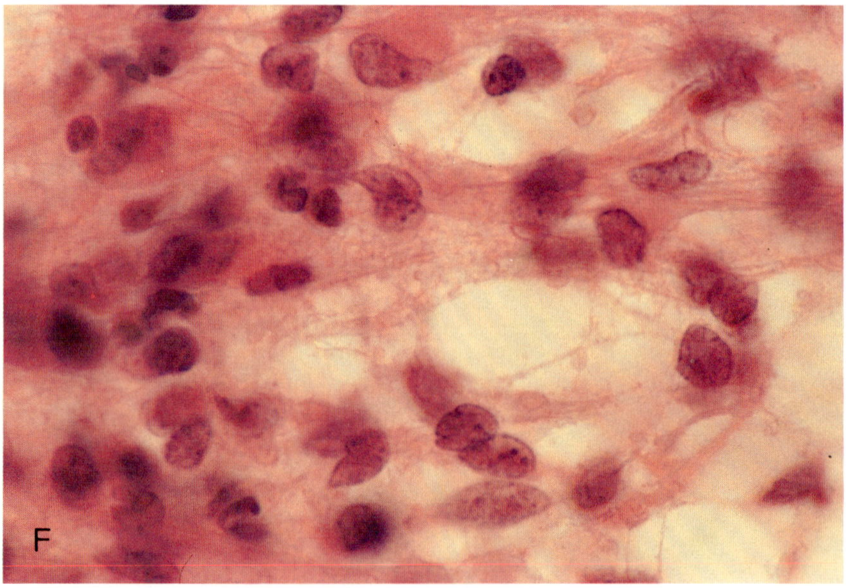

Figure 7.1. F, Anaplastic astrocytoma. Mild to moderate nuclear pleomorphism on a dense fibrillary background. (Smear preparation, H&E, ×320.)

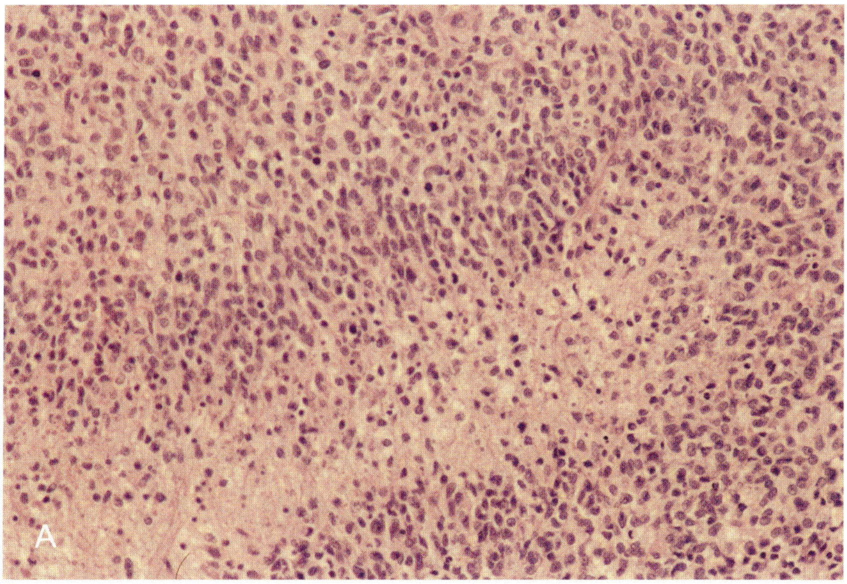

Figure 7.2. **A,** Glioblastoma. Marked cellularity with necrosis and peripheral pseudopalisading of nuclei. (Paraffin section, H&E, ×64.)

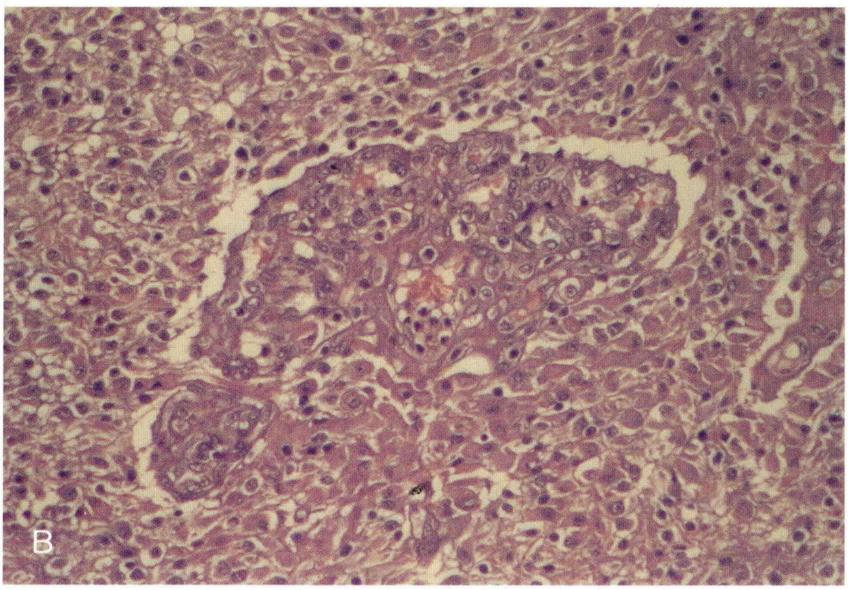

Figure 7.2. **B,** Glioblastoma. Glomeruloid vascular proliferation. (Paraffin section, H&E, ×64.)

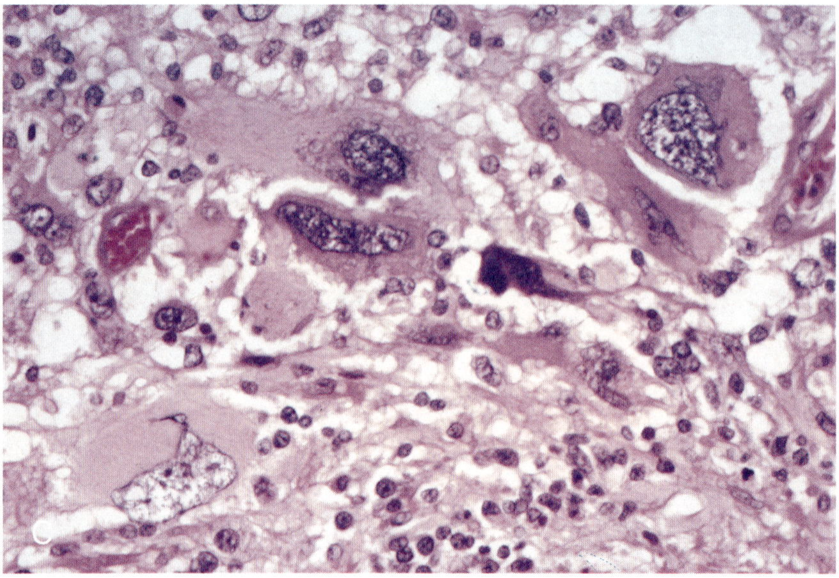

Figure 7.2. C, Glioblastoma with prominent bizarre giant cell formation. Giant cells may occur in both benign and malignant CNS neoplasms (see Table 7.3 and text). (Paraffin section, H&E, ×160.)

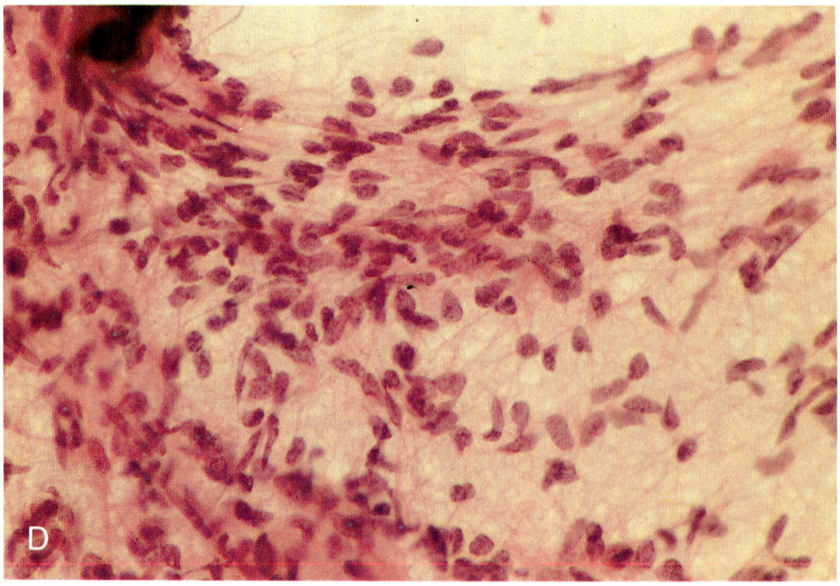

Figure 7.2. D, Glioblastoma. Smear preparation demonstrating fibrillary background, hypercellularity, and moderate pleomorphism. (Smear preparation, H&E, ×128.)

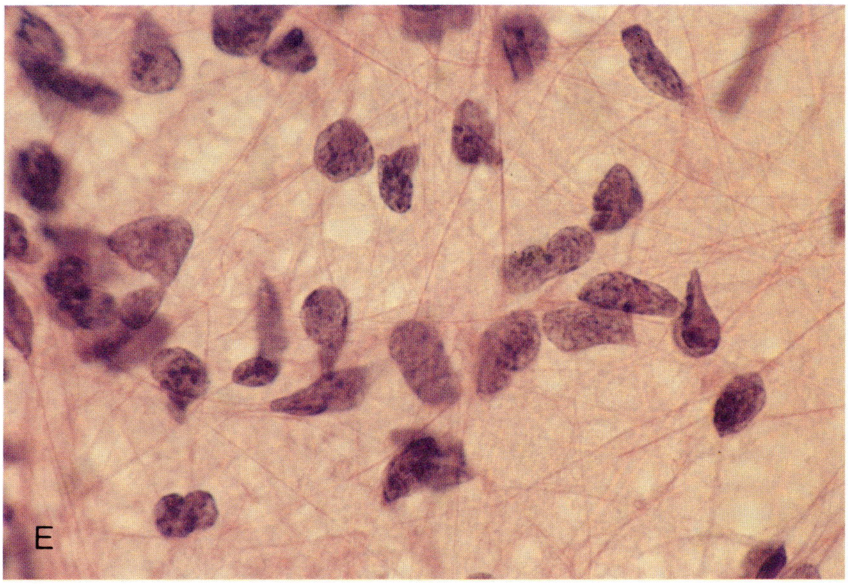

Figure 7.2. E, Glioblastoma. Detail of smear preparation demonstrating nuclear pleomorphism and nuclear membrane irregularities on a fibrillar background. (Smear preparation, H&E, ×320.)

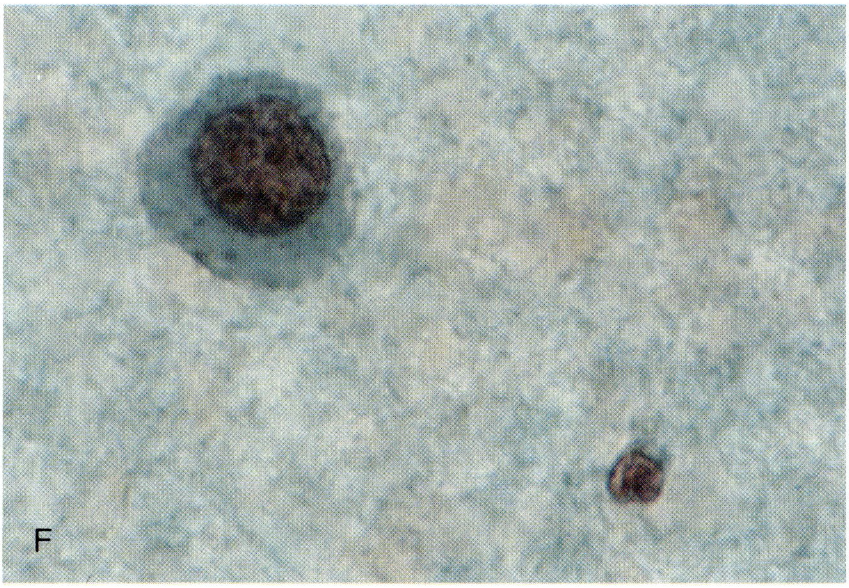

Figure 7.2. F, Glioblastoma. Large neoplastic cell in CSF. Nearby monocyte provides a size comparison. (CSF membrane filter preparation, Pap stain, ×400.)

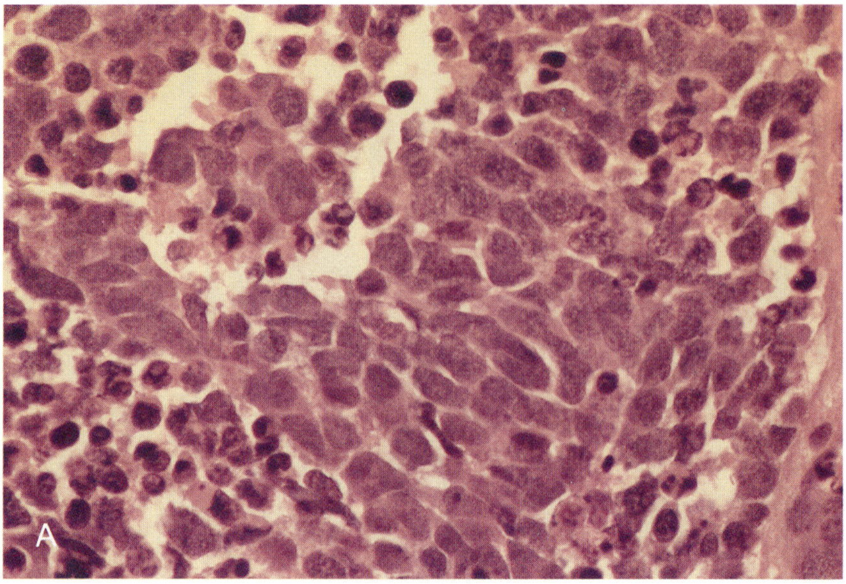

Figure 7.3. A, Epithelioid glioblastoma. Epithelioid area with focal necrosis. Other areas of the tumor were more typical of glioblastoma, with an anaplastic, fibrillary astrocytic component similar to that seen in Figure 7.2**A**. (Paraffin section, H&E, ×128.)

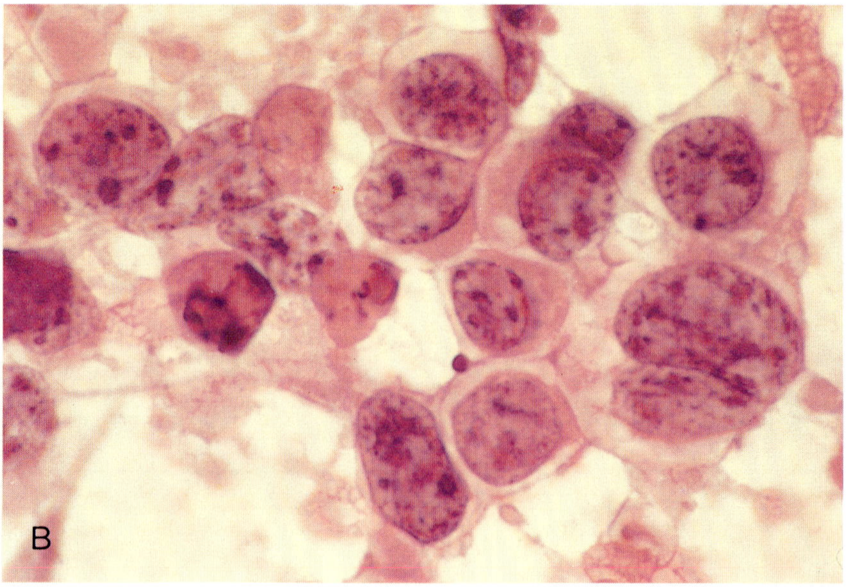

Figure 7.3. B, Epithelioid glioblastoma. Smear preparation, in which the epithelioid component dominates the smear. Marked pleomorphism and epithelial appearance resembles metastatic carcinoma. (Smear preparation, H&E, ×320.)

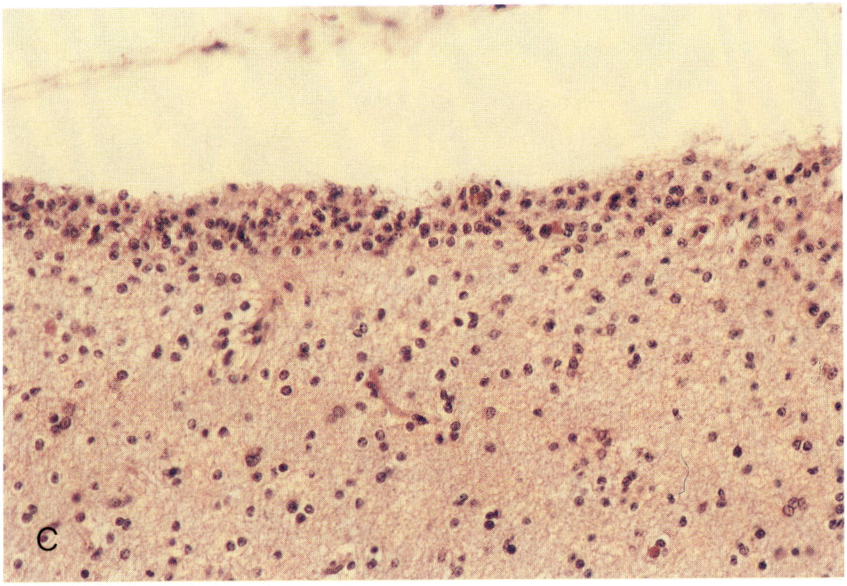

Figure 7.3. C, Scherer's secondary structure. Subpial spread of oligodendroglioma. (Paraffin section, H&E, ×64.)

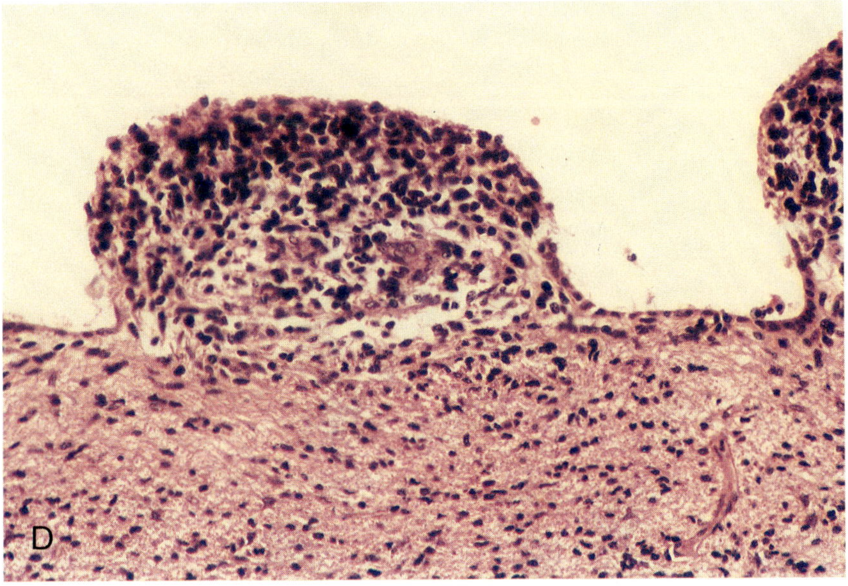

Figure 7.3. D, Scherer's secondary structure. Subependymal spread of glioblastoma. Subependymal and/or subpial spread may be a continuous layer (e.g., Fig. 7.3**C**) or in more irregular fashion, as demonstrated in this example. (Paraffin section, H&E, ×64.)

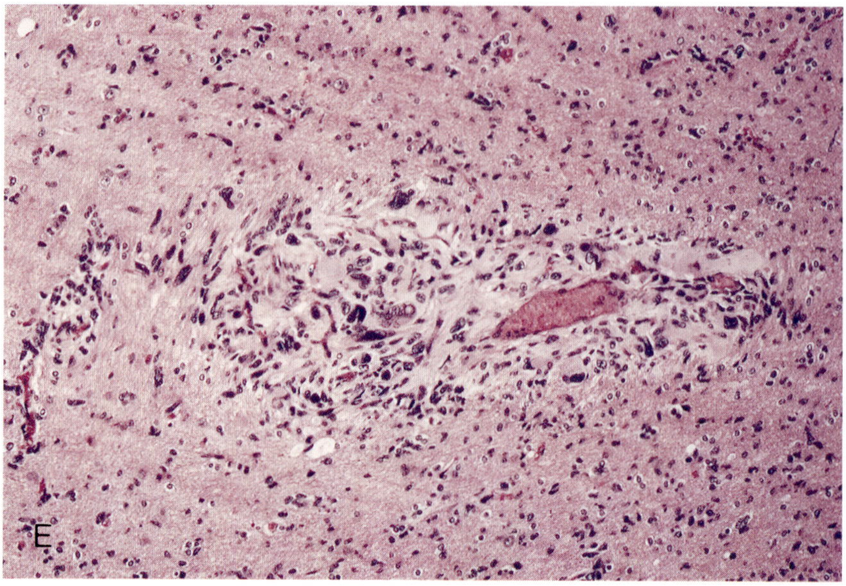

Figure 7.3. **E,** Scherer's secondary structure. Perivascular concentration of anaplastic astrocytoma cells. (Paraffin section, H&E, ×64.)

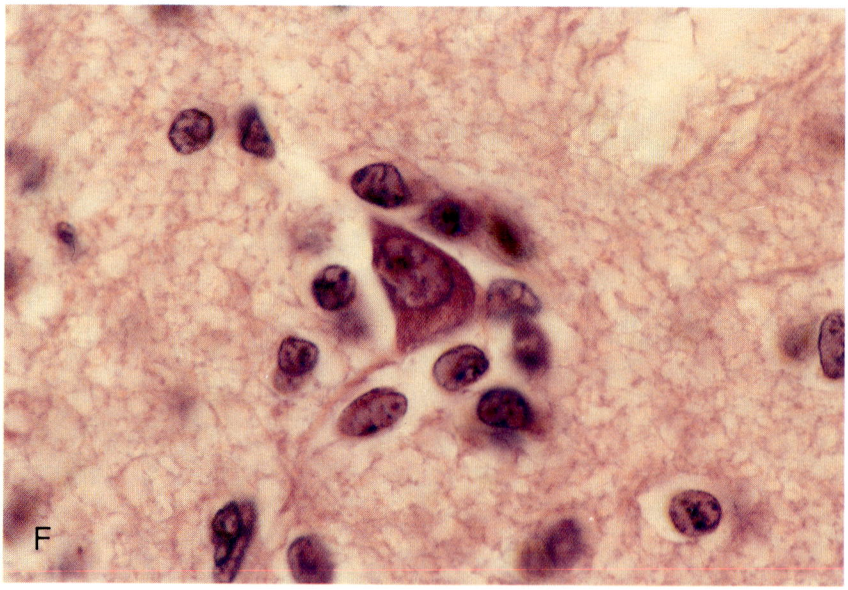

Figure 7.3. **F,** Scherer's secondary structure. Perineuronal satellitosis by neoplastic cells in an oligodendroglioma. Fourteen atypical oligodendroglial nuclei were present around this neuron, only a few of which are seen in this plane of focus. (Paraffin section, H&E, ×320.)

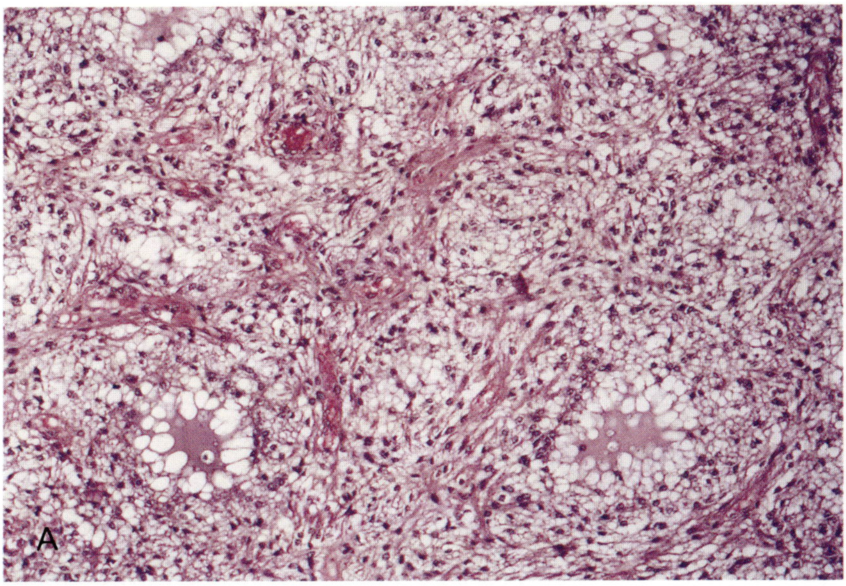

Figure 7.4. A, Juvenile pilocytic astrocytoma. Cystic change in a fibrillary astrocytic background. (Paraffin section, H&E, ×32.)

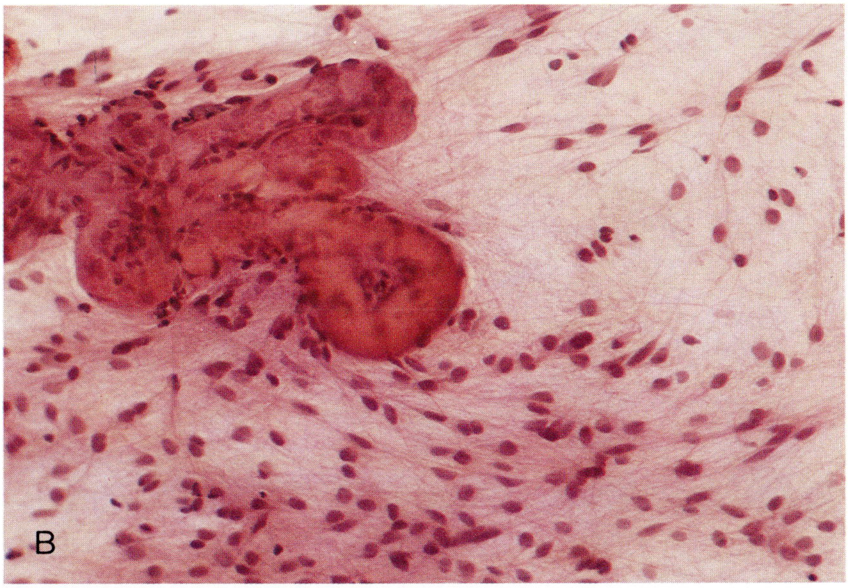

Figure 7.4. B, Pilocytic astrocytoma smear preparation, demonstrating glomeruloid vessels on a background of fibrillary, mildly pleomorphic astrocytes. The glomeruloid vascular formations do not have malignant implications in this tumor (see text). (Smear preparation, H&E, ×64.)

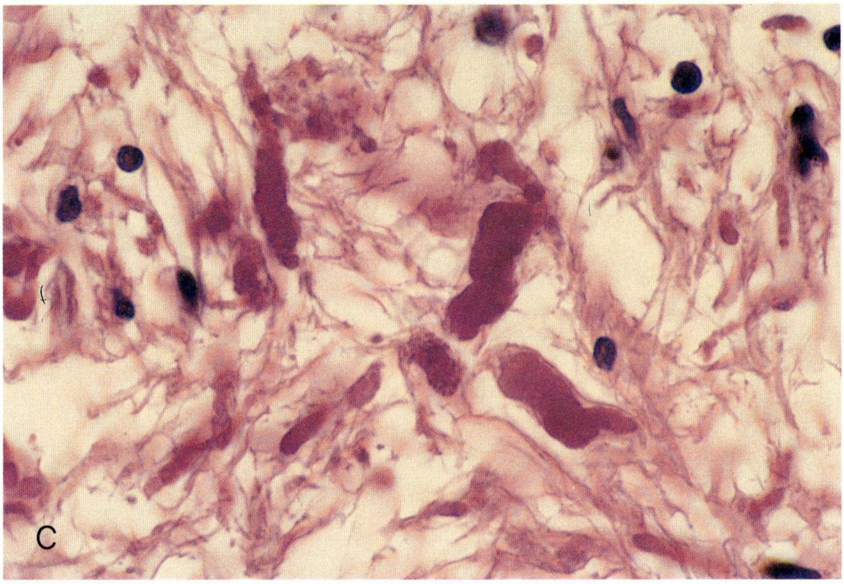

Figure 7.4. **C,** Rosenthal fibers are conspicuous as thick, glassy, slightly refractile eosinophilic structures in an area of fibrillary gliosis. (Paraffin section, H&E, ×320.)

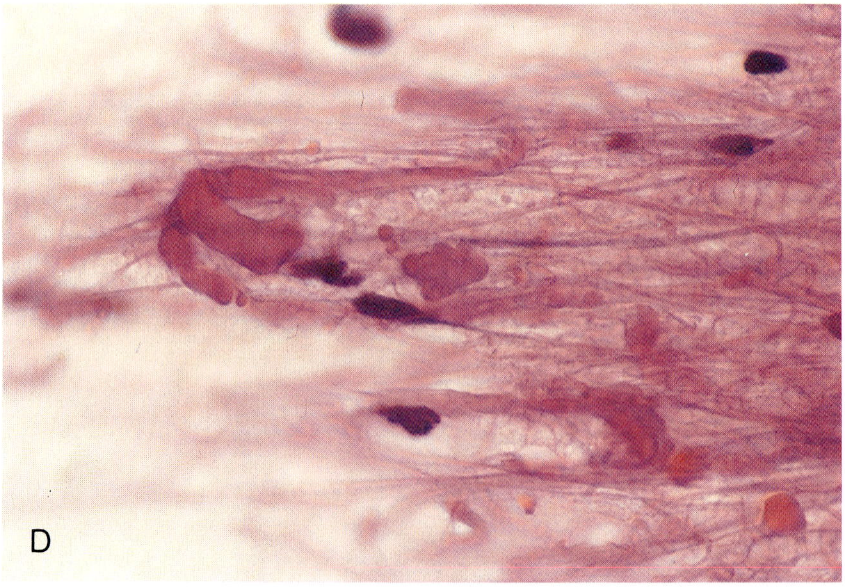

Figure 7.4. **D,** Rosenthal fibers as seen in a smear preparation. Both Figures 7.4**C** and **D** are from a zone of marked gliosis surrounding a craniopharyngioma (see Table 7.6). (Smear preparation, H&E, ×320.)

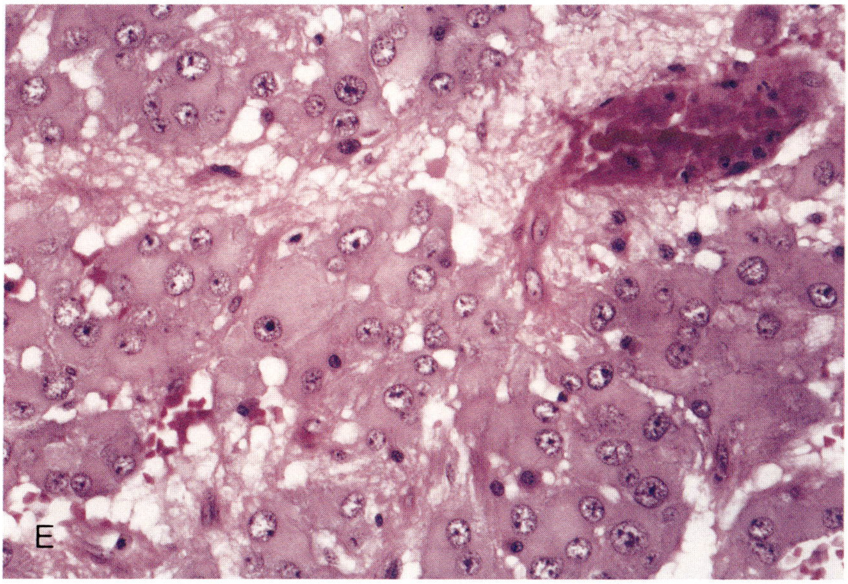

Figure 7.4. **E,** Subependymal giant cell astrocytoma in patient with tuberous sclerosis. (Paraffin section, H&E, ×128.)

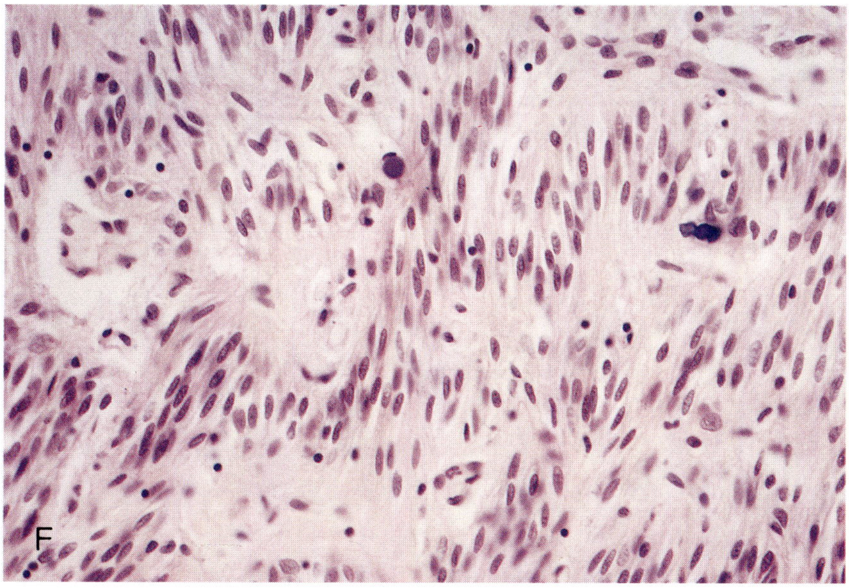

Figure 7.4. **F,** Polar spongioblastoma with prominent nuclear palisades. (Paraffin section, H&E, ×80.)

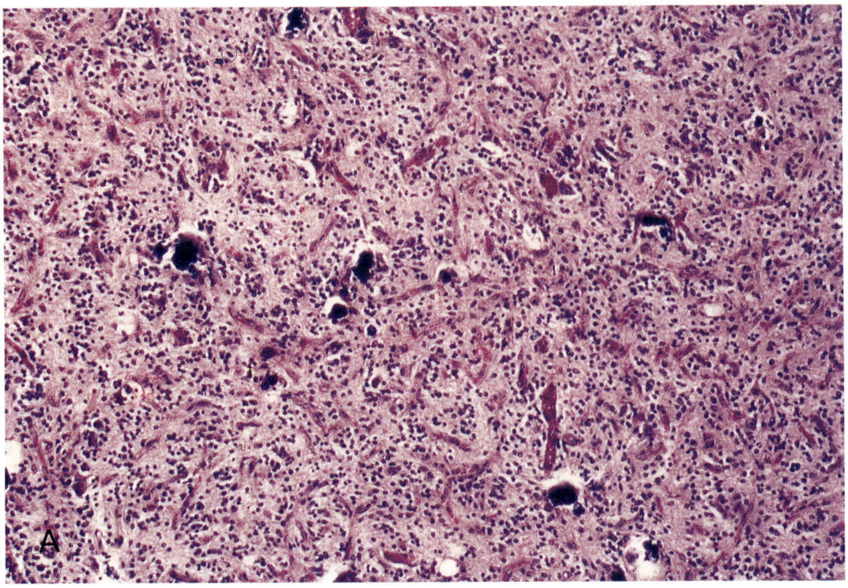

Figure 7.5. A, Oligodendroglioma, with punctate calcification. Note the uniformity of nuclei and the delicate capillary vasculature. (Paraffin section, H&E, ×32.)

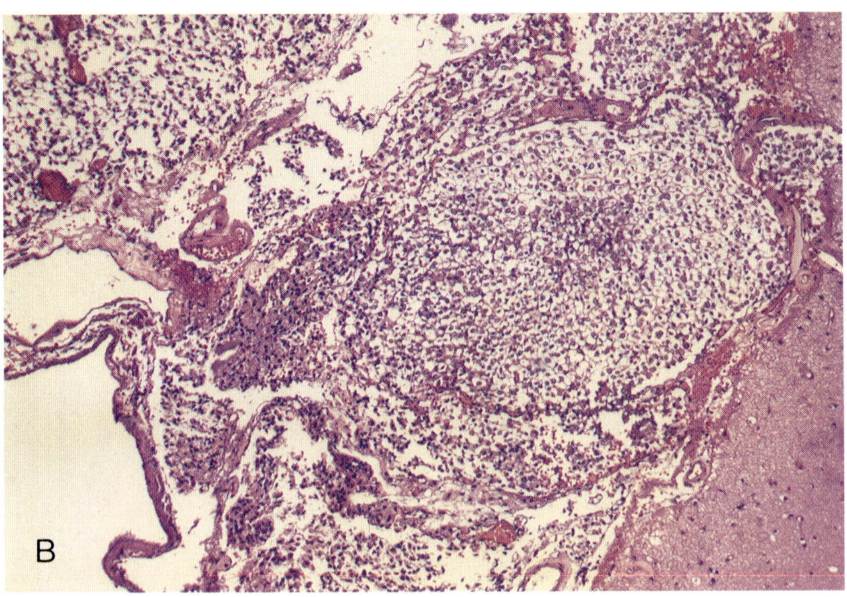

Figure 7.5. B, Oligodendroglioma with diffuse, spontaneous leptomeningeal spread (see Table 7.14). (Paraffin section, H&E, ×32.)

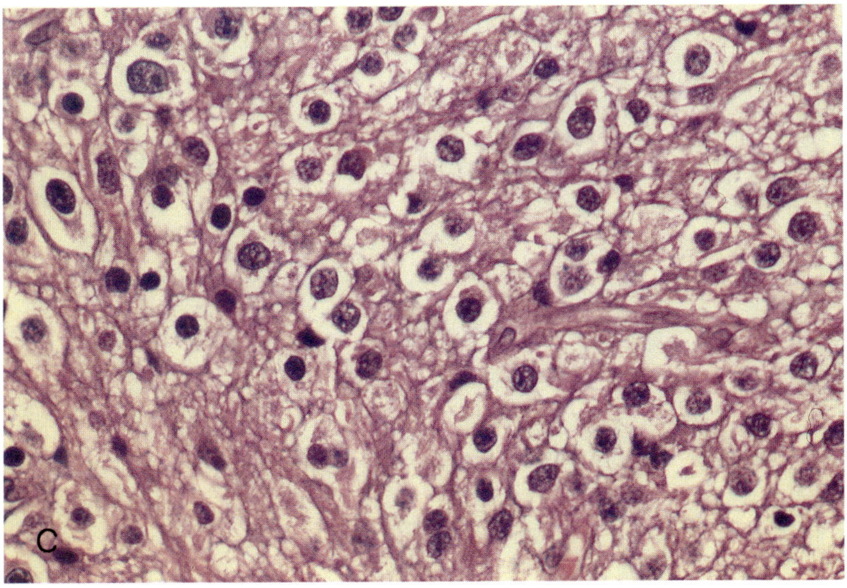

Figure 7.5. C, Oligodendroglioma. Perinuclear halos give a "fried egg" appearance to the cells as a consequence of delayed fixation. (Paraffin section, H&E, ×128.)

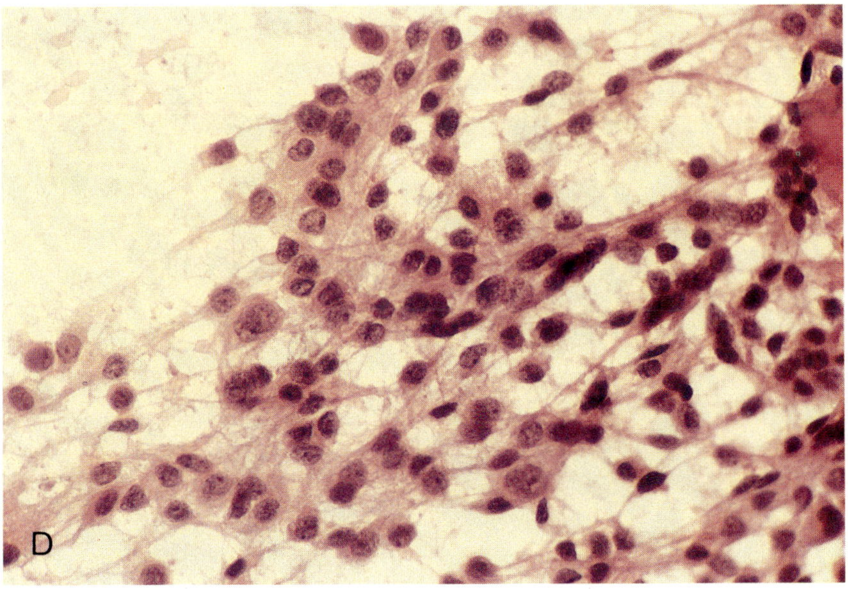

Figure 7.5. D, Oligodendroglioma. A fine fibrillary background is often more conspicuous in smears. (Smear preparation, H&E, ×128.)

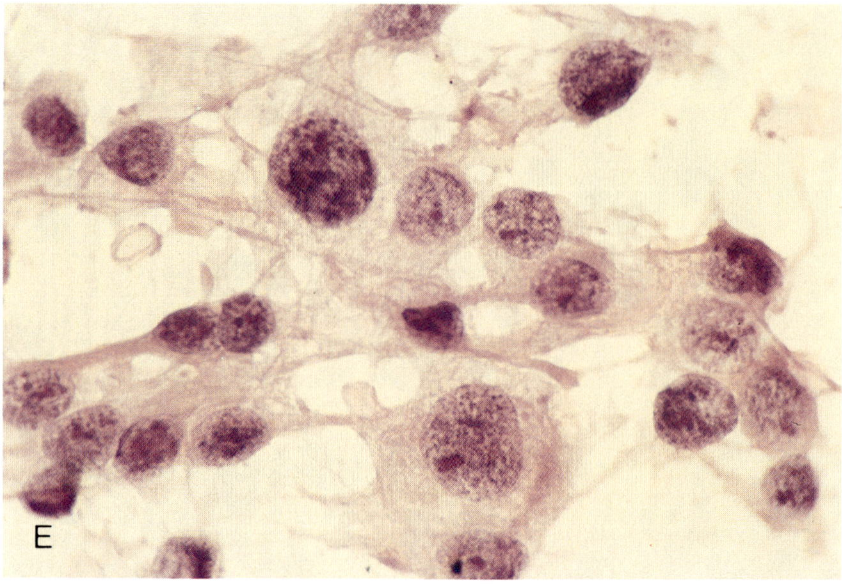

Figure 7.5. E, Oligodendroglioma. Nuclear pleomorphism is often more readily appreciated in smear preparations than in tissue sections. Cytoplasm is more delicate and the background less fibrillar than in most astrocytomas (exception—protoplasmic astrocytoma). (Smear preparation, H&E, ×320.)

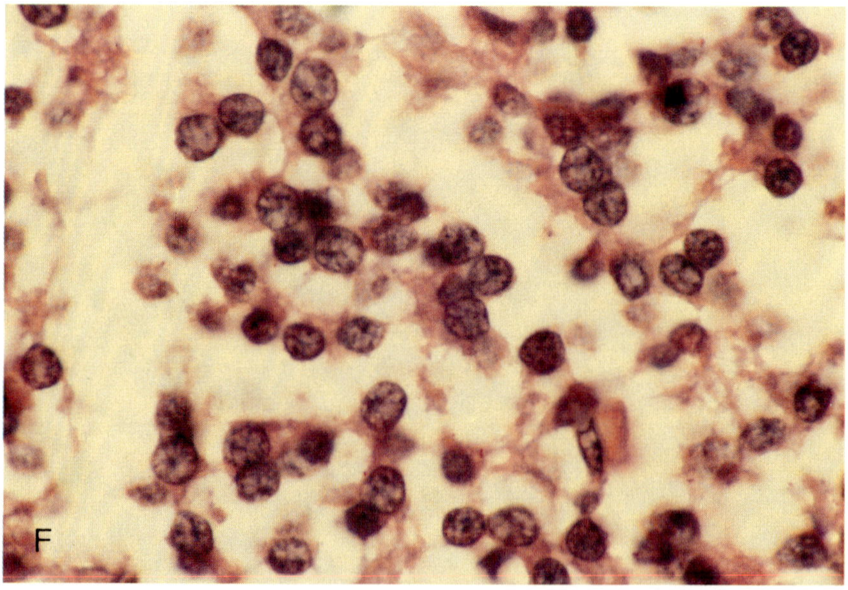

Figure 7.5. F, Central neurocytoma. Although there is some shrinkage artifact as a result of paraffin section processing, note the similarity of appearance of these cells to an oligodendroglioma. Rosettes and indian-file architecture are not always apparent. (Paraffin section, H&E, ×320.)

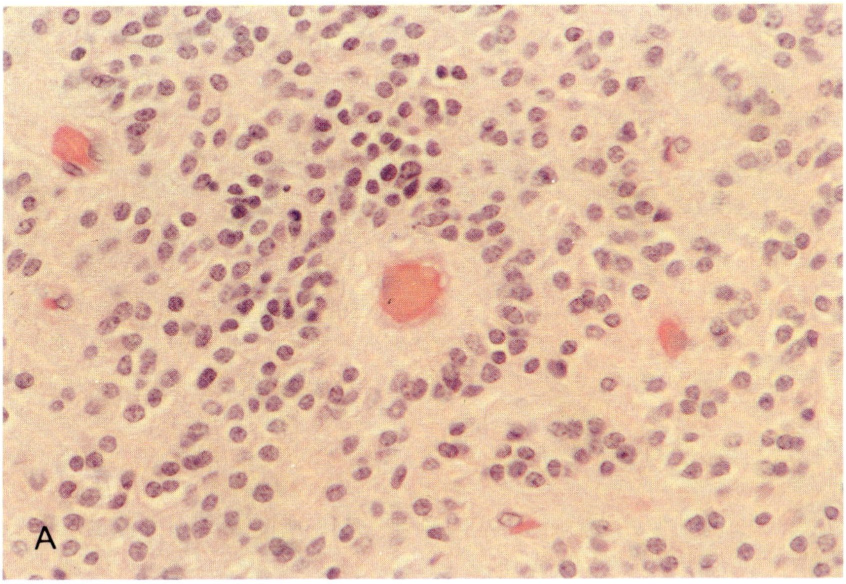

Figure 7.6. **A,** Perivascular pseudorosette in a cellular ependymoma. (Paraffin section, H&E, ×128.)

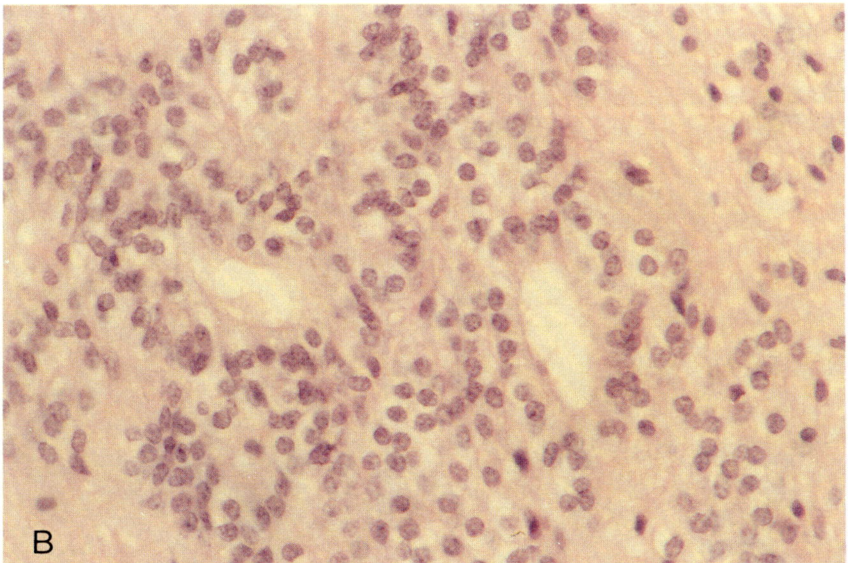

Figure 7.6. **B,** Ependymal "true" rosette, with central lumen, in a cellular ependymoma. (Paraffin section, H&E, ×128.)

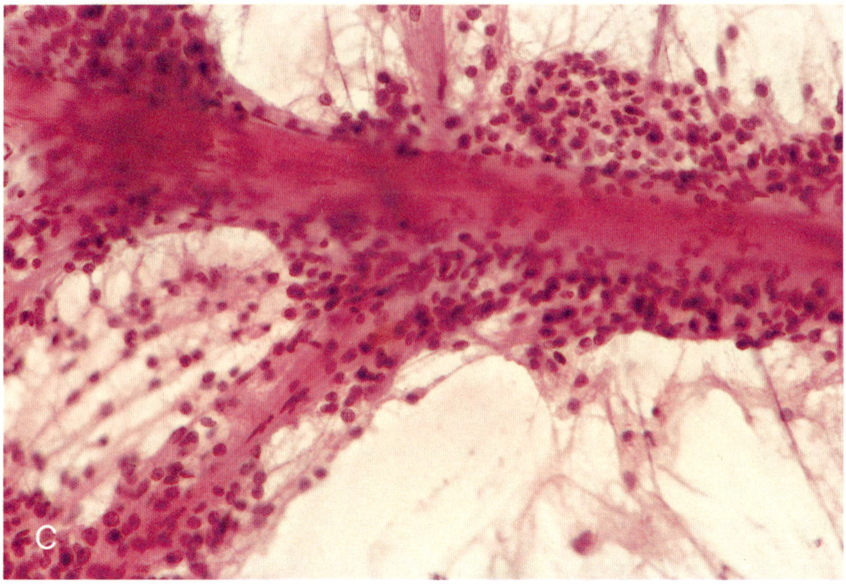

Figure 7.6. C, The perivascular pseudorosettes in a cellular ependymoma are reflected in smear preparations by adherent ependymoma cells around a vessel. (Smear preparation, H&E, ×64.)

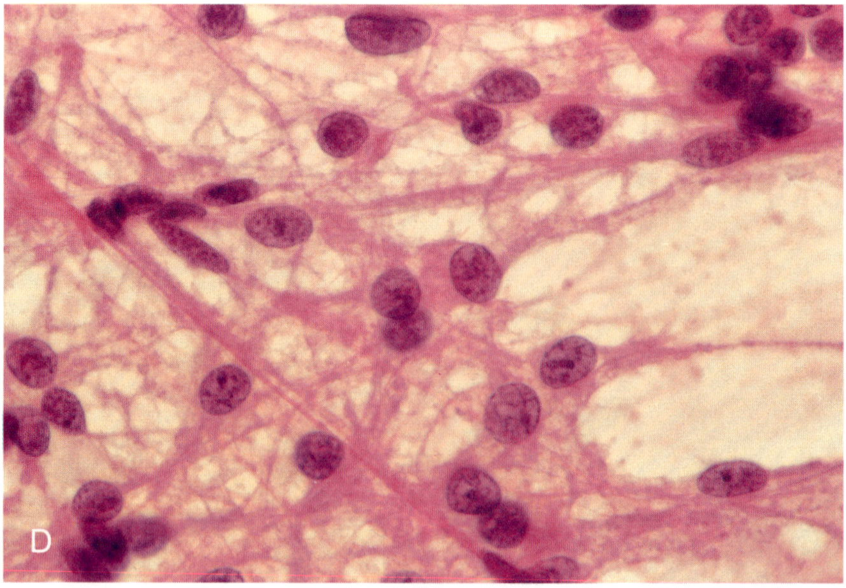

Figure 7.6. D, Detail of cellular ependymoma as demonstrated in a smear preparation. Note the uniformity of bland, ovoid nuclei on a fibrillar background. Small nucleoli are often present, and chromatin is fine. (Smear preparation, H&E, ×320.)

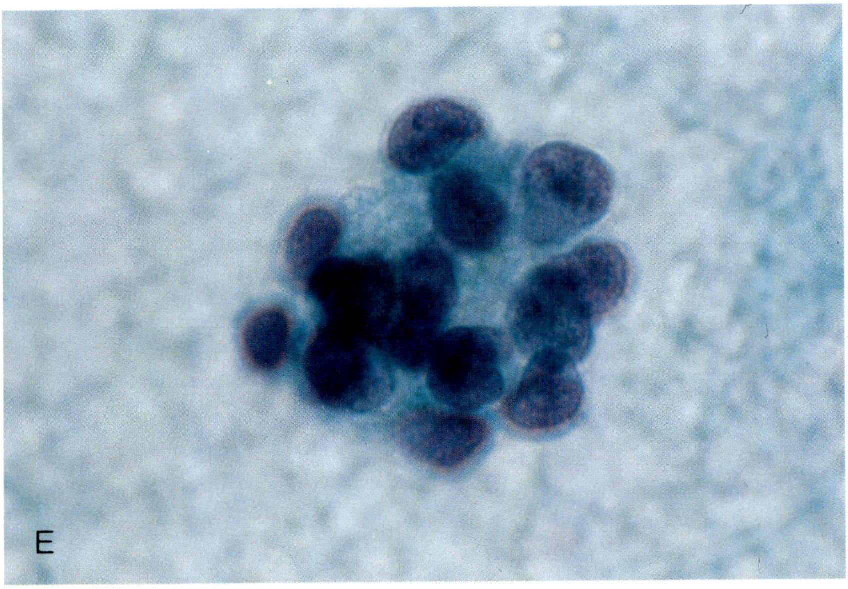

Figure 7.6. E, Ependymoma cells exfoliated in CSF. (CSF membrane filter preparation, Pap stain, ×320.)

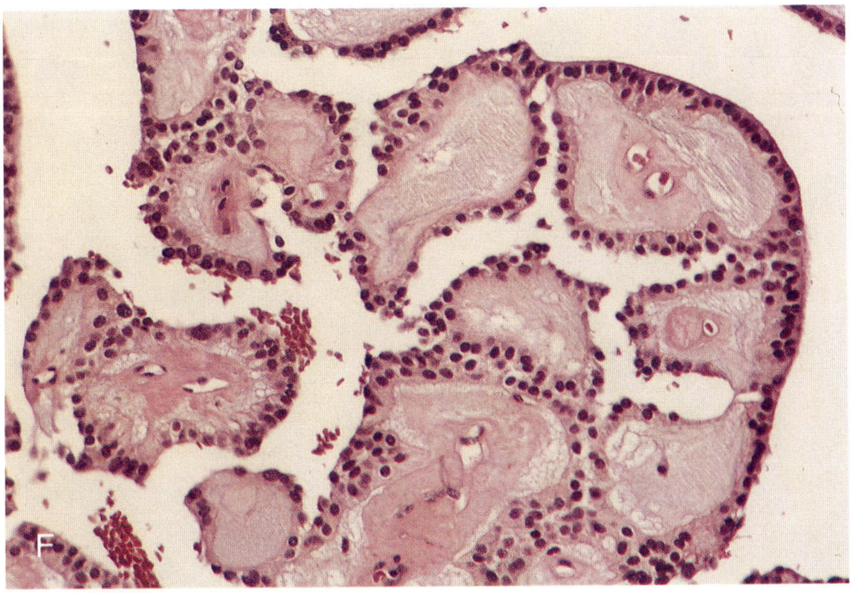

Figure 7.6. F, Myxopapillary ependymoma. Solid portion of tumor fragmenting into papillary structures. The latter are surfaced by ependymoma cells and contain a central hyalinized vessel and surrounding myxoid material. (Paraffin section, H&E, ×64.)

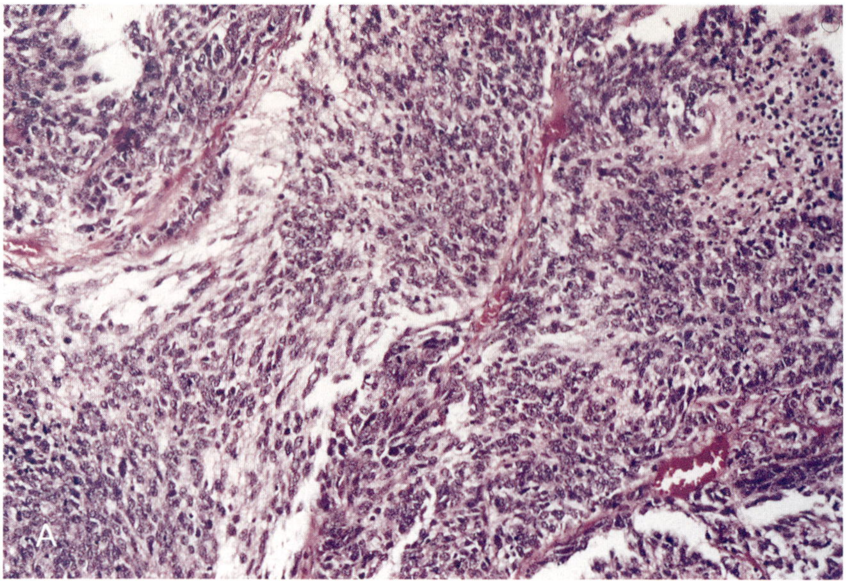

Figure 7.7. **A,** Medulloblastoma. Sheets of poorly differentiated small cells dominate the histologic field. (Paraffin section, H&E, ×40.)

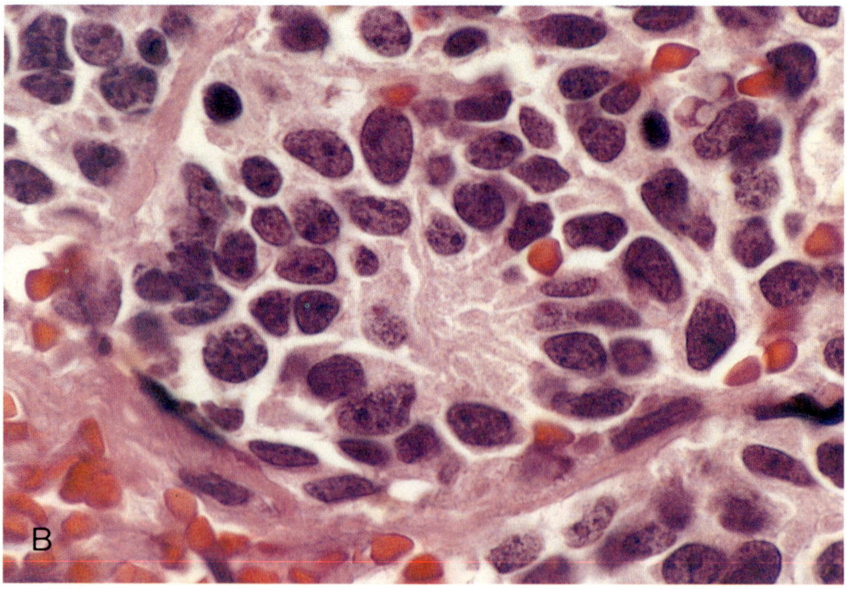

Figure 7.7. **B,** Detail of medulloblastoma cells demonstrating nuclear molding and a fairly well-formed Homer Wright rosette. (Paraffin section, H&E, ×320.)

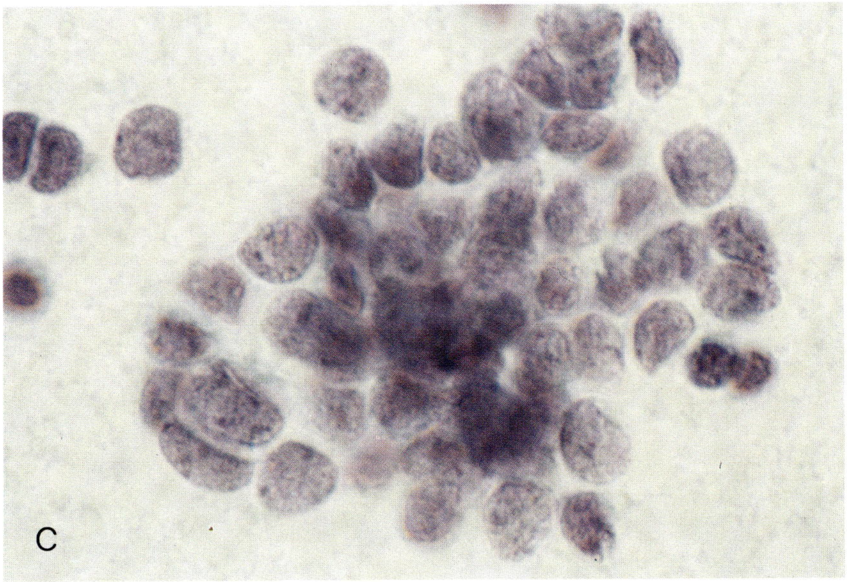

Figure 7.7. **C,** Medulloblastoma cells exfoliated in CSF. (CSF membrane filter preparation, Pap stain, ×400.)

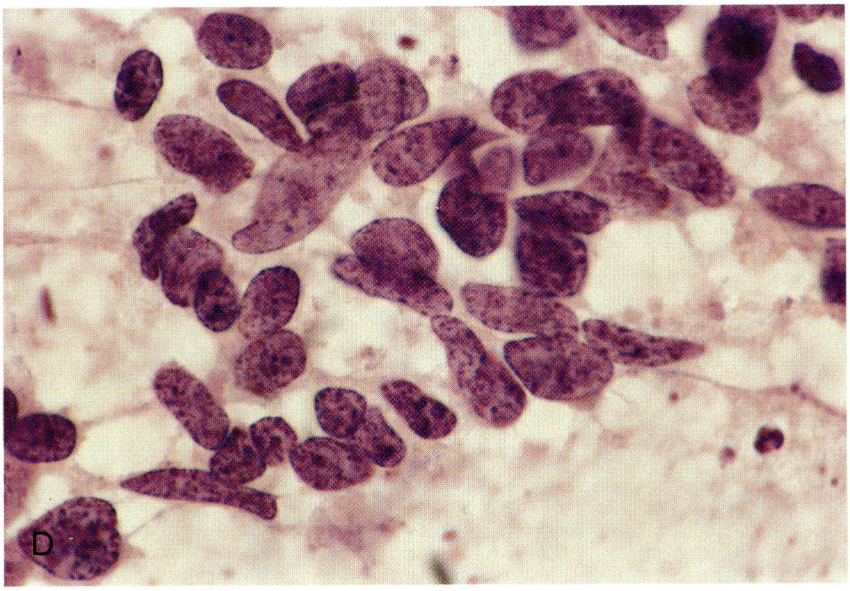

Figure 7.7. **D,** Lung small cell carcinoma cells metastatic to cerebellum (see text). Note necrotic debris in background. (Smear preparation, H&E, ×320.)

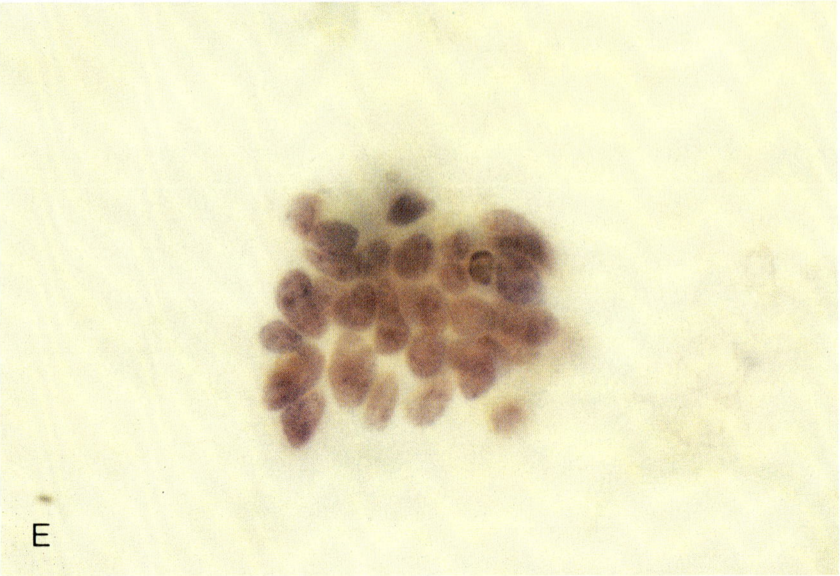

Figure 7.7. E, Retinoblastoma cells exfoliated in CSF. (CSF membrane filter preparation, Pap stain, ×400.)

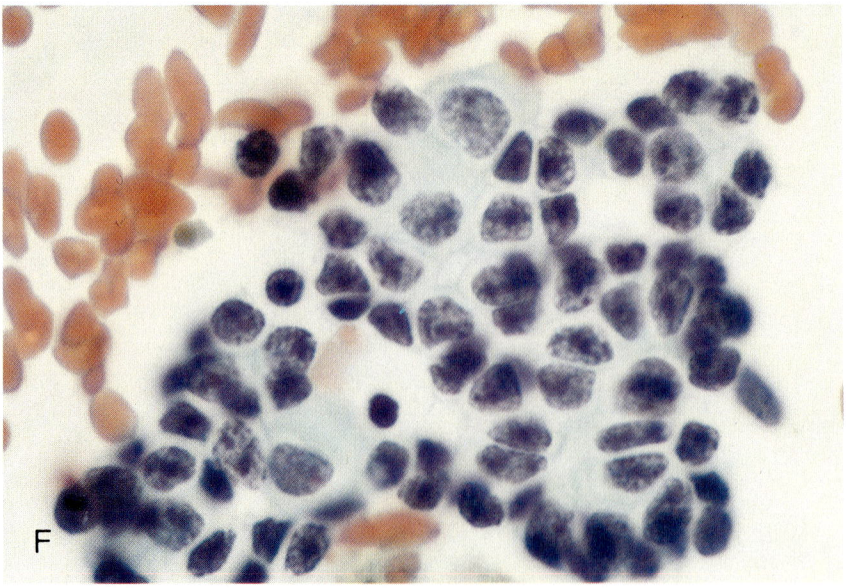

Figure 7.7. F, Retinal dysplasia from a case of Norrie's disease. Vitreous aspirate. (CSF membrane filter preparation, H&E, ×400.)

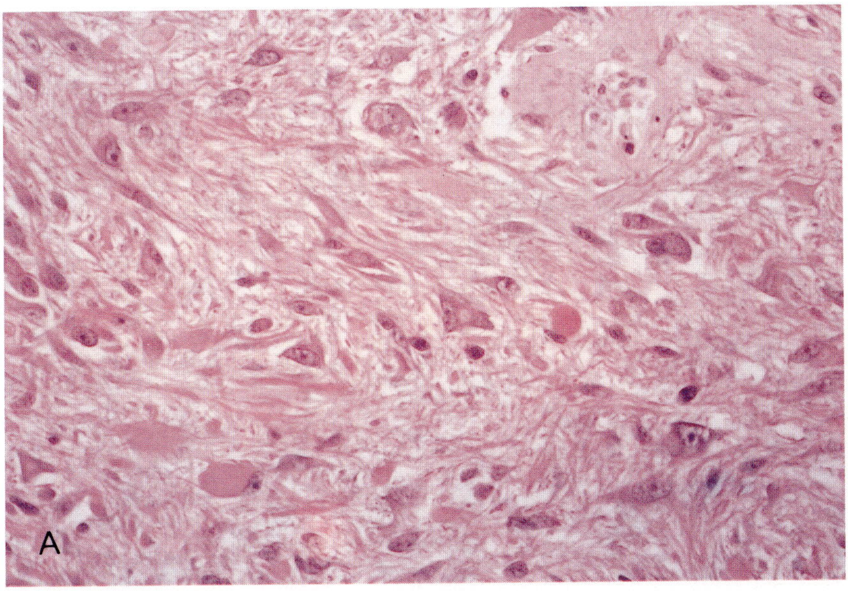

Figure 7.8. **A,** Ganglioglioma of cerebrum. Atypical ganglion cells are admixed with a predominantly fibrillary astrocytoma background. (Paraffin section, H&E, ×100.)

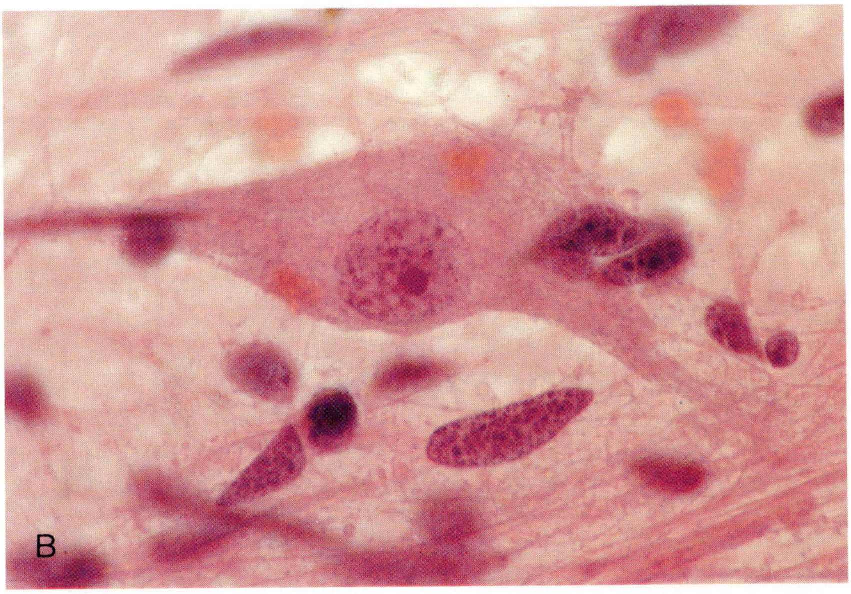

Figure 7.8. **B,** Ganglioglioma. Smear preparation shows nuclear detail of neoplastic astrocytes and a neuron. Differential diagnosis should include normal neurons entrapped within an astrocytoma (see text). (Smear preparation, H&E, ×320.)

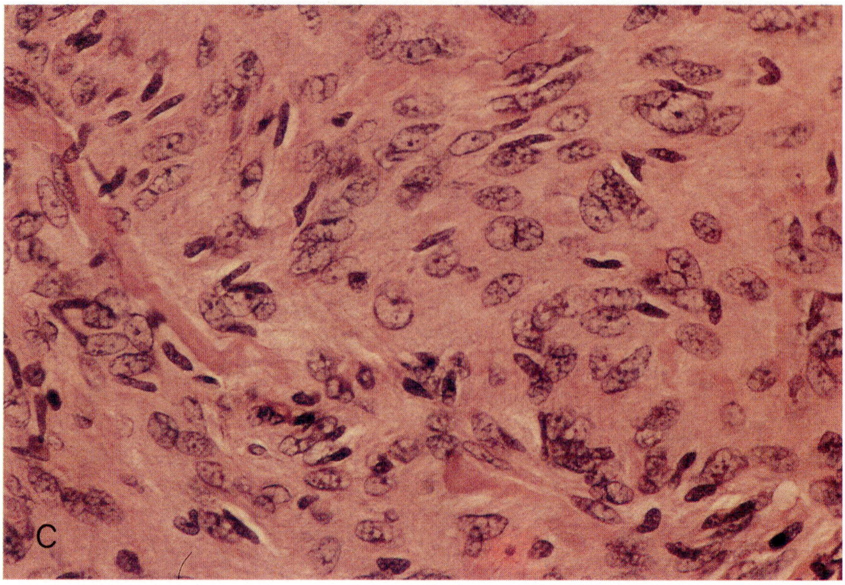

Figure 7.8. C, Syncytial (meningotheliomatous) meningioma. Cell membranes are not well visualized. (Paraffin section, H&E, ×128.)

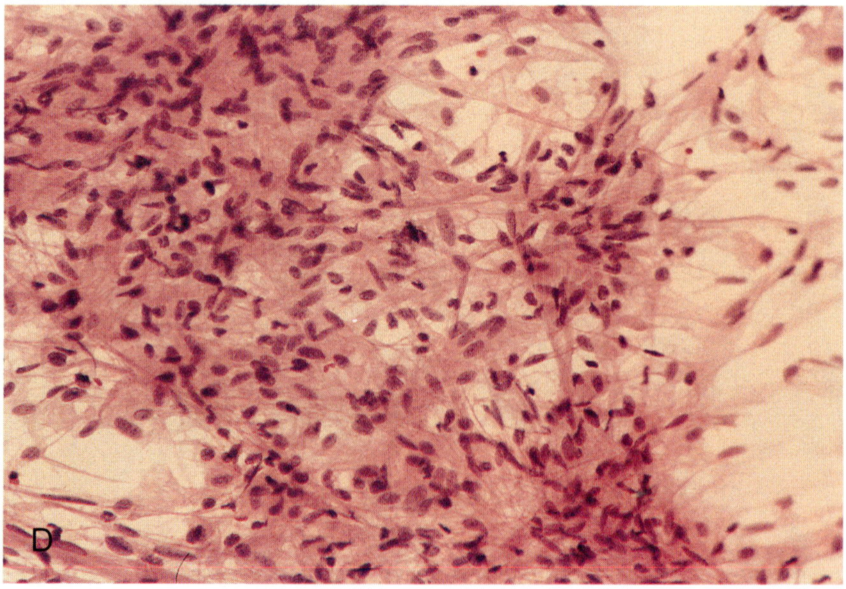

Figure 7.8. D, Syncytial (meningotheliomatous) meningioma. Most cases smear readily, allowing study of cytologic detail. (Smear preparation, H&E, ×64.)

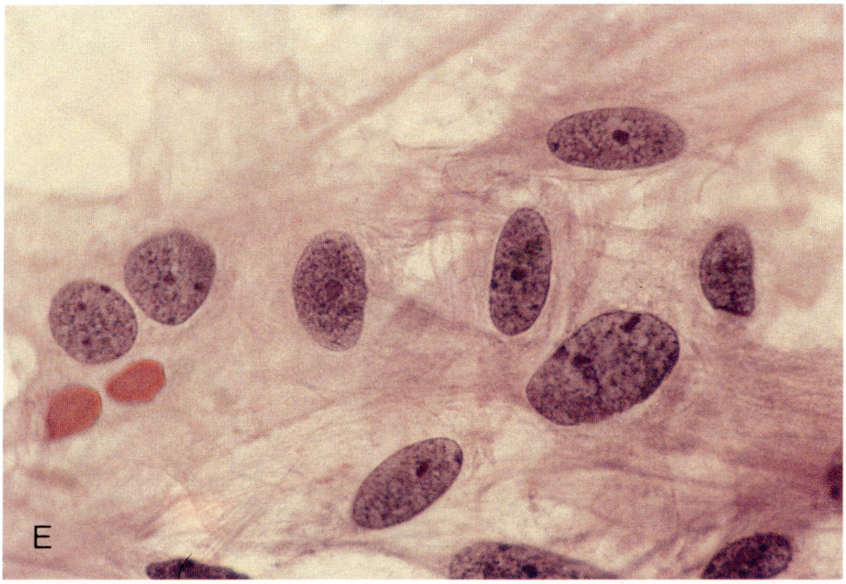

Figure 7.8. E, Syncytial meningioma cellular detail. Compare with normal pia-arachnoid cells (Fig. 2.10**A**, **B**, **C**, and **D**). (Smear preparation, H&E, x320.)

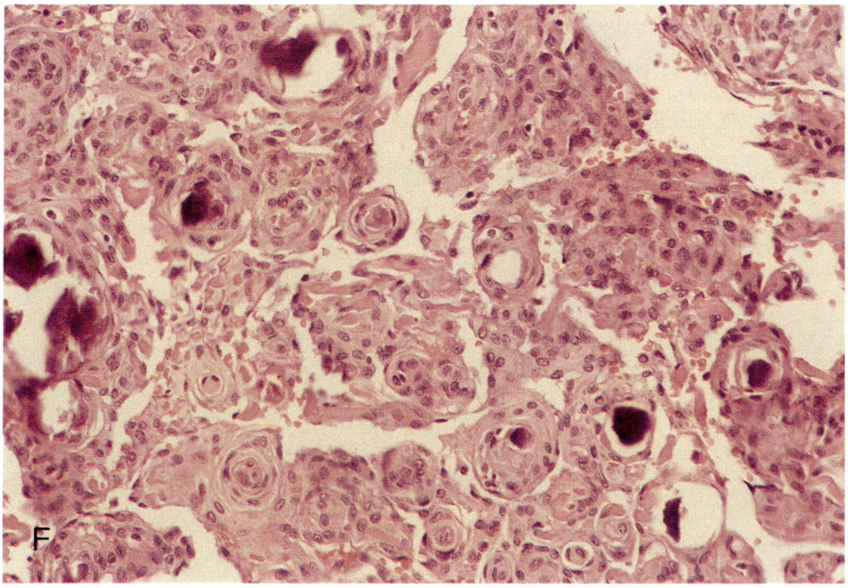

Figure 7.8. F, Transitional meningioma demonstrating whorls and psammoma bodies. (Paraffin section, H&E, ×64.)

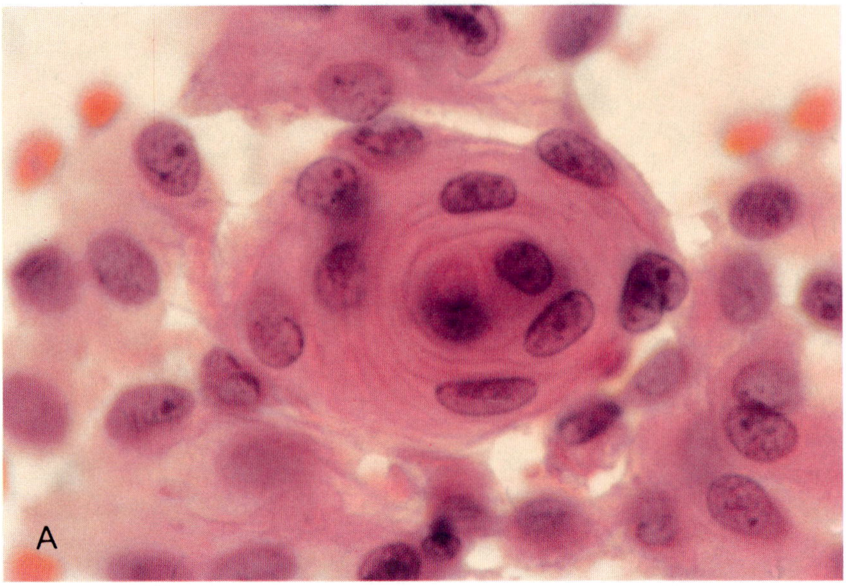

Figure 7.9. **A,** Meningothelial whorl from transitional meningioma. (Smear preparation, H&E, ×320.)

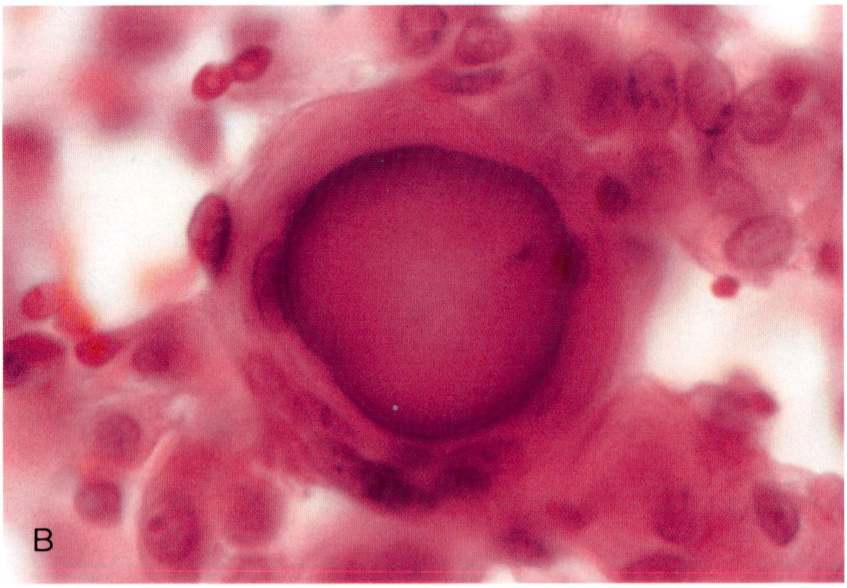

Figure 7.9. **B,** Psammoma body from transitional meningioma. (Smear preparation, H&E, ×320.)

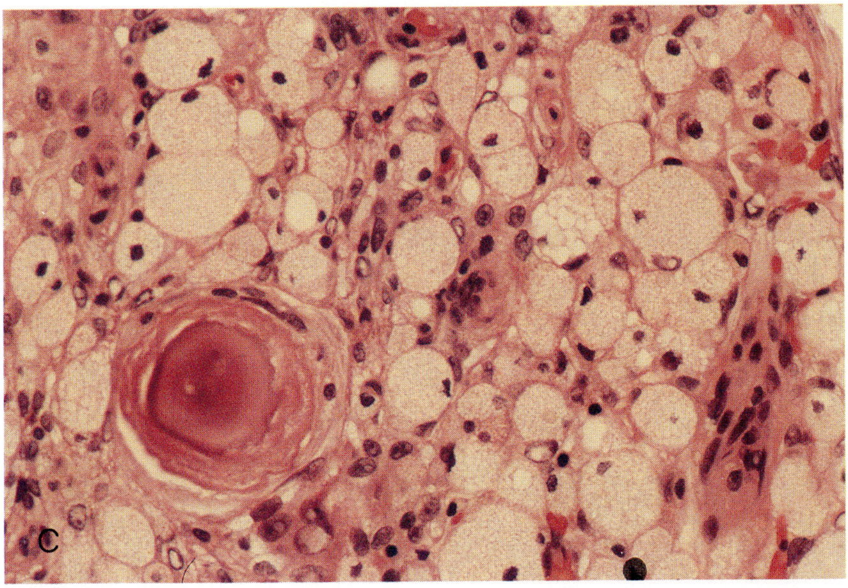

Figure 7.9. **C,** Xanthomatous meningioma area. Other portions of the tumor demonstrated a transitional meningioma pattern. A psammoma body is present. (Paraffin section, H&E, ×128.)

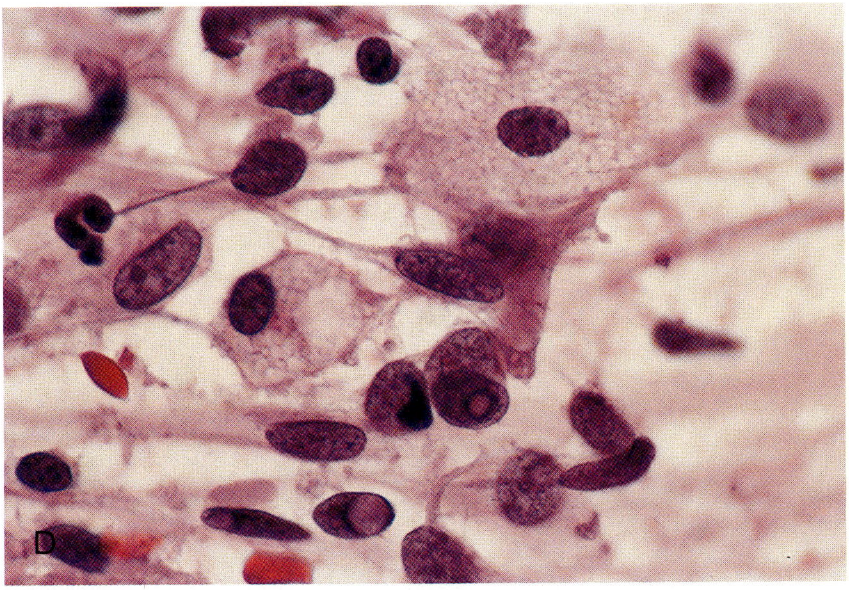

Figure 7.9. **D,** Xanthomatous meningioma area, from same case seen in **C**. Smear preparation demonstrates foam cells admixed with more typical meningothelial cells. (Smear preparation, H&E, ×320.)

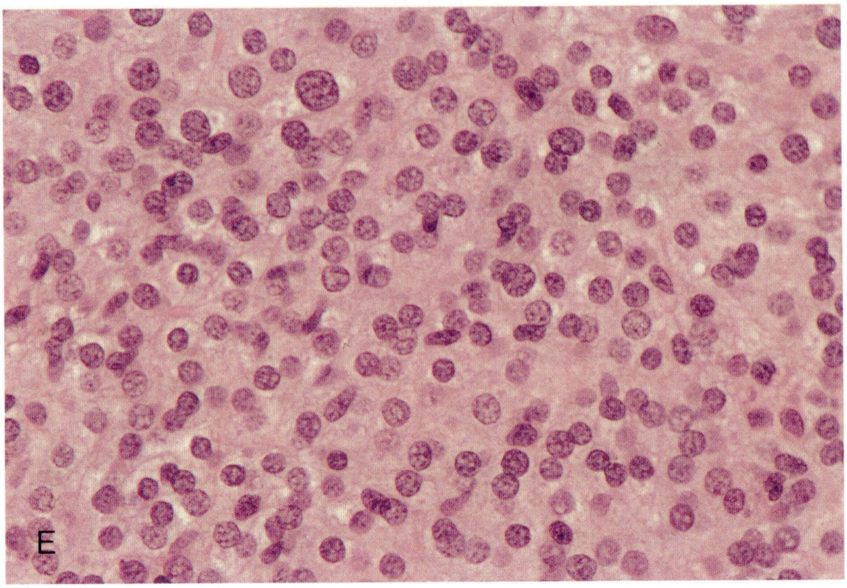

Figure 7.9. **E,** Atypical meningioma demonstrating hypercellularity, mild to moderate pleomorphism, and many cells with prominent nucleoli. (Paraffin section, H&E, ×128.)

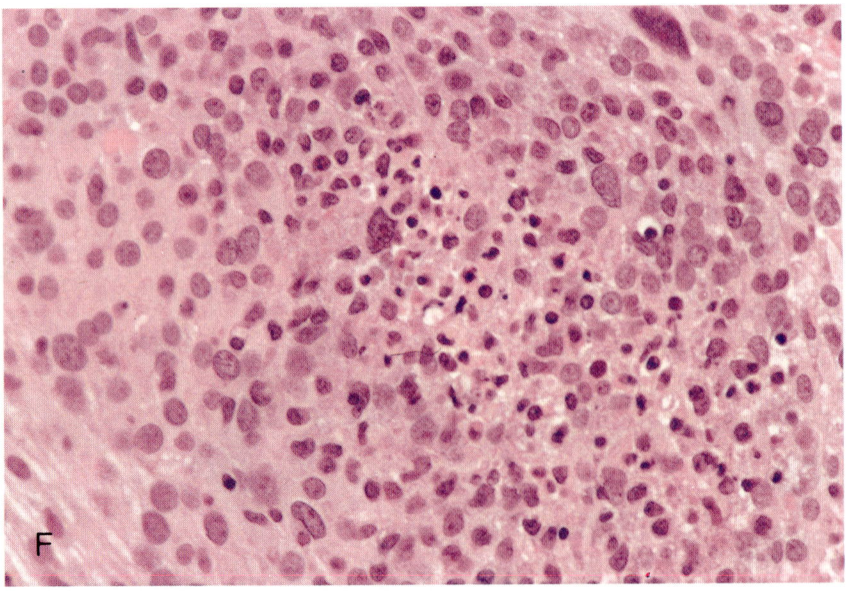

Figure 7.9. **F,** Atypical meningioma, focus of necrosis. Mitoses (up to three per 10 high-power fields) were present elsewhere in this tumor. (Paraffin section, H&E, ×128.)

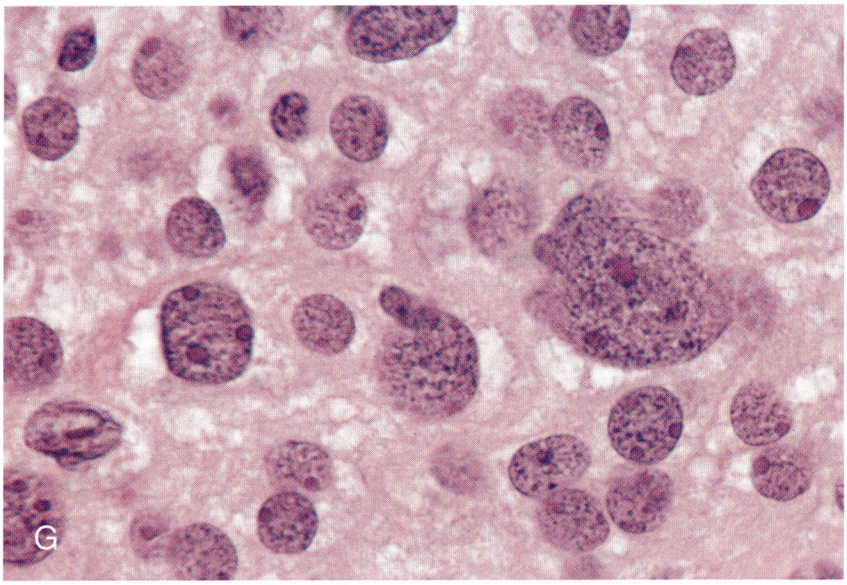

Figure 7.9. **G,** Atypical meningioma. Detail of cytologic features demonstrating pleomorphism, nuclear irregularity, hyperchromatism, coarse chromatin, and prominent nucleoli. (Paraffin section, H&E, ×320.)

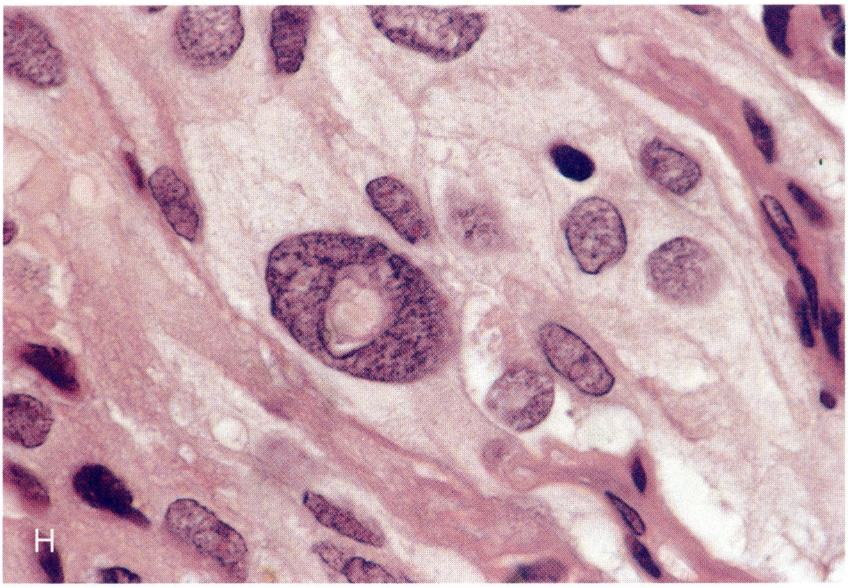

Figure 7.9. **H,** Benign cystic meningioma with "degenerative" nuclear atypia. Compare with **G**. Note less cellularity, less nucleolar prominence, and less chromatin coarseness in most cells. No necrosis or mitoses were present. (Paraffin section, H&E, ×320.)

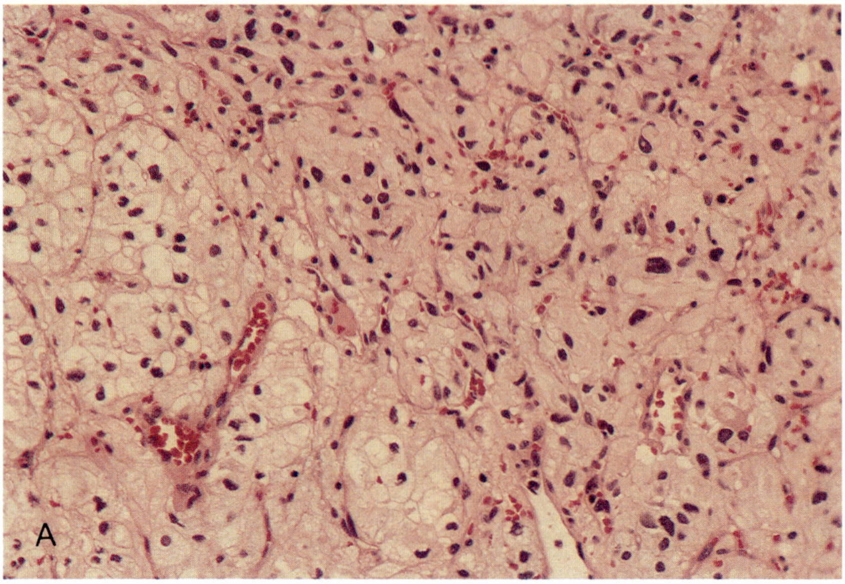

Figure 7.10. **A,** Capillary hemangioblastoma of cerebellum. Stromal cells are more vacuolated in the left lower portion of the field. (Paraffin section, H&E, ×64.)

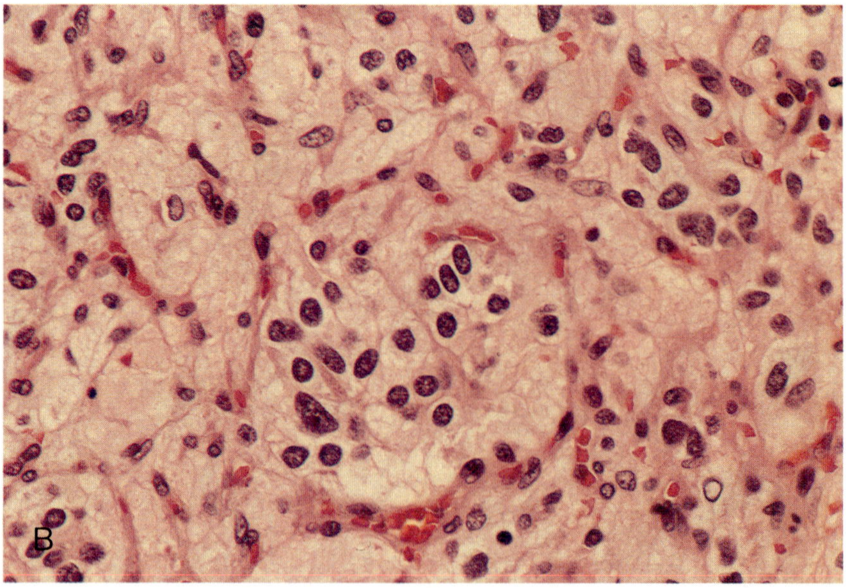

Figure 7.10. **B,** Capillary hemangioblastoma of cerebellum. Detail of delicate vascular pattern and nests of stromal cells. This field demonstrates moderate pleomorphism. (Paraffin section, H&E, ×128.)

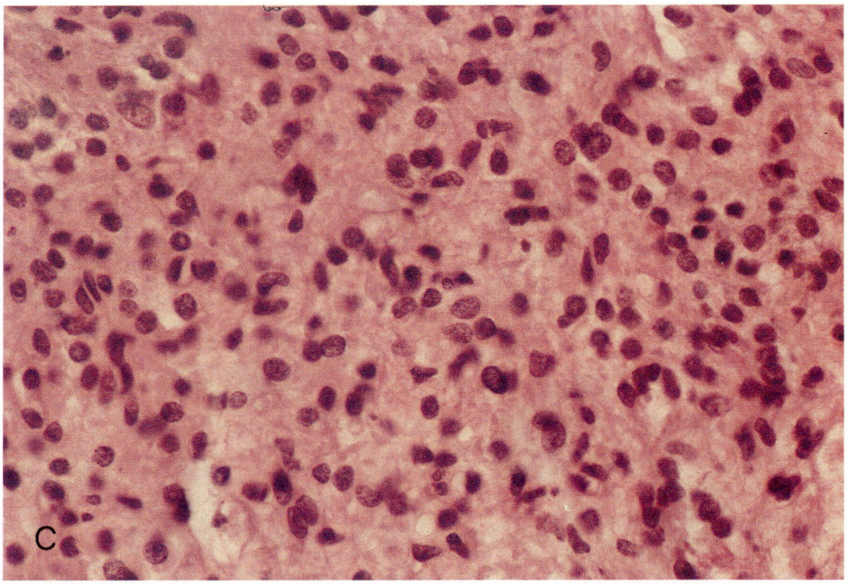

Figure 7.10. C, Capillary hemangioblastoma of cerebellum. The foamy cells and capillary pattern are often less conspicuous in frozen sections, and the appearance may be very similar to that of an astrocytoma. (Frozen section, H&E, ×128.)

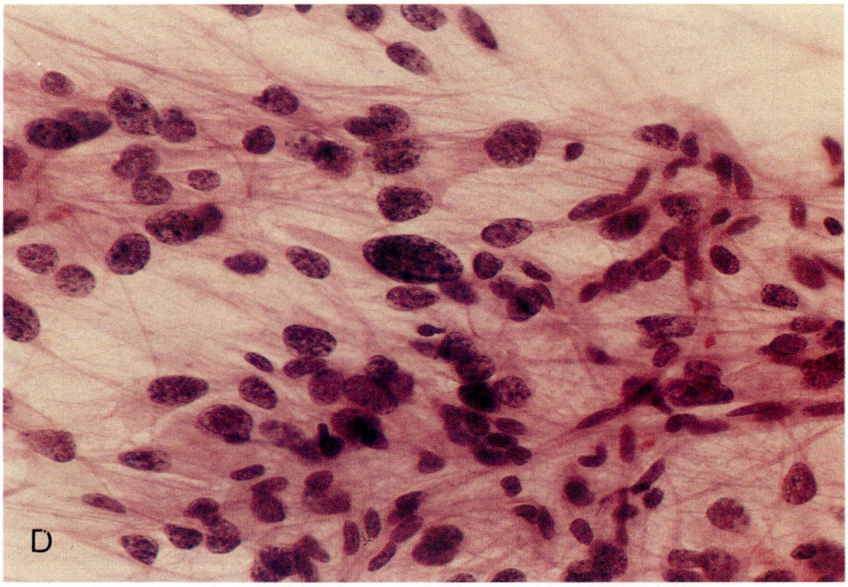

Figure 7.10. D, Capillary hemangioblastoma of cerebellum. Smear preparations tend to emphasize the fibrillary background as well as the pleomorphism. Although vasculature is well seen, foamy cells are more difficult to define. Note the resemblance to smear preparations of anaplastic astrocytomas and glioblastomas (Figs. 7.1 and 7.2). (Smear preparation, H&E, ×160.)

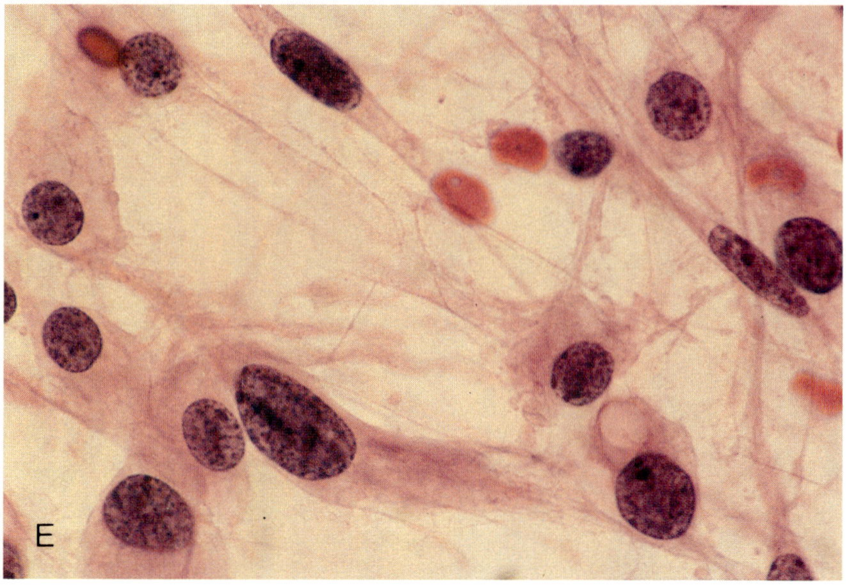

Figure 7.10. E, Capillary hemangioblastoma of cerebellum. Both fibrillar and vacuolated cells are demonstrated. The stromal cell cytoplasm is more membranous, or filmy, than fibrillar in some cells. Obvious cytoplasmic vacuoles are found infrequently. (Smear preparation, H&E, ×320.)

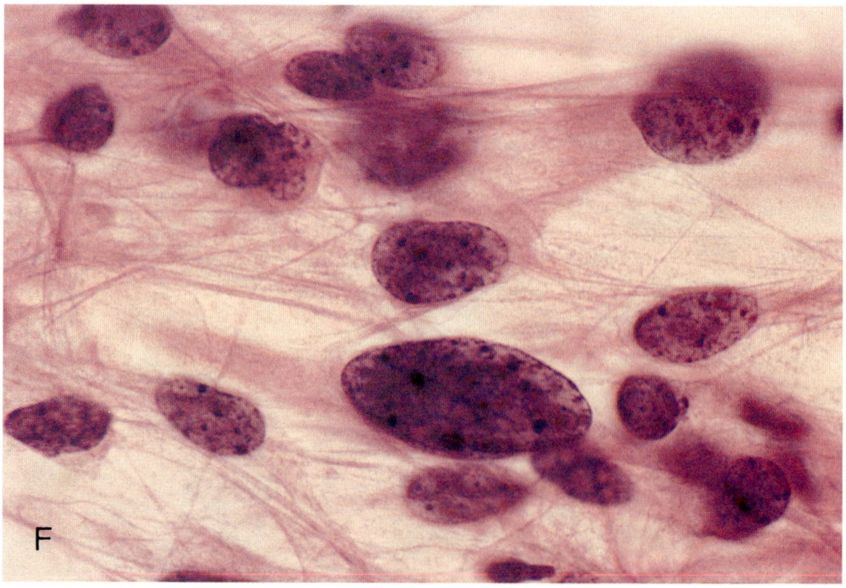

Figure 7.10. F, Capillary hemangioblastoma of cerebellum. The nuclear appearance, pleomorphism, and fibrillar background in this area can resemble an anaplastic astrocytoma, but mitoses are sparse or absent in hemangioblastomas. (Smear preparation, H&E, ×320.)

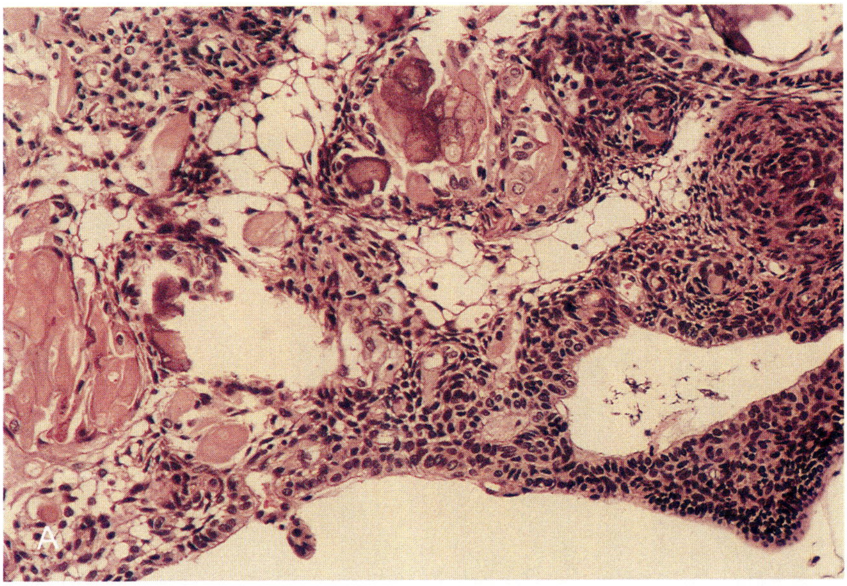

Figure 7.11. **A,** Craniopharyngioma demonstrating basaloid cells, stellate reticulum, squamous differentiation, calcification, and cystic change. (Paraffin section, H&E, ×64.)

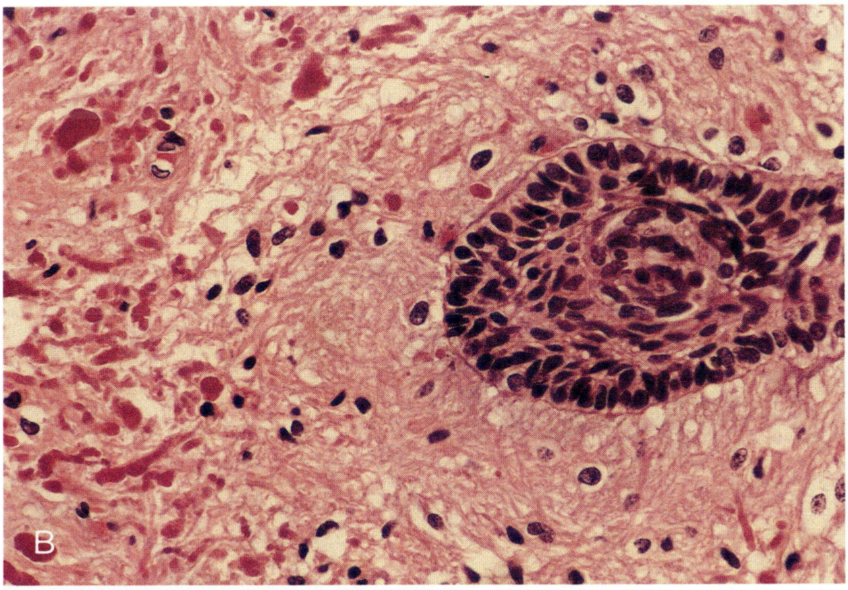

Figure 7.11. **B,** Craniopharyngioma. Extension of tumor (right side of figure) into surrounding brain tissue (left side of figure) elicits prominent fibrillary gliosis and Rosenthal fiber formation. (Paraffin section, H&E, ×128.)

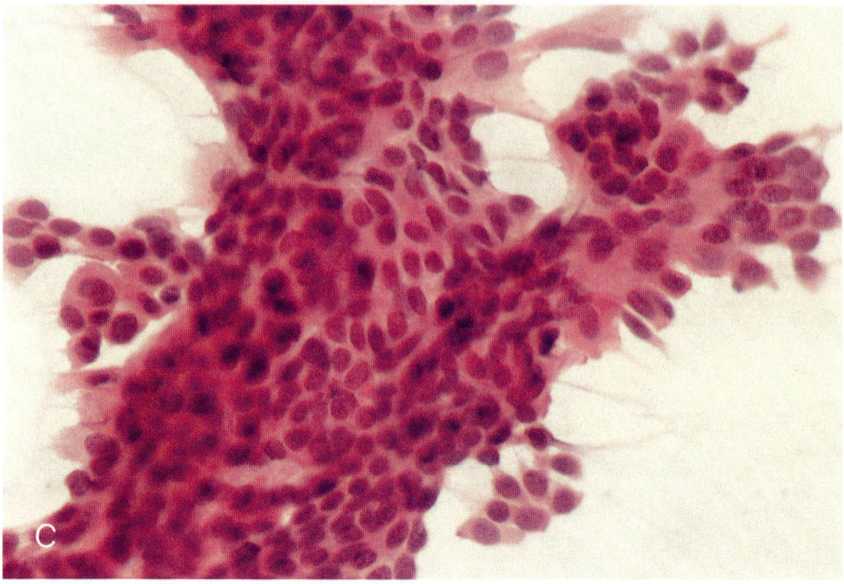

Figure 7.11. **C,** Craniopharyngioma. Squamous cells demonstrated in smear preparations. (Smear preparation, H&E, ×128.)

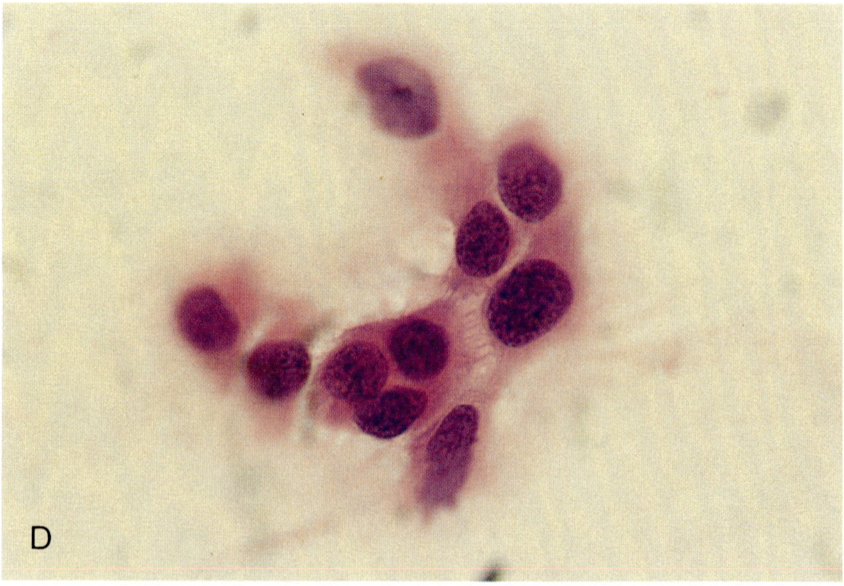

Figure 7.11. **D,** Craniopharyngioma. Detail of squamous cells with visible desmosomes in smear preparation. (Smear preparation, H&E, ×320.)

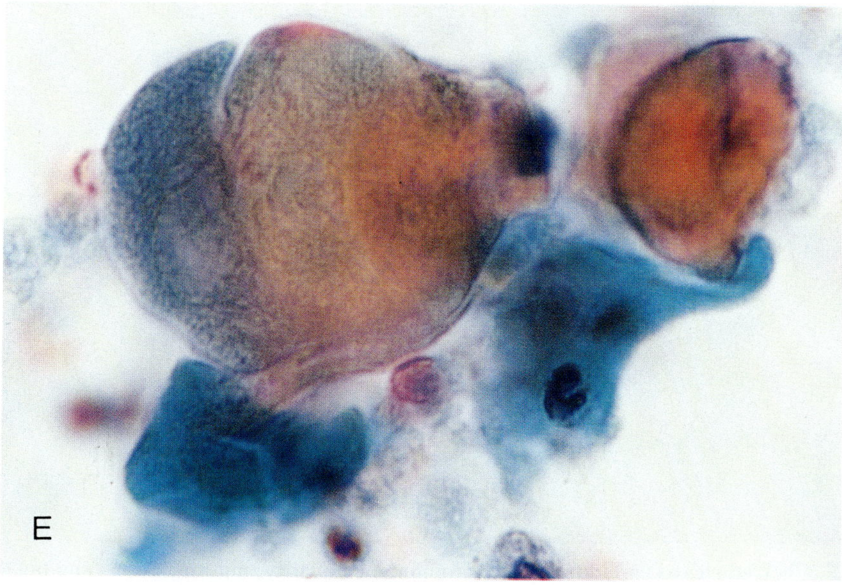

Figure 7.11. **E,** Craniopharyngioma cyst aspirate, demonstrating keratinized squamous cells, leukocytes, and necrotic debris. (Membrane filter preparation, Pap stain, ×400.)

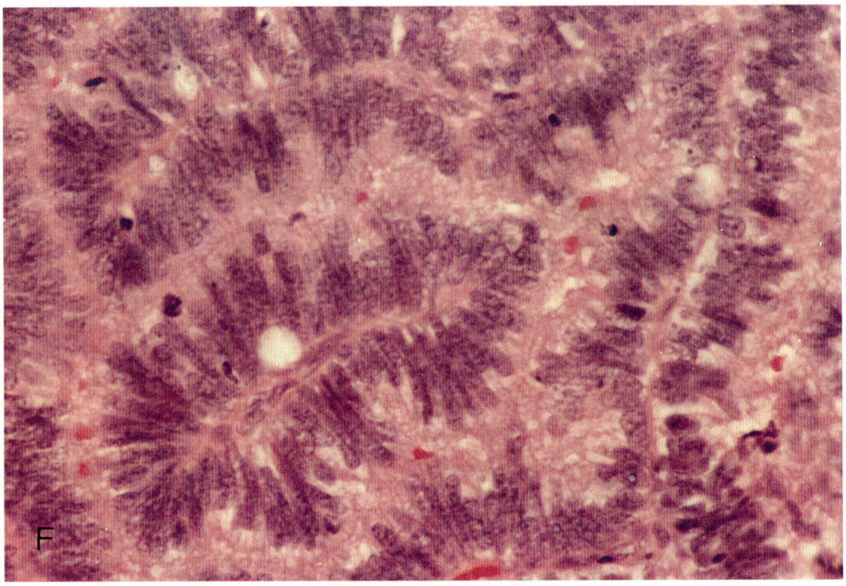

Figure 7.11. **F,** Choroid plexus carcinoma. Note prominent cellularity, mitotic figures, and tightly packed papillary architecture. (Paraffin section, H&E, ×128.)

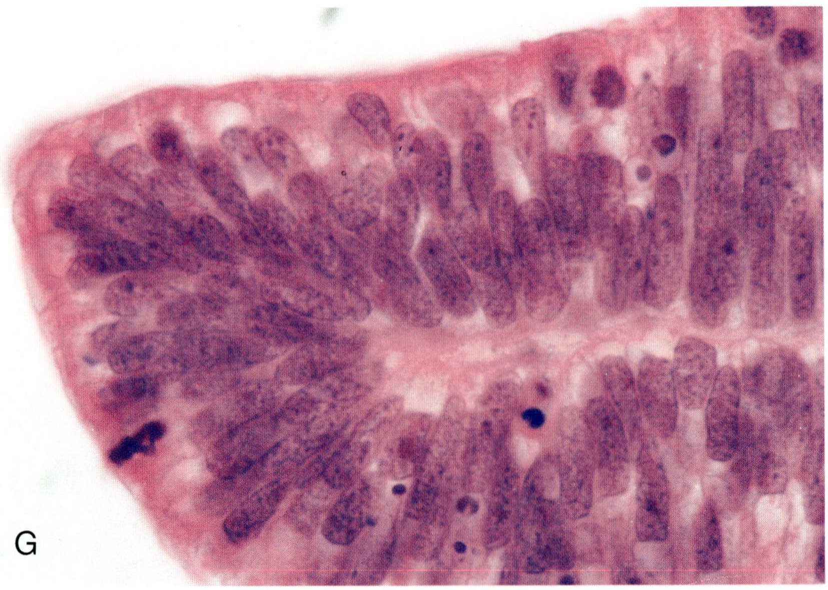

Figure 7.11. **G,** Choroid plexus carcinoma. Note tall columnar epithelium with nuclear stratification, atypia, mitotic figures, and autophagic vacuoles. Compare with normal choroid plexus (see Figs. 2.8 and 2.9). (Paraffin section, H&E, ×320.)

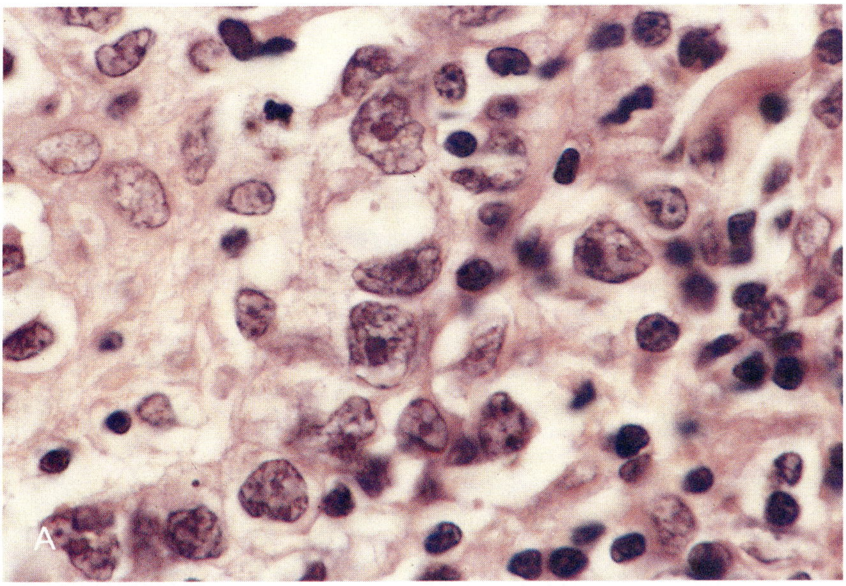

Figure 7.12. **A,** Pineal germinoma. Larger, primitive-appearing neoplastic cells with prominent nucleoli, admixed with small lymphocytes. (Paraffin section, H&E, ×160.)

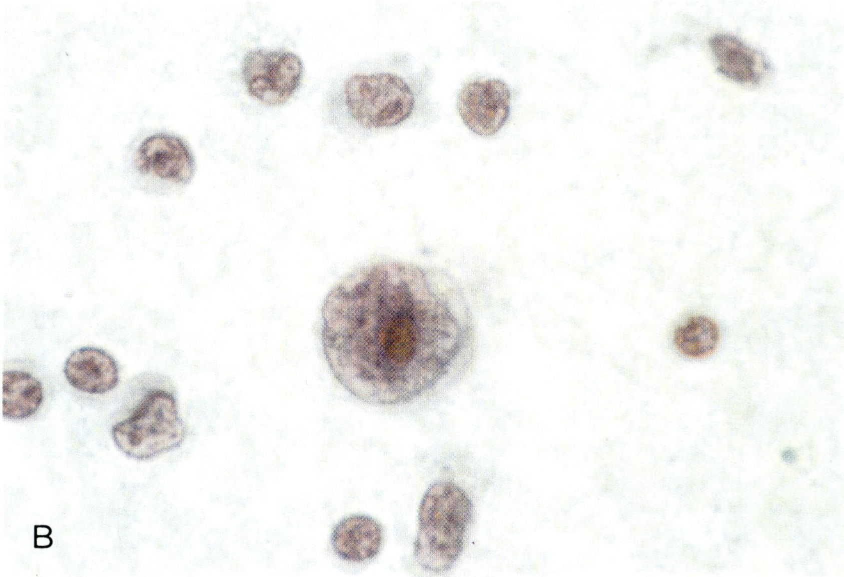

Figure 7.12. **B,** Pineal germinoma. Large neoplastic cell and several smaller surrounding lymphocytes and monocytes in CSF. (CSF membrane filter preparation, Pap stain, ×400.)

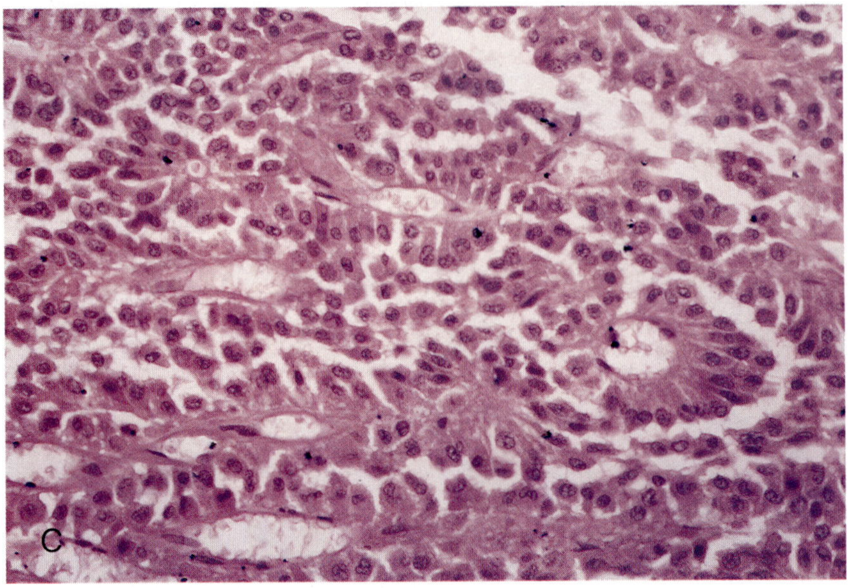

Figure 7.12. **C,** Pituitary chromophobe adenoma. A trabecular pattern is prominent in this field. (Paraffin section, H&E, ×64.)

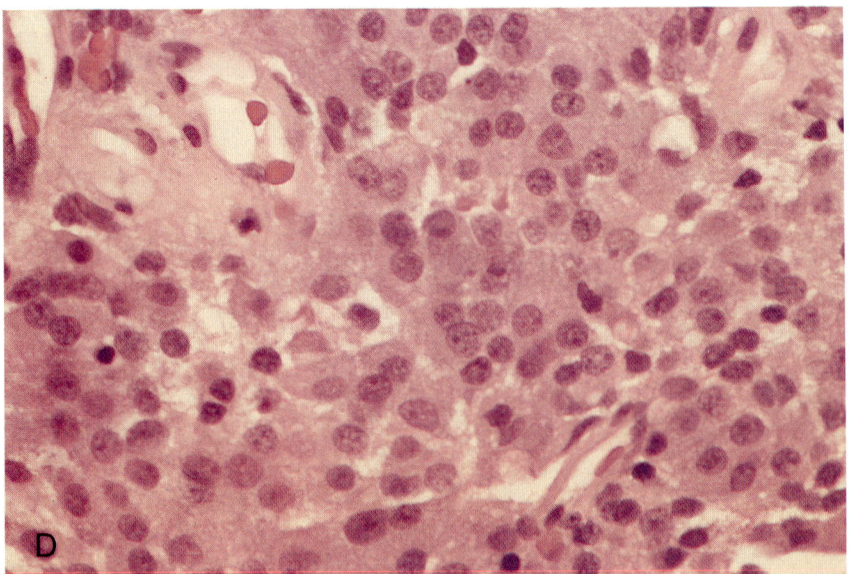

Figure 7.12. **D,** Pituitary chromophobe adenoma. Field showing diffuse architectural pattern. (Paraffin section, H&E, ×160.)

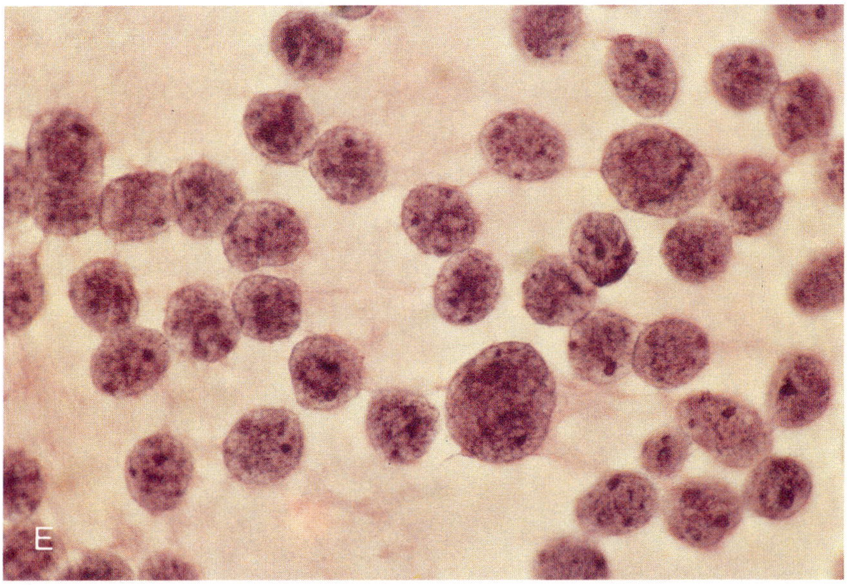

Figure 7.12. E, Pituitary chromophobe adenoma. In smear preparations, a "dirty"-appearing background with bare nuclei resembles smears of the normal pituitary (see Fig. 2.13**B**). Pleomorphism is often more conspicuous in smears. Nuclei have a dusty appearance, with more punctate chromatin superimposed. Nucleoli are seen in some cells. (Smear preparation, H&E, ×320.)

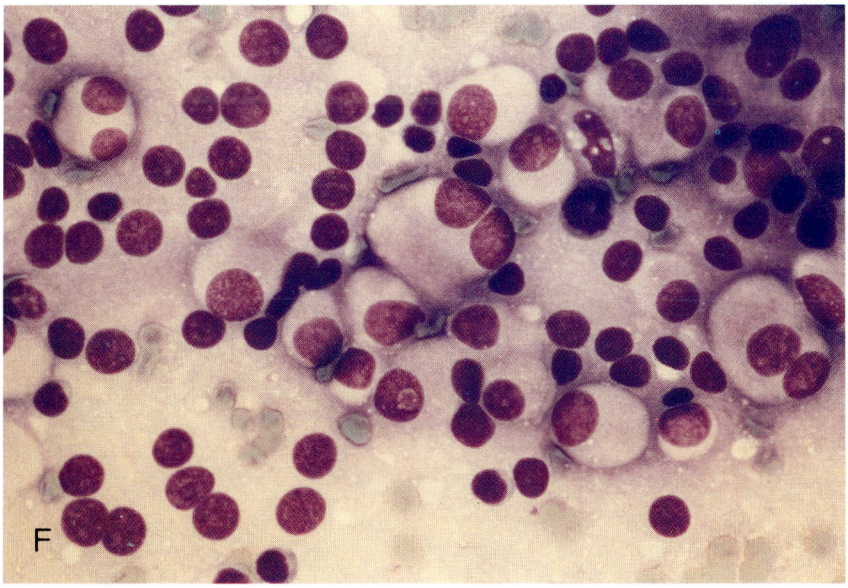

Figure 7.12. F, Pituitary chromophobe adenoma, as seen with Diff-Quik stain. Cells with still-intact cytoplasm stand out in the background of bare nuclei. (Smear preparation, ×128.)

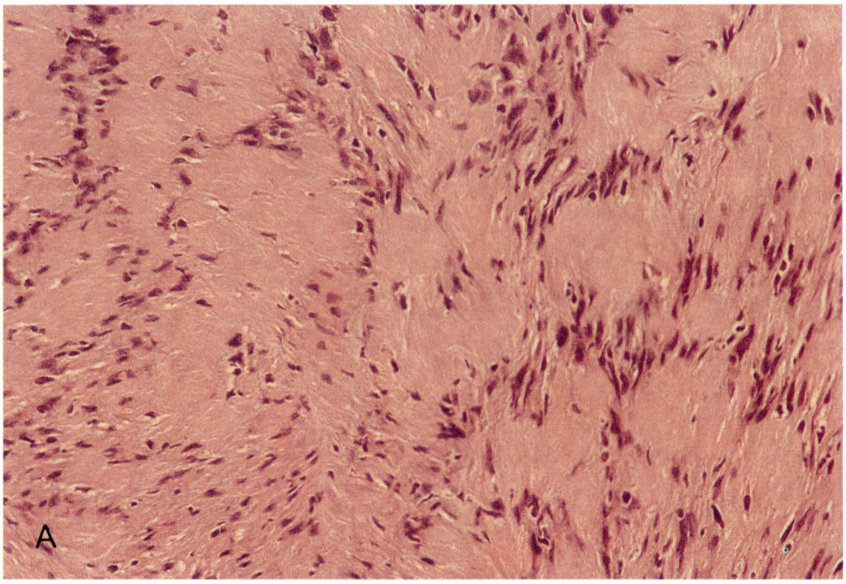

Figure 7.13. A, Schwannoma of spinal nerve root. Antoni type A zone, with Verocay bodies. (Paraffin section, H&E, ×64.)

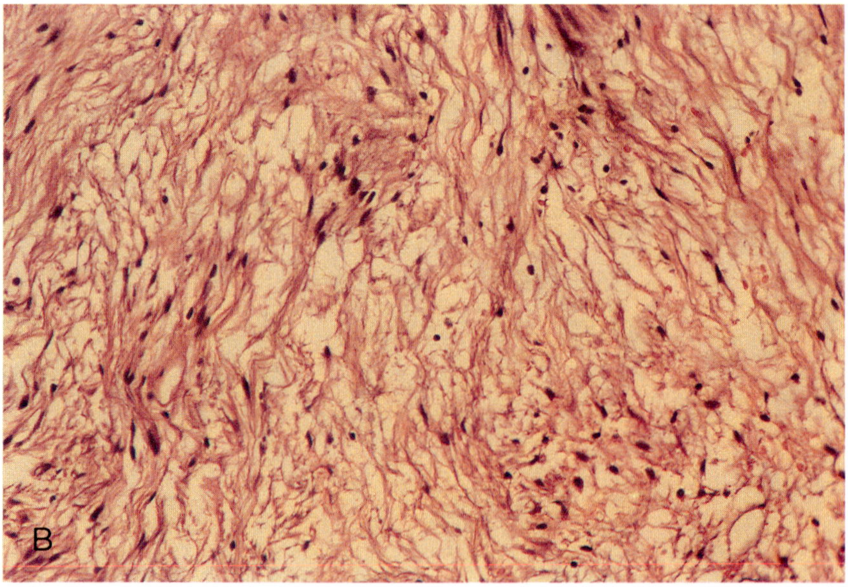

Figure 7.13. B, Schwannoma of spinal nerve root. Antoni type B area. (Paraffin section, H&E, ×64.)

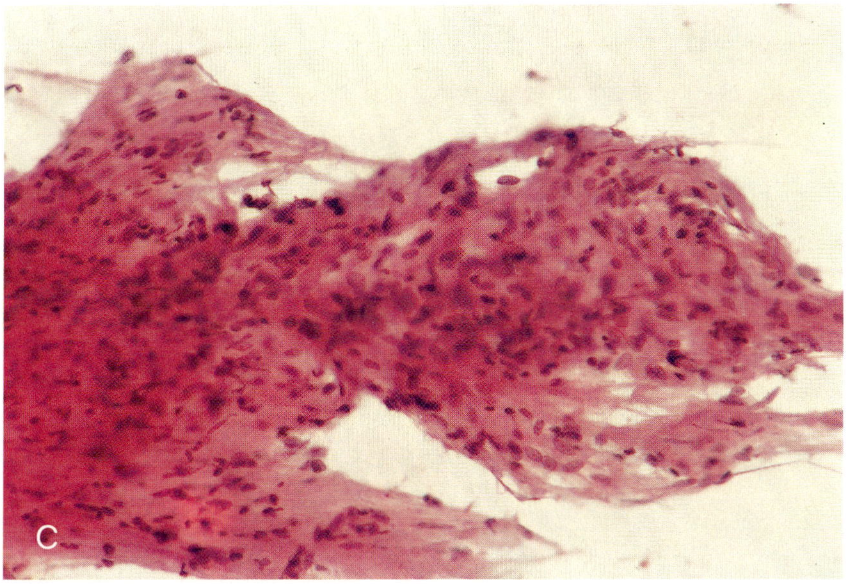

Figure 7.13. **C,** Schwannoma of spinal nerve root. This fibrous tumor smears poorly, with resultant thick cellular aggregates. (Smear preparation, H&E, ×128.)

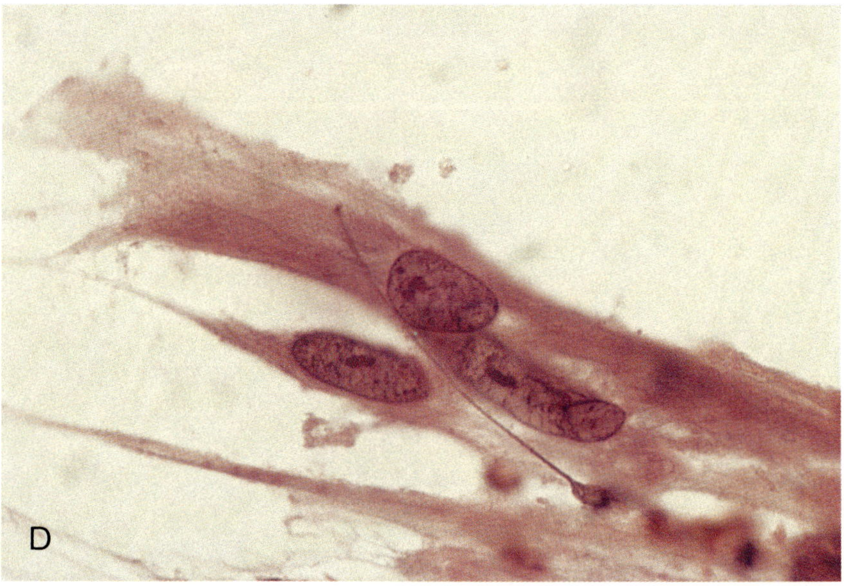

Figure 7.13. **D,** Schwannoma of spinal nerve root. Smear preparation demonstrating cytologic detail at the periphery of a cellular aggregate. (H&E, ×320.)

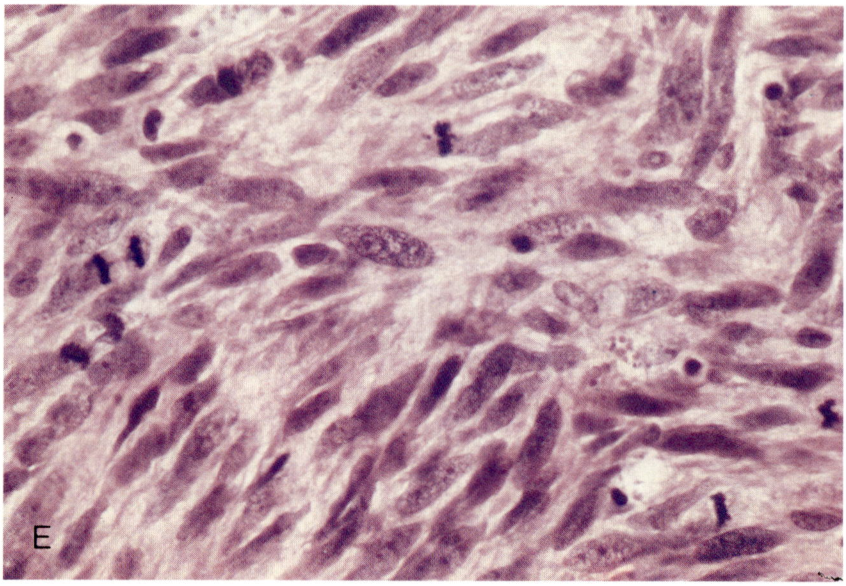

Figure 7.13. E, Malignant peripheral nerve sheath tumor in patient with von Recklinghausen's disease. This cellular spindle cell lesion demonstrates numerous mitotic figures. (Paraffin section, H&E, ×128.)

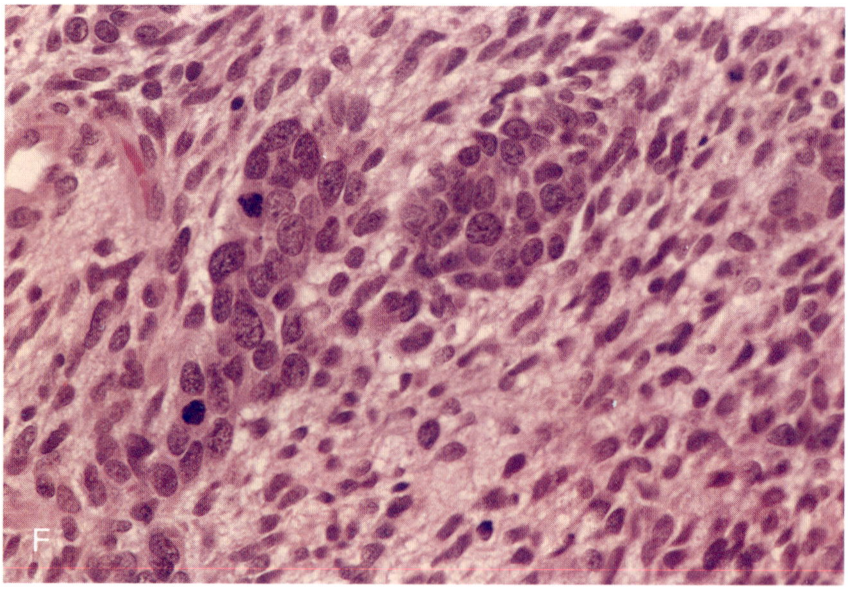

Figure 7.13. F, Malignant peripheral nerve sheath tumor in patient with von Recklinghausen's disease. Epithelial-like areas may be seen, particularly in the vicinity of blood vessels. (Paraffin section, H&E, ×128.)

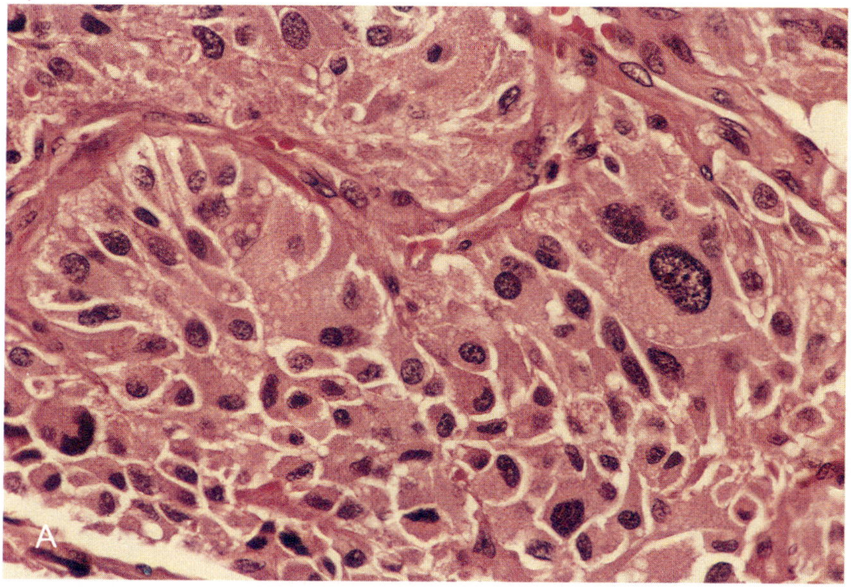

Figure 7.14. A, Paraganglioma from para-aortic area. Although the nesting pattern of cells persists, surrounded by capillaries, this tumor demonstrates more prominent pleomorphism than is found in many paragangliomas. (Paraffin section, H&E, ×128.)

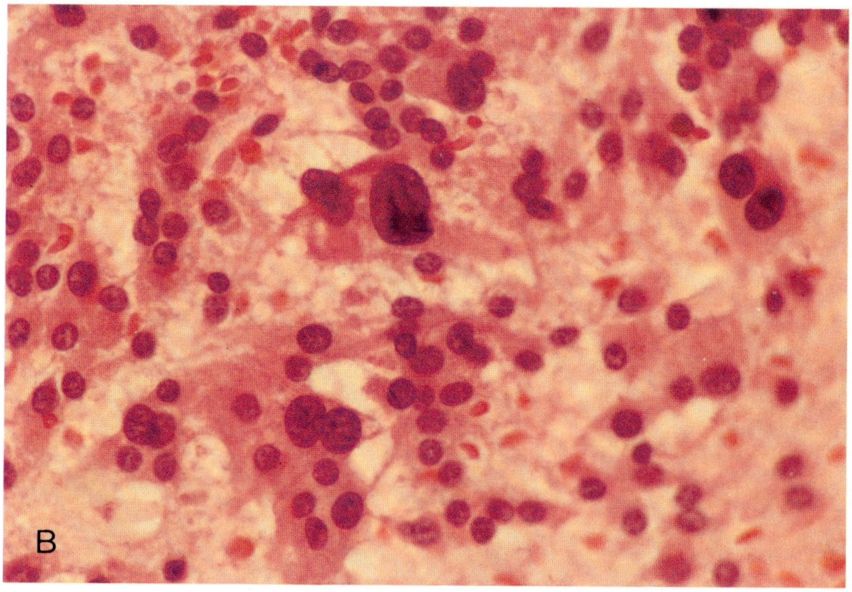

Figure 7.14. B, Paraganglioma. Smear preparations demonstrate prominent cellularity, pleomorphism, and a dirty-appearing background. (Smear preparation, H&E, ×128.)

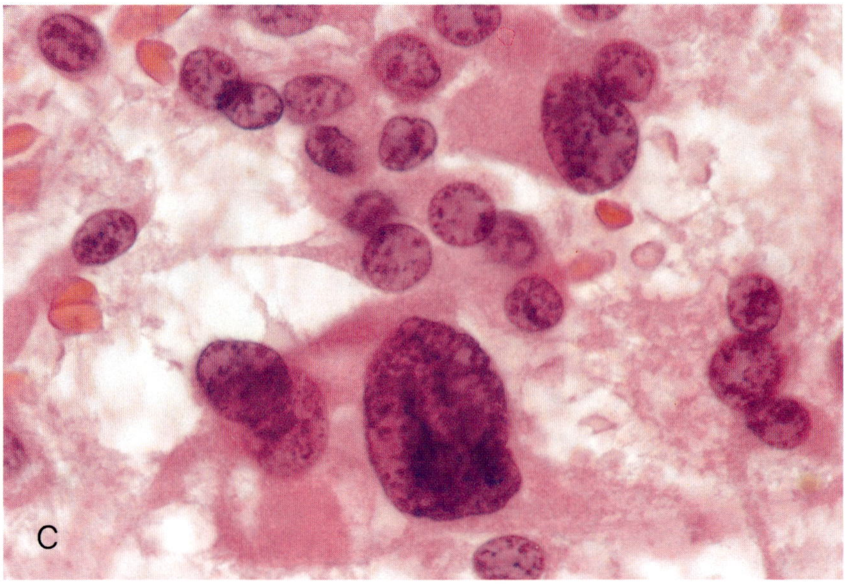

Figure 7.14. **C,** Paraganglioma. Same case as demonstrated in **A** and **B**. Marked nuclear atypia and pleomorphism. (Smear preparation, H&E, ×320.)

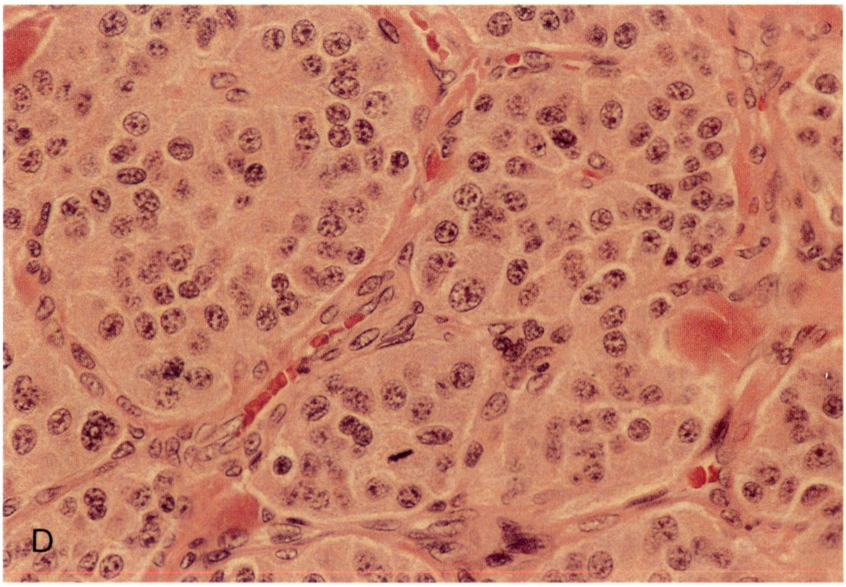

Figure 7.14. **D,** Carcinoid tumor, lung. Nests of tumor cells surrounded by capillaries, and punctate "salt and pepper" chromatin are evident. (Paraffin section, H&E, ×128.)

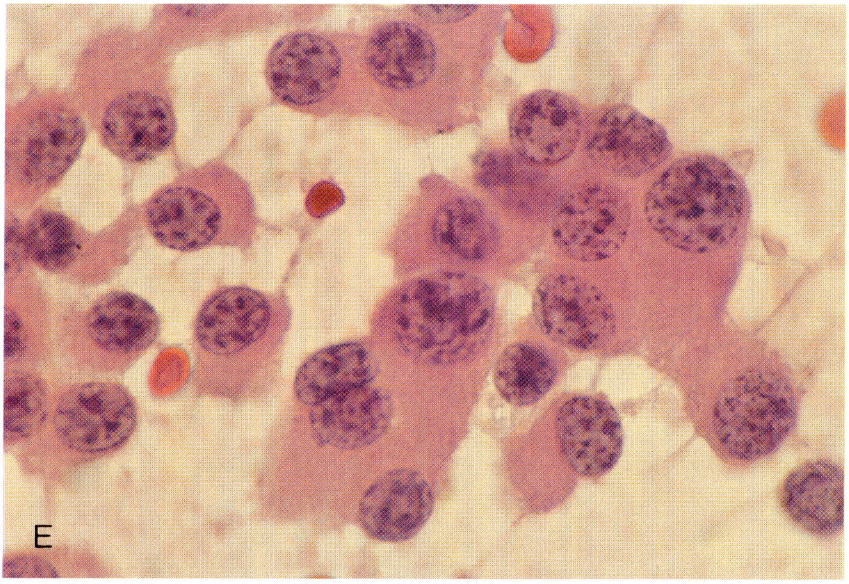

Figure 7.14. E, Carcinoid tumor, lung. In smear preparations, carcinoid tumor cells cling to their cytoplasm with moderate tenacity. (Smear preparation, H&E, ×320.)

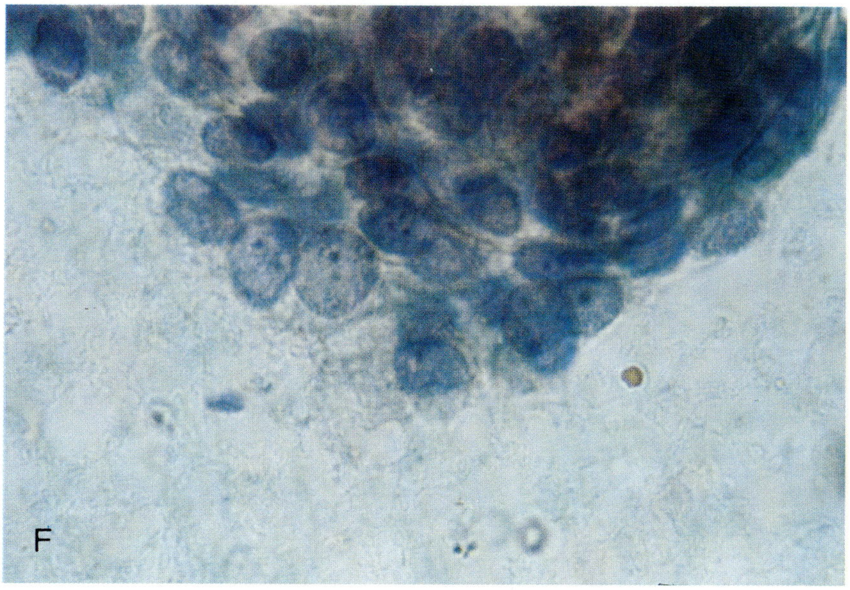

Figure 7.14. F, Carcinoid tumor metastatic to the leptomeninges. (CSF membrane filter preparation, Pap stain, ×320.)

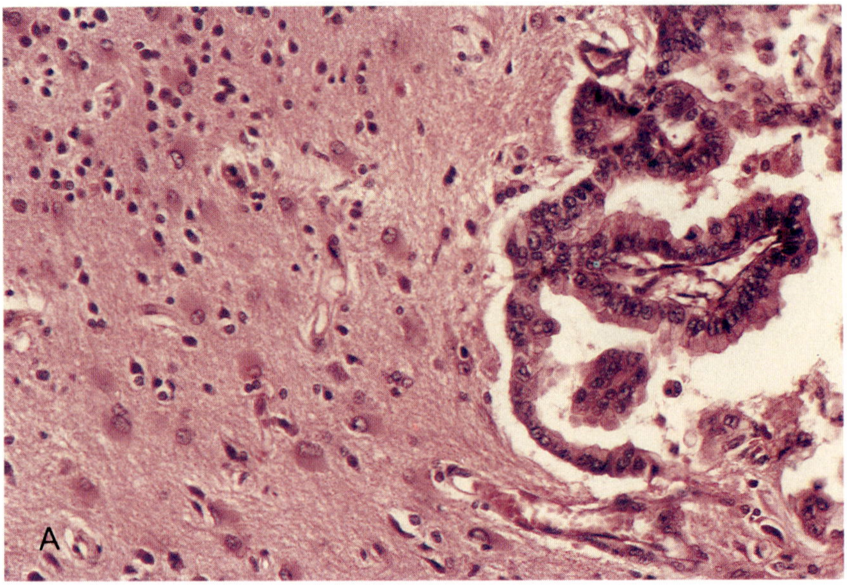

Figure 7.15. A, Metastatic adenocarcinoma to brain, demonstrating abrupt tumor-neuropil interface and glial response, with prominent reactive astrocytes in surrounding neuropil. (Paraffin section, H&E, ×64.)

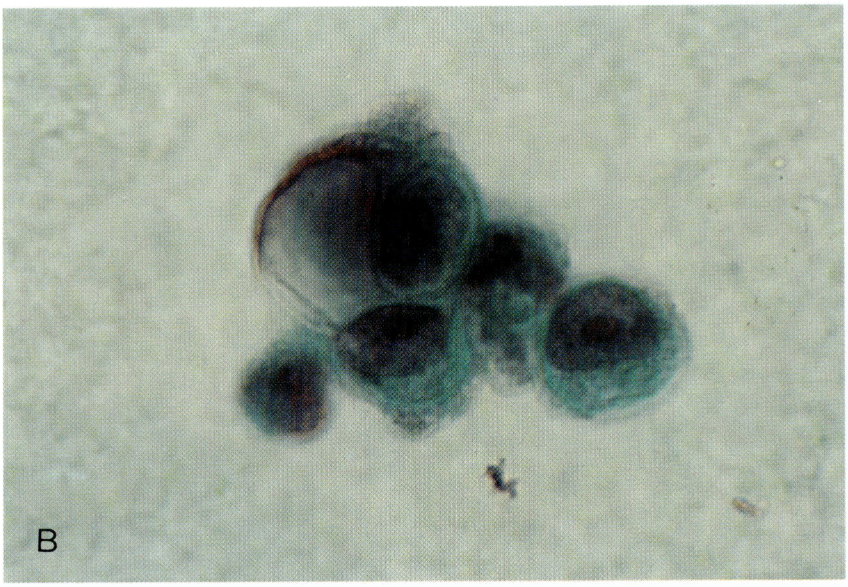

Figure 7.15. B, Metastatic breast carcinoma in CSF. (CSF membrane filter preparation, Pap stain, ×400.)

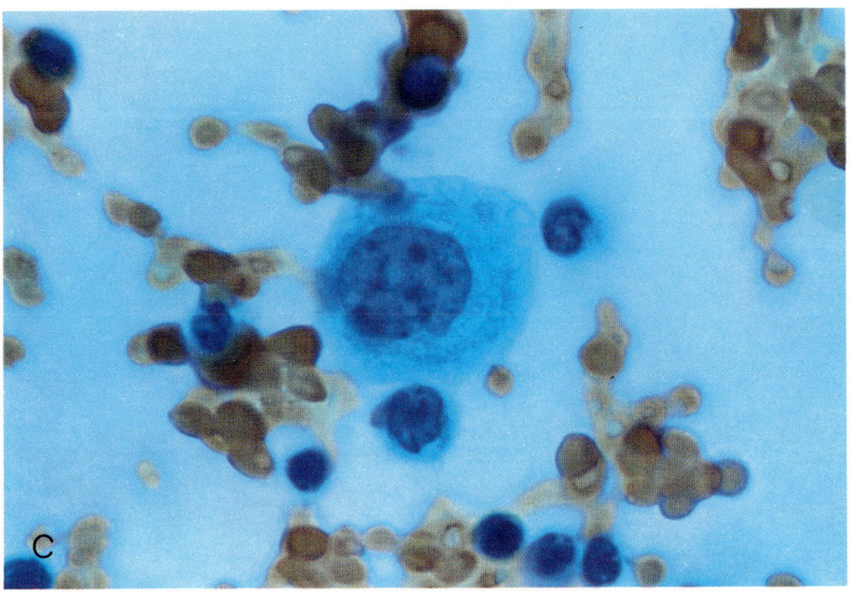

Figure 7.15. C, Metastatic transitional cell carcinoma to CSF. (CSF membrane filter preparation, Pap stain, ×400.)

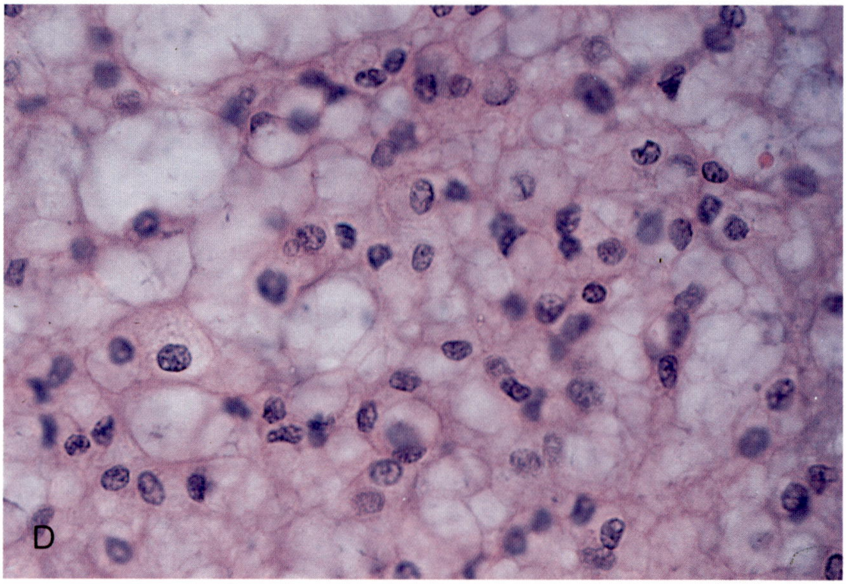

Figure 7.15. D, Chordoma, demonstrating relatively bland nuclei with bubbly cytoplasm and well-defined cell membranes. (Paraffin section, H&E, ×160.)

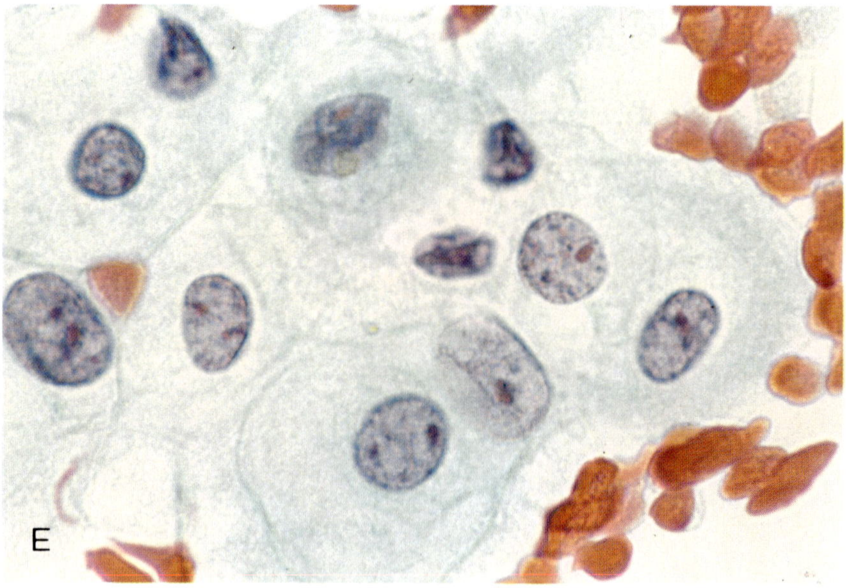

Figure 7.15. E, Chordoma metastatic to subarachnoid space. (CSF membrane filter preparation, Pap stain. ×400.)

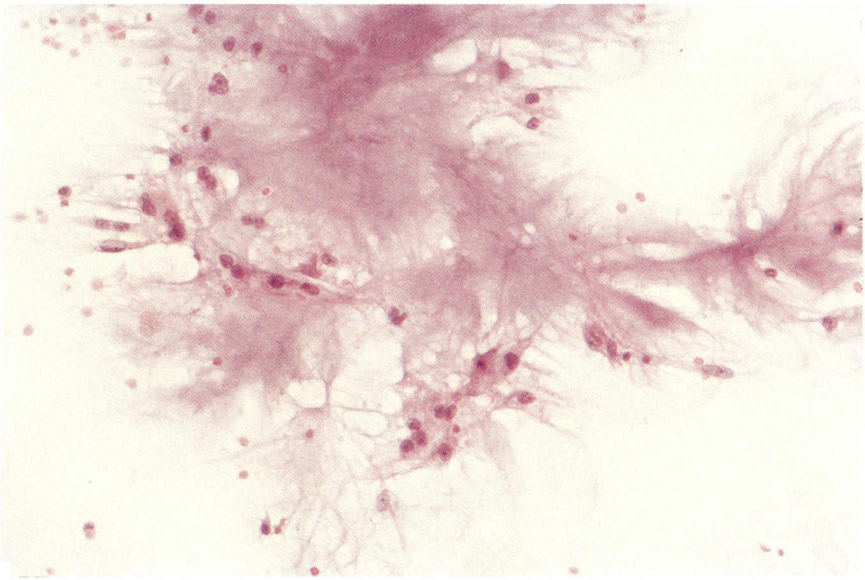

Figure 7.15. F, Chordoma, sacrococcygeal area. Smear preparation of zone with prominent myxoid change and sparse cellularity. (Smear preparation, H&E, ×64.)

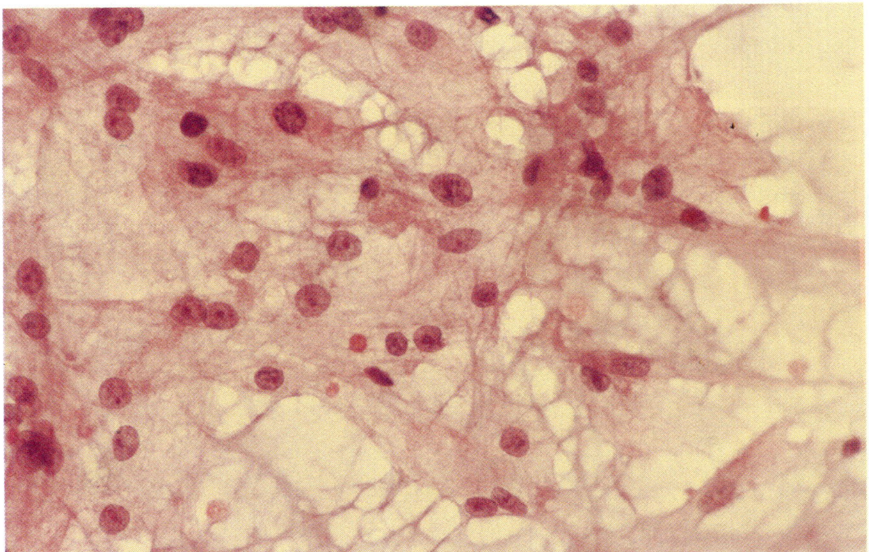

Figure 7.15. G, Chordoma. Same case as in **F**. Moderately cohesive cells with filmy, often vacuolated cytoplasm on a myxoid background. (Smear preparation, H&E, ×128.)

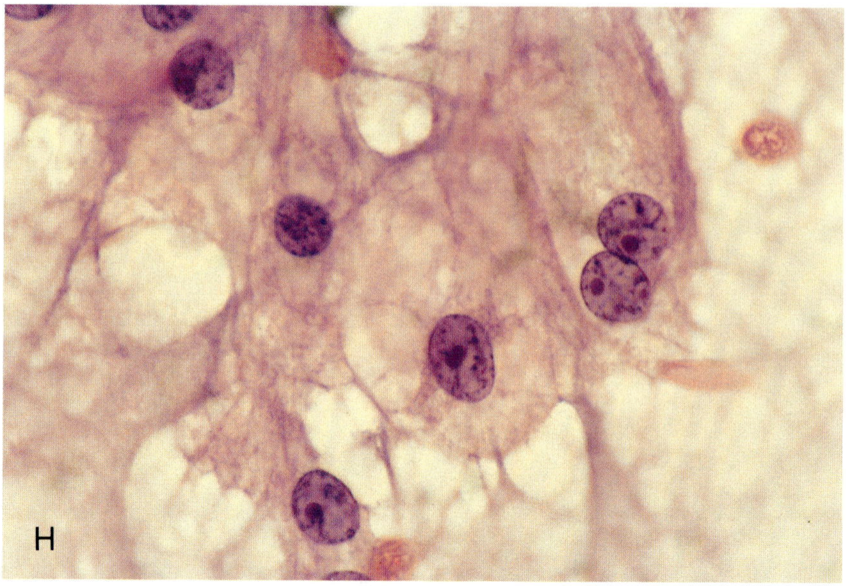

Figure 7.15. **H,** Chordoma. Same case as in **F** and **G**. Detail of cytologic features. Rather uniform, ovoid nuclei with distinct eosinophilic nucleoli, and vacuolated, delicate-appearing cytoplasm. Occasional binucleate cells are present. (Compare with cells exfoliated in CSF in another case, Fig. 7.15**E**.)

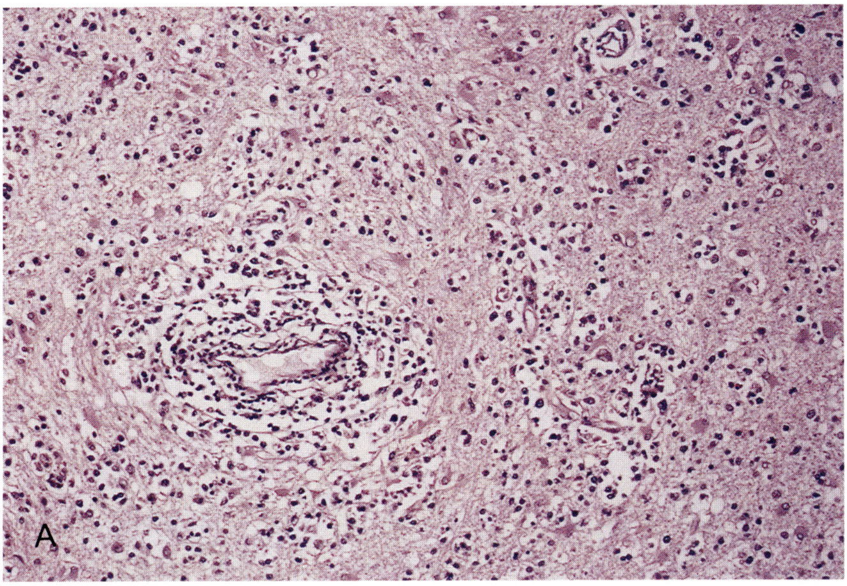

Figure 7.16. **A,** Primary CNS lymphoma. Note the tendency of cells to form concentric layers around the blood vessel. (Paraffin section, H&E, ×40.)

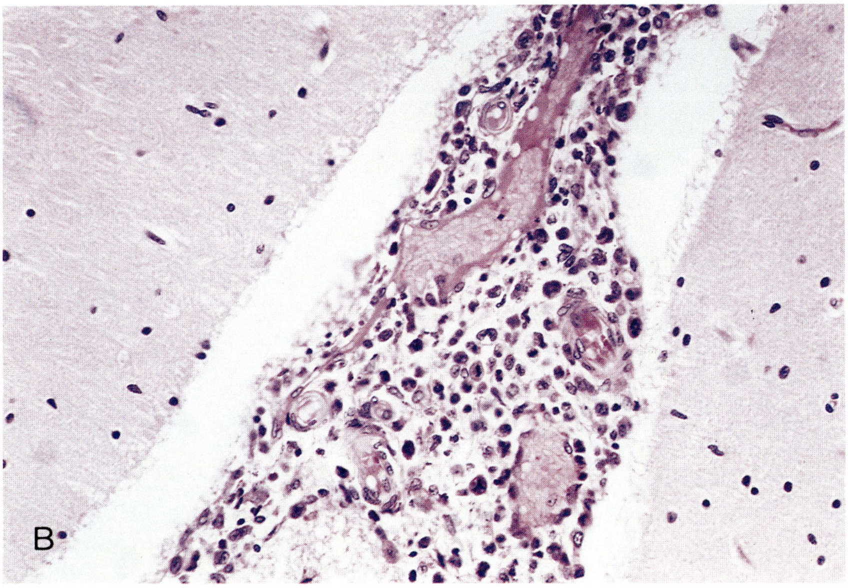

Figure 7.16. **B,** Lymphoma spread to subarachnoid space. (Paraffin section, H&E, ×100.)

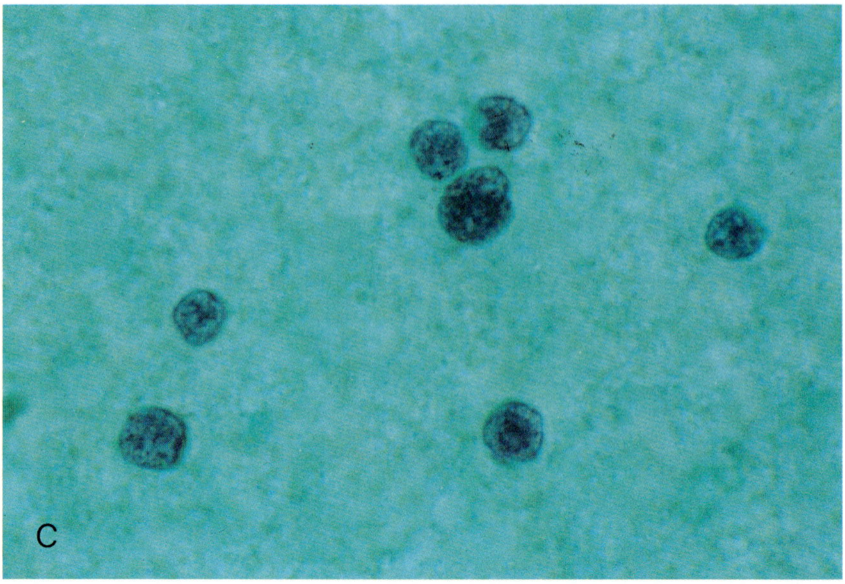

Figure 7.16. **C,** Burkitt's lymphoma spread to subarachnoid space. (CSF membrane filter preparation, Pap stain, ×400.)

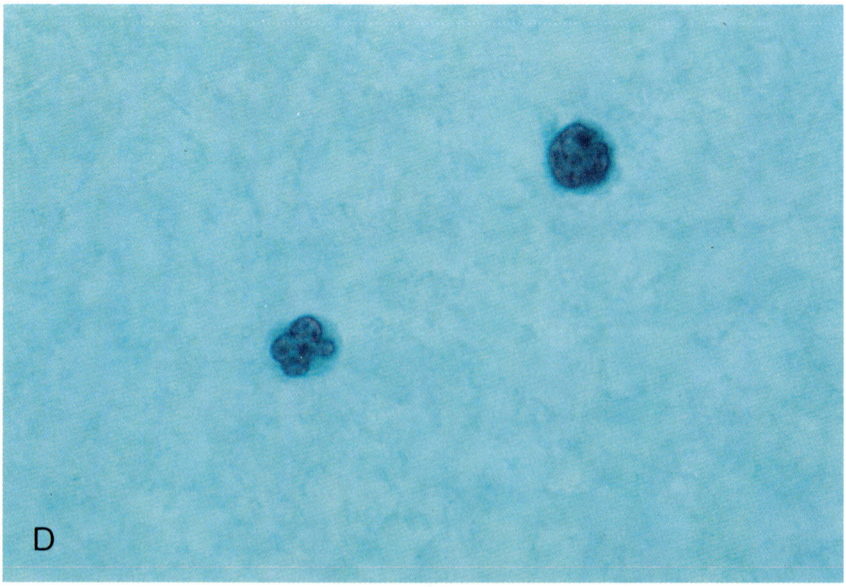

Figure 7.16. **D,** Diffuse large-cell lymphoma with spread to CSF. Note high N/C ratio and nuclear membrane irregularities. (CSF membrane filter preparation, Pap stain, ×400.)

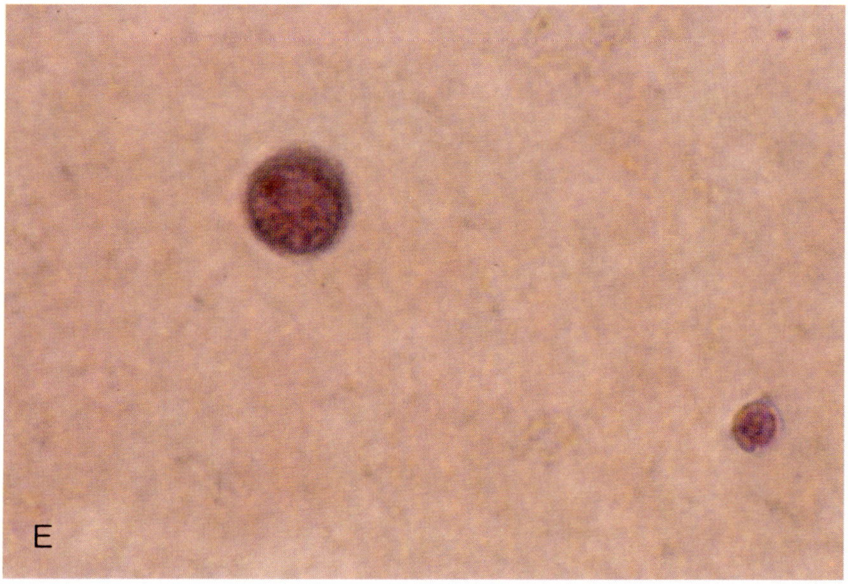

Figure 7.16. E, Immunoblastic lymphoma in CSF. (CSF membrane filter preparation, Pap stain, ×400.)

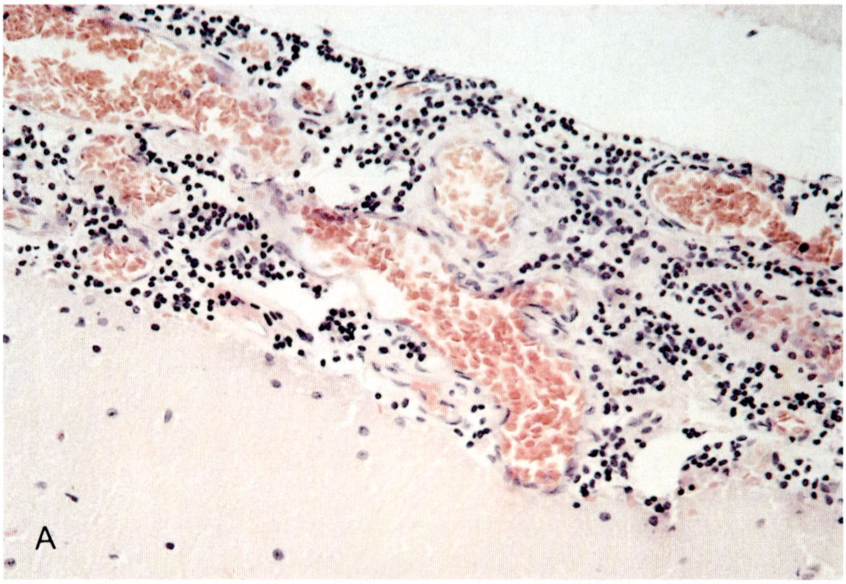

Figure 7.17. **A,** Acute lymphoblastic leukemia spread in subarachnoid space. Cerebral cortex is in the lower portion of the field. (Paraffin section, H&E, ×40.)

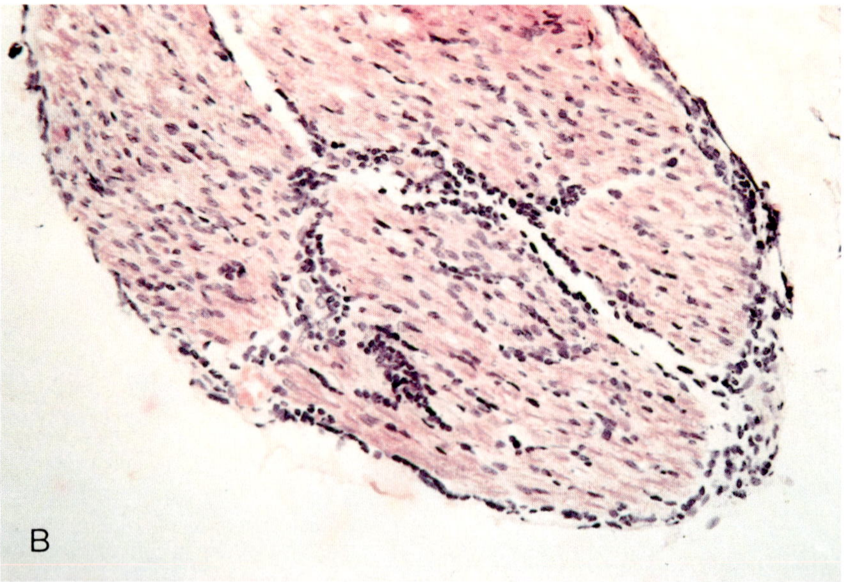

Figure 7.17. **B,** Acute lymphoblastic leukemia permeating a spinal nerve root. (Paraffin section, H&E, ×40.)

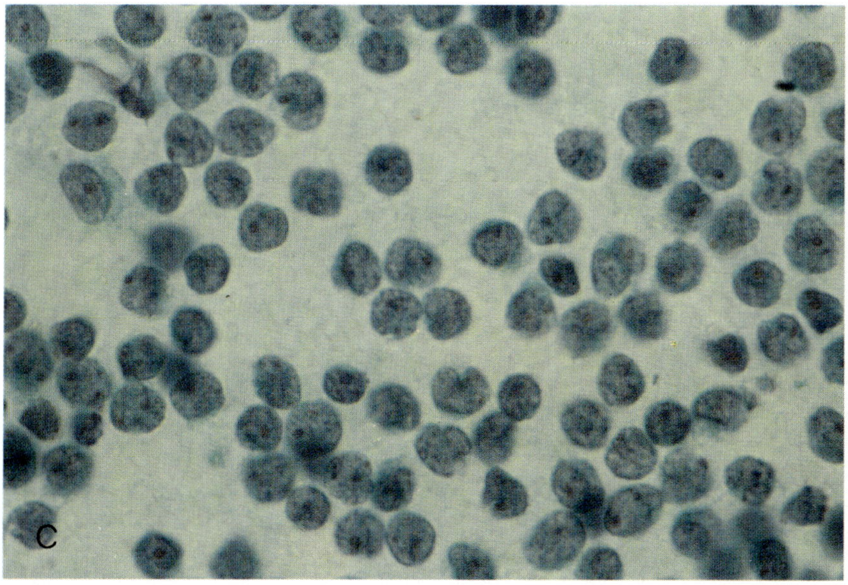

Figure 7.17. C, Acute myeloblastic leukemia with CSF involvement. (CSF membrane filter preparation, Pap stain, ×400.)

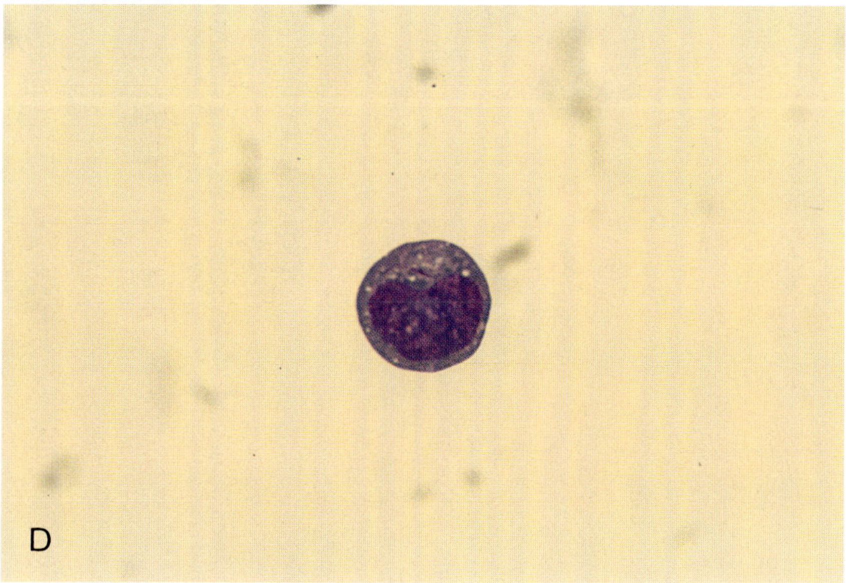

Figure 7.17. D, Acute myelogenous leukemia involving CSF. Immature myeloid cell with Auer rod. (Air-dried cytospin preparation, Wright's stain, ×320.)

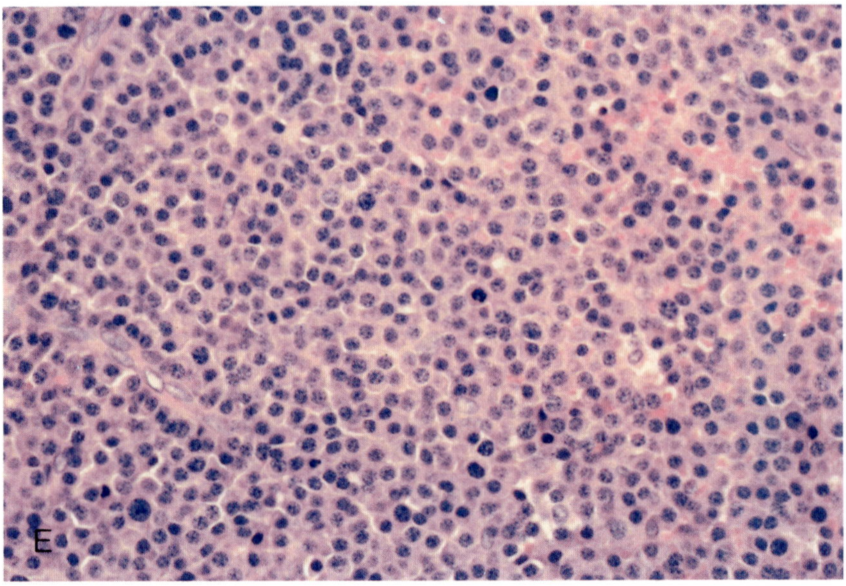

Figure 7.17. **E,** Multiple myeloma with cerebral involvement. Monotonous field of plasma cells. (Paraffin section, H&E, ×100.)

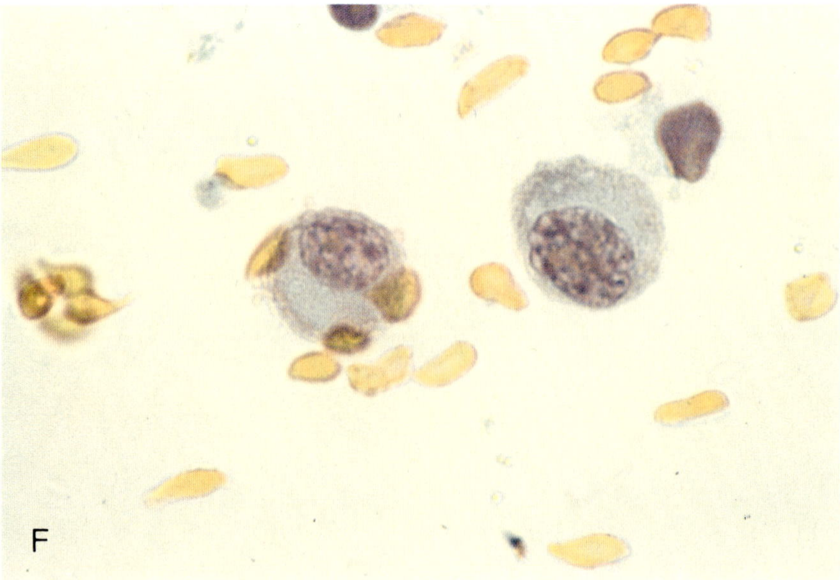

Figure 7.17. **F,** Multiple myeloma with subarachnoid space spread. (CSF membrane filter preparation, Pap stain, ×400.)

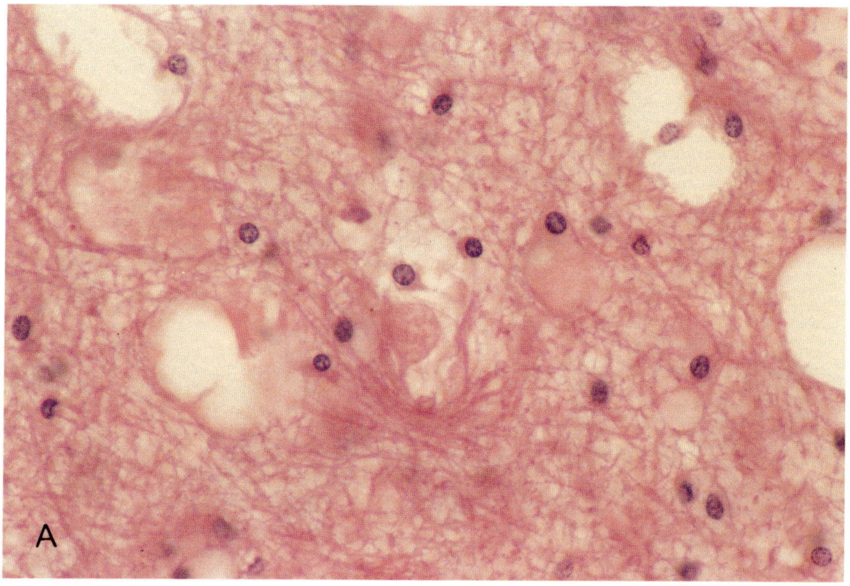

Figure 8.1. A, Fibrillary gliosis in the zone of chronic edema surrounding a focus of metastatic carcinoma. The edema is reflected in the vacuoles present. Note the dense fibrillar neuropil. A rare gemistocytic astrocyte is present, but most do not have obvious paranuclear cytoplasm. (Paraffin section, H&E, ×128.)

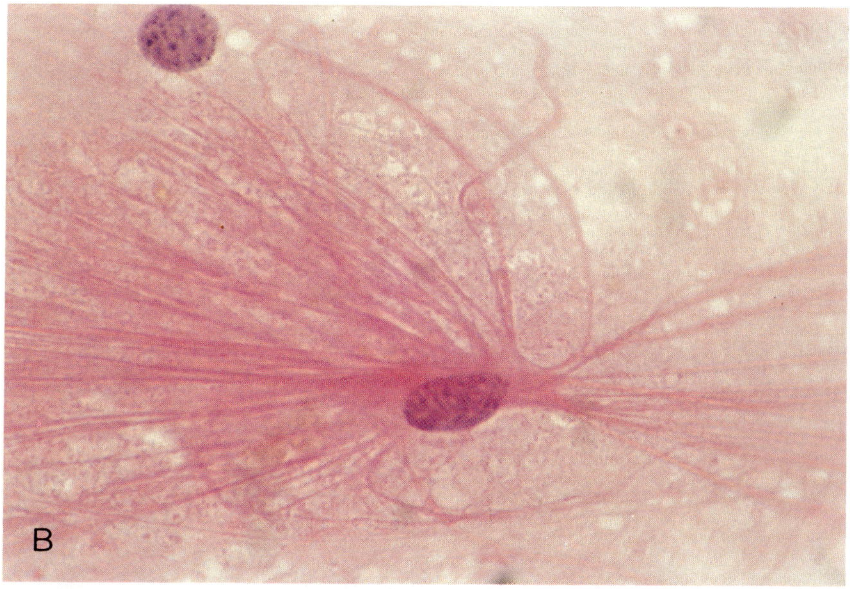

Figure 8.1. B, The stellate radiation of fibrillary astrocyte processes is much more apparent in smear preparations of zones of chronic gliosis. (Smear preparation, H&E, ×320.)

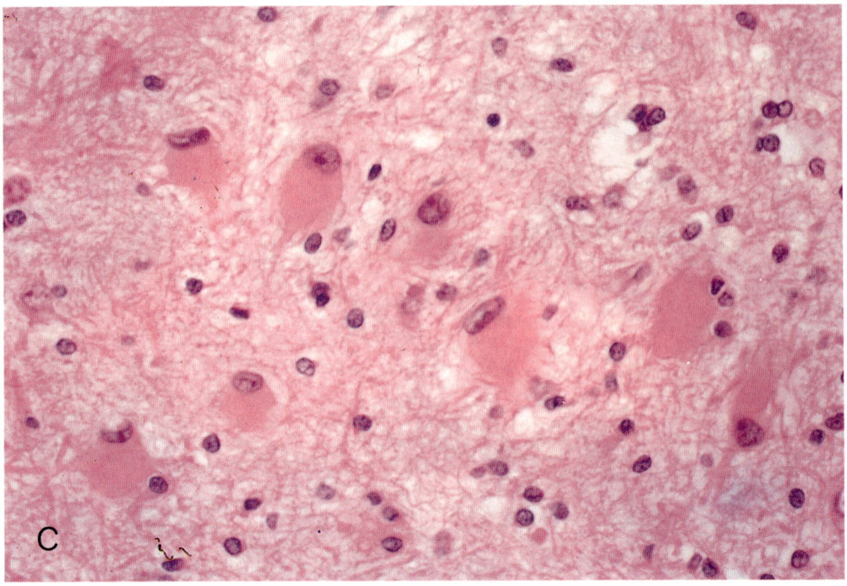

Figure 8.1. **C,** Gemistocytic astrocytes, with prominent glassy eosinophilic cytoplasm around the nucleus. These represent an earlier and more easily recognized stage in the evolution of gliosis than the later stages seen in Figure 8.1**A** and **B**. (Paraffin section, H&E, ×128.)

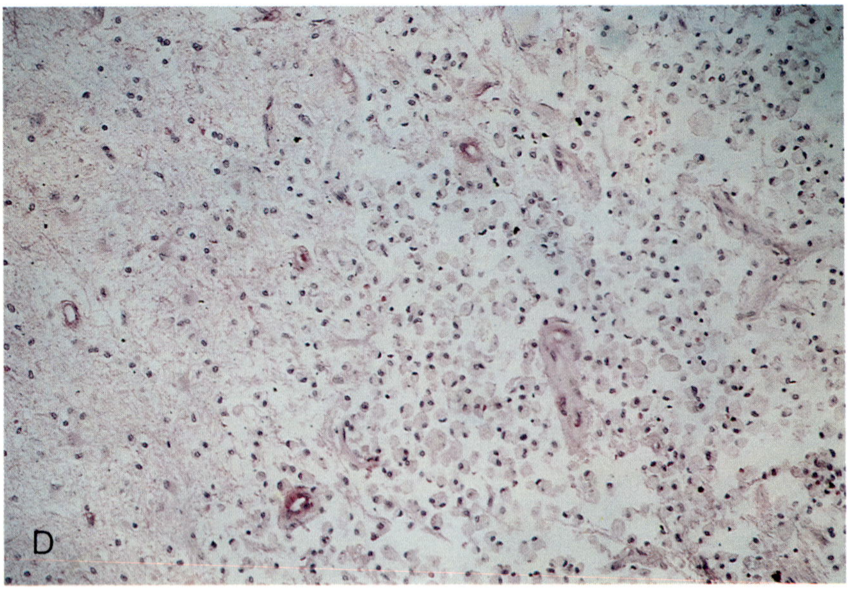

Figure 8.1. **D,** Thalamic infarction with gliotic neuropil on the left side and encephalomalacia and numerous foamy macrophages in the necrotic zone to the right side of the field. (Paraffin section, H&E, ×64.)

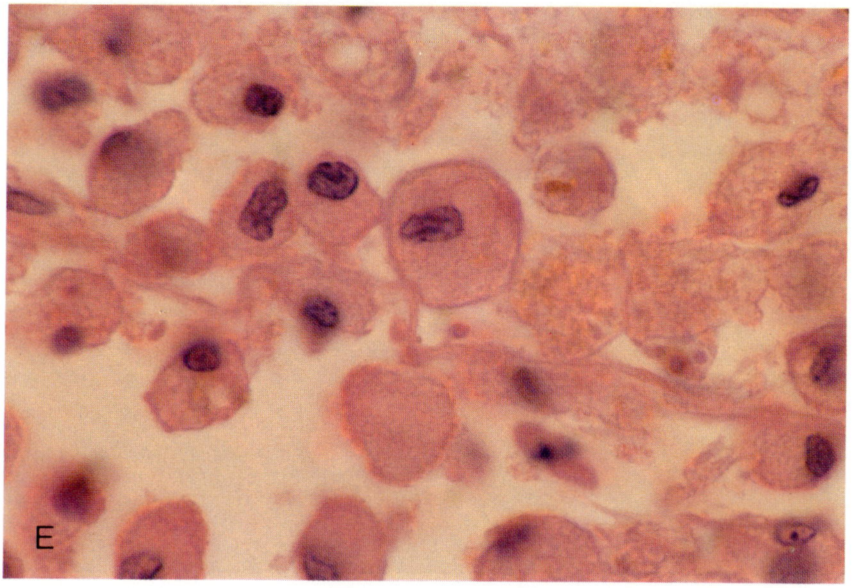

Figure 8.1. **E,** Foamy macrophages in the zone of infarction. Their cytoplasm often appears more granular than vacuolated in paraffin sections. The golden brown granules in the cytoplasm of cells in the right center of the field are hemosiderin pigment. (Paraffin section, H&E, ×320.)

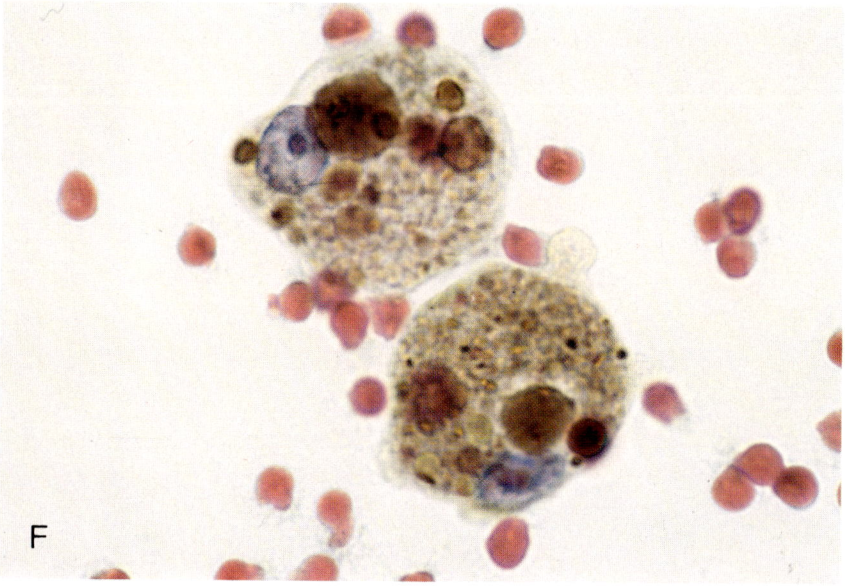

Figure 8.1. **F,** Hemosiderin-laden macrophage as demonstrated in fine-needle aspiration preparation from necrotic area of brain adjacent to carcinoma. (Cytospin preparation, Pap stain, ×400.)

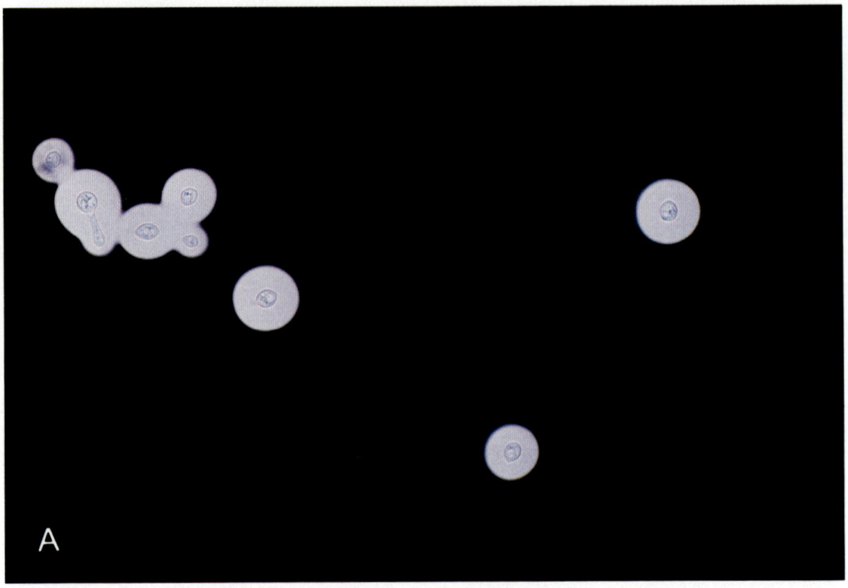

Figure 8.2. A, *Cryptococcus neoformans* meningoencephalitis. India ink preparation of CSF. Budding of organisms is readily demonstrated, as is the thick mucopolysaccharide capsule. (×320.)

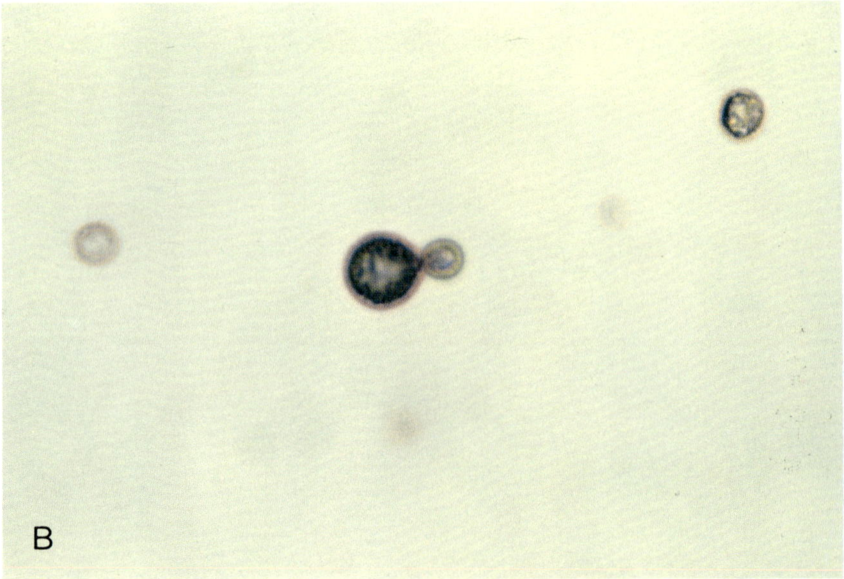

Figure 8.2. B, *Cryptococcus neoformans* in CSF. Budding is evident. (Membrane filter preparation, Pap stain, ×400.)

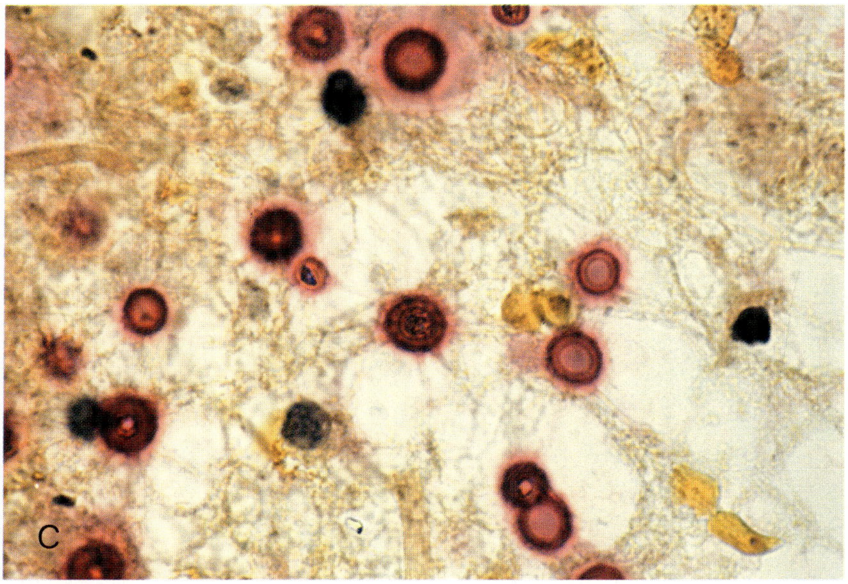

Figure 8.2. **C,** *Cryptococcus neoformans* in CSF. (Cytospin preparation, mucicarmine stain, ×400.)

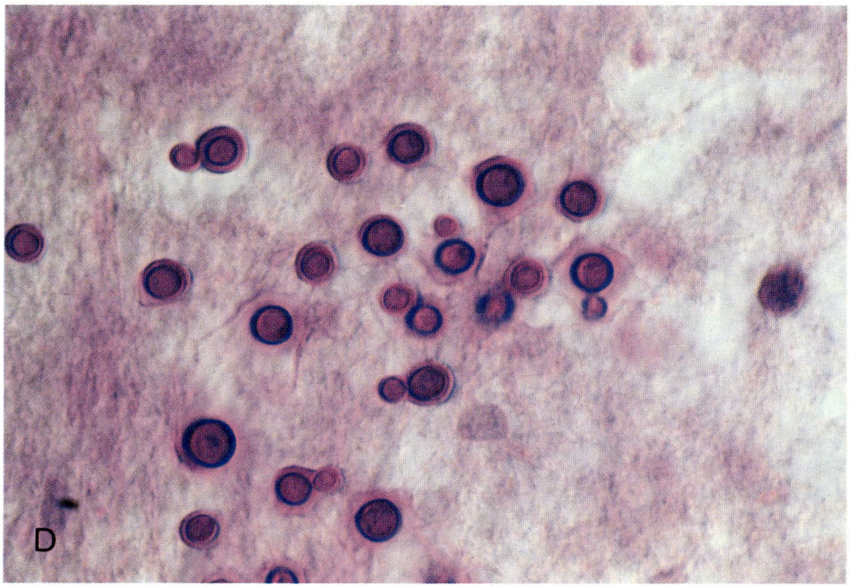

Figure 8.2. **D,** *Cryptococcus neoformans* in CSF. (Cytospin preparation, PAS stain, ×320.)

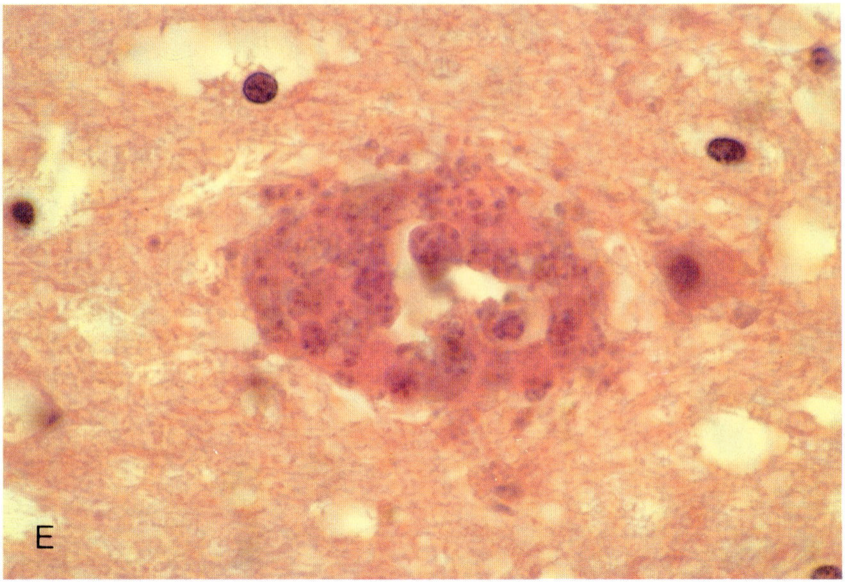

Figure 8.2. E, Toxoplasmosis in CNS. Punctate organisms are visible with H&E staining, but are difficult to see within macrophages. (Paraffin section, ×320.)

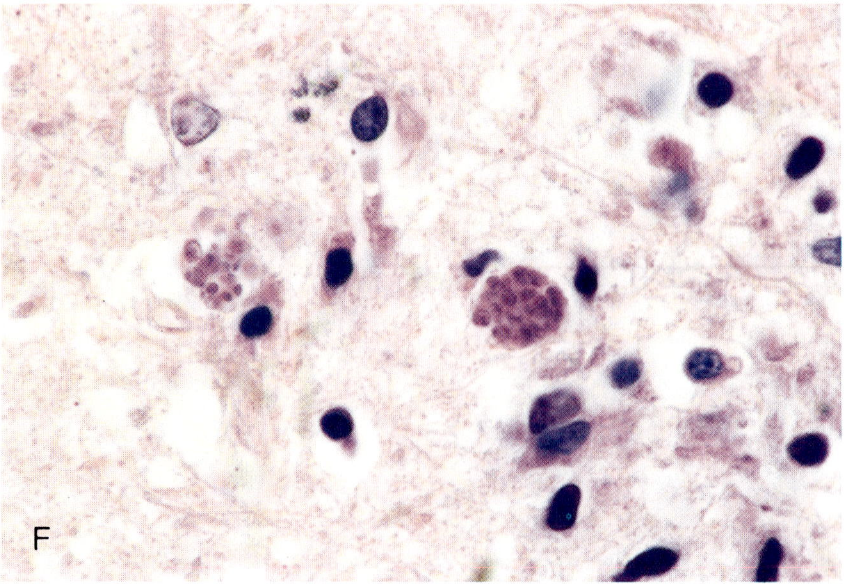

Figure 8.2. F, Toxoplasmosis in CNS. Giemsa stain enhances the ability to locate organisms seen in clusters to the left and right of center. (Paraffin section, Giemsa, ×400.)

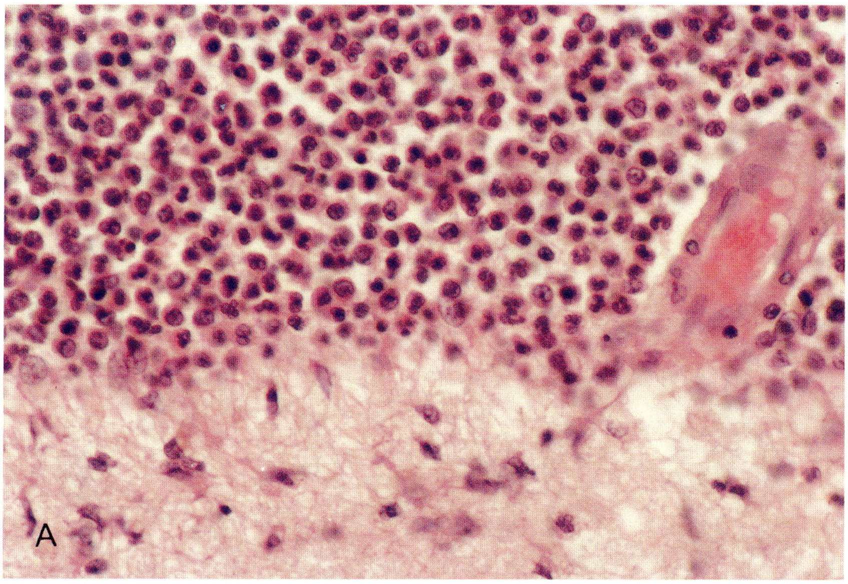

Figure 8.3. **A,** Meningococcal meningitis with purulent exudate. Brain tissue below, subarachnoid space above. Neutrophils fill the subarachnoid space. (Paraffin section, H&E, ×128.)

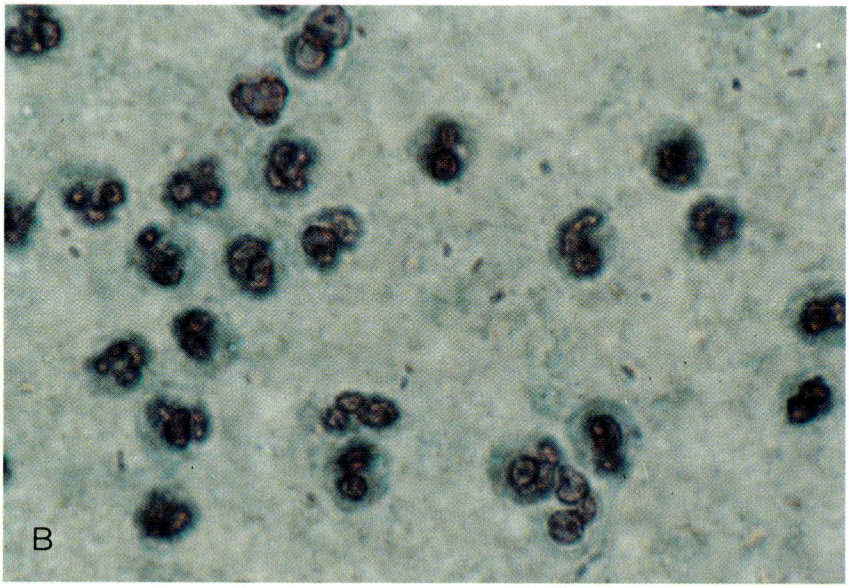

Figure 8.3. **B,** Purulent meningitis, with neutrophils in CSF. (Membrane filter preparation, Pap stain, ×400.)

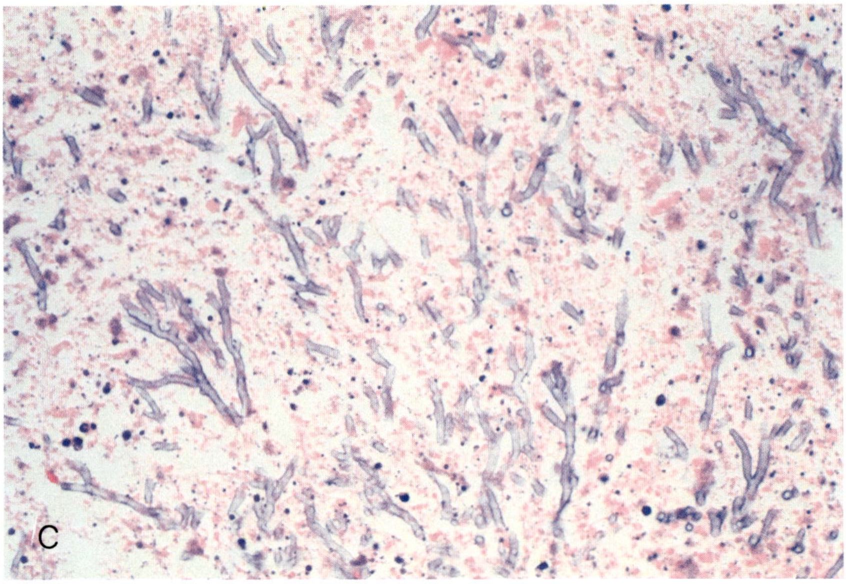

Figure 8.3. C, Aspergillosis causing CNS abscess. (Paraffin section, ×160.)

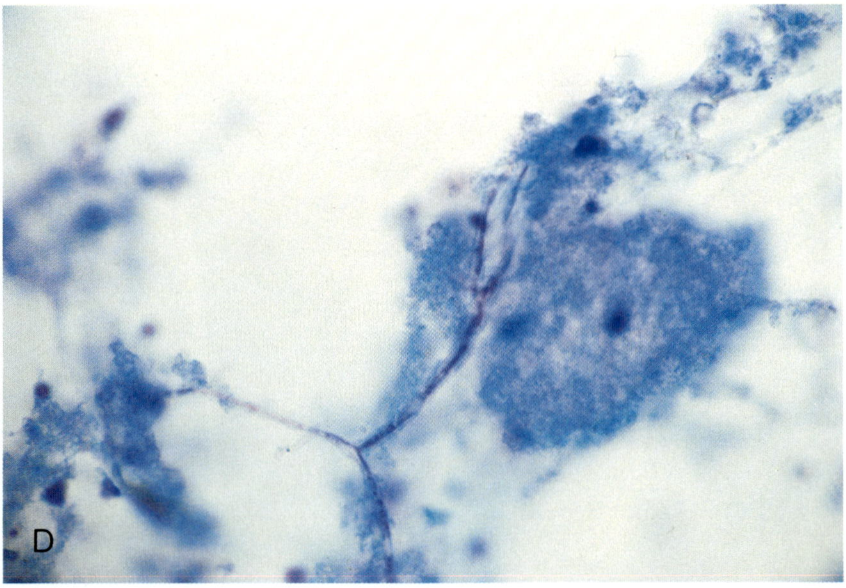

Figure 8.3. D, Aspergillosis. (Cytospin preparation, Pap stain, ×430.)

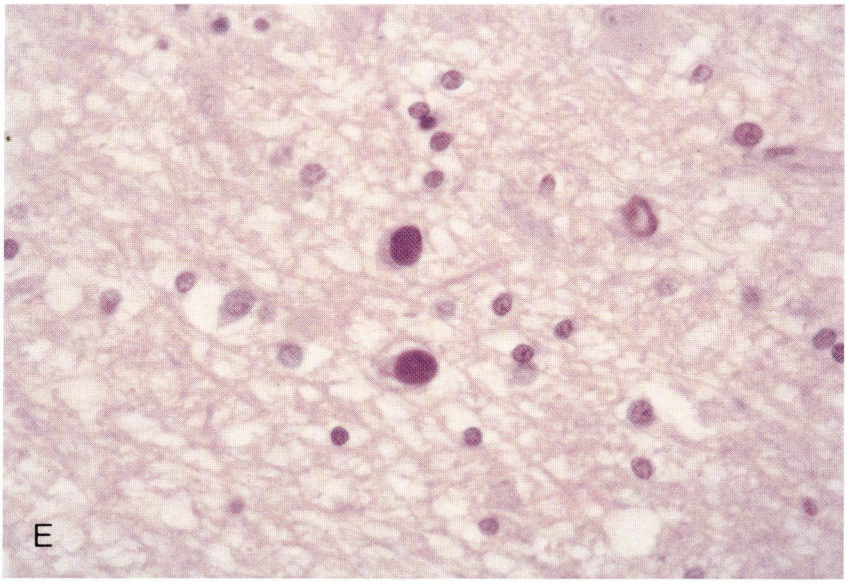

Figure 8.3. E, Progressive multifocal leukoencephalopathy. Enlarged, smudged-appearing intranuclear inclusions in oligodendrocytes (the two cells in the center of the field) in the margin of the area of demyelination. More normal-appearing glial nuclei are in the adjacent neuropil. (Paraffin section, H&E, ×160.)

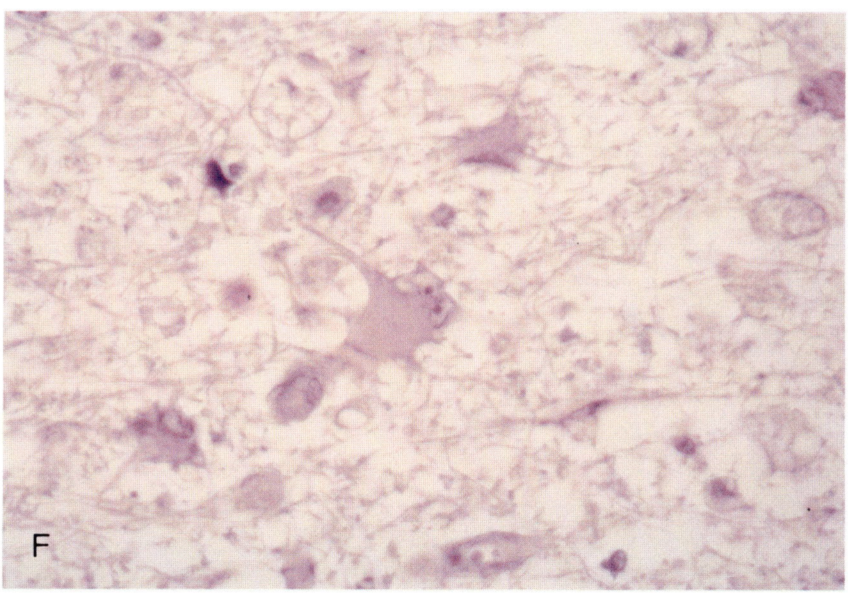

Figure 8.3. F, Progressive multifocal leukoencephalopathy. Enlarged, bizarre binucleate astrocyte within an area of demyelination. (Paraffin section, H&E, ×160.)

Index

Page numbers in *italics* denote figures; those followed by "t" denote tables.